W9-BSN-849

Coronary Artery Disease

Gregory W. Barsness • David R. Holmes Jr.
Editors

Coronary Artery Disease

New Approaches without Traditional Revascularization

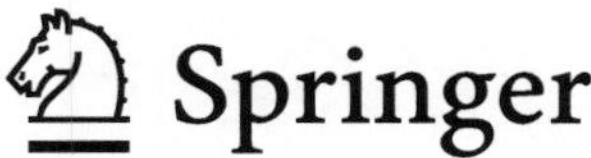

Editors
Gregory W. Barsness, MD
Mayo Clinic College of Medicine
Rochester, MN
USA

David R. Holmes Jr., MD
Mayo Clinic College of Medicine
Rochester, MN
USA

ISBN 978-1-84628-460-1 e-ISBN 978-1-84628-712-1
DOI 10.1007/978-1-84628-712-1
Springer London Dordrecht Heidelberg New York

British Library Cataloguing in Publication Data
A catalogue record for this book is available from the British Library

Library of Congress Control Number: 2011944198

Printed on acid-free paper

Springer is part of Springer Science+Business Media (www.springer.com)

For Samuel and Joseph, who have demonstrated patience and understanding far beyond their years during the completion of this book.

In addition, we wish to dedicate this book to all of our colleagues throughout the cardiology community who have continued to encourage us in this important endeavor.

Most importantly, we want to thank our patients who have brought these clinical issues to the forefront of our practice and served as the impetus to bring this project to fruition.

Preface

While the majority of patients with symptomatic coronary artery disease achieve acceptable angina relief through the standard armamentarium of medical therapy, coronary artery bypass grafting and percutaneous coronary intervention, a growing number are not candidates for standard revascularization procedures. Standard revascularization procedures are largely palliative, and symptom recurrence is relatively common particularly as patients live longer following revascularization earlier in life in an aging population. In addition, the rapid worldwide increase in obesity and type 2 diabetes sets the stage for a potential explosion of patients with severe, diffuse coronary disease. As these trends continue, the population of patients who fail to achieve adequate symptomatic improvement through standard medical and revascularization strategies will certainly grow exponentially. Because the therapeutic options for patients with "unrevascularizable" symptomatic coronary artery disease are currently limited, there is a growing need for development of novel, effective and safe methods of symptom relief. Experimental and developing strategies have included transmyocardial laser revascularization (TMR), therapeutic angiogenesis, spinal cord stimulation, external counterpulsation (ECP), novel medical therapies and complex percutaneous and surgical revascularization strategies. To date, there is no central repository for data regarding these developing therapeutic strategies and a resulting lack of direction and focus in clinical management and research. Patients and clinicians alike are then left with a sense of helplessness and resignation that "nothing can be done."

A growing recognition of past failures in the treatment of "untreatable" patients and expanding awareness of the need for development of safe and effective therapies makes this an ideal time for the development of a textbook detailing current approaches and future directions in the management of the unrevascularizable patient. Through a comprehensive and clinically oriented review of the epidemiology and basic science foundation for studies in this population, current treatment strategies can be put in the context of past failures and future directions. As the first textbook of its kind, this book provides a framework within which the practicing clinician can expand on current practice, and experienced and young researchers alike can find an insightful resource, thereby addressing an entirely unmet need. We hope it is met with the enthusiasm with which it was developed and provides a reliable reference for clinical and basic researchers interested in this topic, as well as affected patients and their families.

Rochester, MN, USA

Gregory W. Barsness, MD
David R. Holmes Jr., MD

Contents

Contributors

Romero Corral Abel, M.D. Cardiovascular Division, Mayo Clinic Rochester, Rochester, MN, USA

Cardiovascular Department, Albert Einstein Medical Center, Philadelphia, PA, USA

Gregory W. Barsness, M.D. Mayo Clinic College of Medicine, Rochester, MN, USA

Bradley A. Bart, M.D. Hennepin County Medical Center, University of Minnesota, Minneapolis, MN, USA

Brent A. Bauer, M.D. Complementary and Integrative Medicine Program, Mayo Clinic, Rochester, MN, USA

Piero O. Bonetti, M.D. Division of Cardiology, Kantonsspital Graubuenden, Chur, Switzerland

Martial G. Bourassa, M.D. Montreal Heart Institute, Université de Montréal, Montreal, QC, Canada

Noel Caplice, M.D., Ph.D. Division of Cardiovascular Diseases, Department of Internal Medicine, Mater Private Hospital, Cork, Ireland

Mauricio G. Cohen, M.D. Cardiovascular Division, Department of Medicine, University of Miami Miller School of Medicine, Miami, FL, USA

Cardiac Catheterization Laboratory, University of North Carolina at Chapel Hill, Chapel Hill, NC, USA

Brendan Doyle, M.D., BCh Division of Cardiovascular Diseases, Department of Internal Medicine, Mater Private Hospital, Cork, Ireland

Lopez Jimenez Francisco, M.D., M.Sc. Cardiovascular Division, Mayo Clinic College of Medicine, Rochester, MN, USA

Timothy D. Henry, M.D. Minneapolis Heart Institute Foundation at Abbott Northwestern Hospital, University of Minnesota, Minneapolis, MN, USA

Joerg Herrmann, M.D. Department of Internal Medicine, Mayo Clinic Rochester, Rochester, MN, USA

David R. Holmes Jr., M.D. Mayo Clinic College of Medicine, Rochester, MN, USA

E. Marc Jolicoeur, M.D., M.Sc., MHS Montreal Heart Institute, Université de Montréal, Montreal, QC, Canada

Karen E. Joynt, M.D. Cardiovascular Division, Brigham and Women's Hospital, Boston, MA, USA

David E. Kandzari, M.D. Duke Clinical Research Institute, Duke University Medical Center, Durham, NC, USA

Thomas J. Kiernan, M.D. Division of Cardiovascular Diseases, Mayo Clinic, Rochester, MN, USA

Josef Korinek, M.D. Cardiovascular Division, Mayo Clinic Rochester, Rochester, MN, USA

Thomas E. Kottke, M.D. MSPH Cardiovascular Division, HealthPartners Research Foundation, Minneapolis, MN, USA

Roger J. Laham, M.D. Cardiovascular Division, Beth Israel Deaconess Medical Center and Harvard Medical School, Boston, MA, USA

Shahar Lavi, M.D. Division of Cardiovascular Diseases, Mayo Clinic, Rochester, MN, USA

Amir Lerman, M.D. Department of Internal Medicine, Mayo Clinic Rochester, Rochester, MN, USA

Robroy H. Mac Iver, M.D. Division of Cardiothoracic Surgery, Bluhm Cardiovascular Institute, Northwestern Memorial Hospital, Northwestern University's Feinberg School of Medicine, Chicago, IL, USA

Patrick M. McCarthy, M.D. Division of Cardiothoracic Surgery, Bluhm Cardiovascular Institute, Northwestern Memorial Hospital, Northwestern University's Feinberg School of Medicine, Chicago, IL, USA

Edwin C. McGee Jr., M.D. Division of Cardiothoracic Surgery, Bluhm Cardiovascular Institute, Northwestern Memorial Hospital, Northwestern University's Feinberg School of Medicine, Chicago, IL, USA

Christopher M. O'Connor, M.D. Division of Clinical Pharmacology, Departments of Medicine and Psychiatry and Behavioral Sciences, Duke University Medical Center, Durham, NC, USA

E. Magnus Ohman, M.D. Division of Cardiology, Department of Medicine, Duke University Medical Center, Durham, NC, USA

Daniel Satran, M.D. Department of Internal Medicine, University of Minnesota, Minneapolis, MN, USA

Jignesh S. Shah, M.D. Cardiovascular Division, Beth Israel Deaconess Medical Center and Harvard Medical School, Boston, MA, USA

Virend Somers, M.D., Ph.D. Cardiovascular Division, Mayo Clinic College of Medicine, Rochester, MN, USA

Joanna J. Wykrzykowska, M.D. Cardiovascular Division, Beth Israel Deaconess Medical Center and Harvard Medical School, Boston, MA, USA

1 Epidemiology of Cardiovascular Disease and Refractory Angina

Shahar Lavi, David E. Kandzari, and Gregory W. Barsness

Against the background of increasing health care expenditures, coronary heart disease has a significant impact on global economics as a leading cause of disability and loss of productivity. Over 70 million Americans suffer from cardiovascular disease, contributing to approximately 900,000 deaths annually. Coronary heart disease and cerebrovascular disease account for more than six million hospitalizations every year in the USA alone [1]. As treatment outcomes of acute coronary syndromes continue to improve, more patients survive the acute event and thus their disease state changes into a chronic phase. The increasing incidence of cardiovascular risk factors such as diabetes mellitus and obesity combined with the increasing number of revascularization procedures and decreased cardiac mortality rate have transformed the demographic of patients with ischemic heart disease into a steadily increasing population of patients with chronic, and occasionally refractory, angina pectoris.

S. Lavi (✉)
Division of Cardiovascular Diseases, Mayo Clinic, Rochester, MN, USA
e-mail: lavi.shahar@mayo.edu

D.E. Kandzari
Duke Clinical Research Institute, Duke University Medical Center, Durham, NC, USA

G.W. Barsness
Mayo Clinic College of Medicine, Rochester, MN, USA

Trends in Mortality from Cardiovascular Disease

One hundred years ago, cardiovascular disease accounted for less than 10% of death. As the risk of dying from communicable diseases decreased and the population aged, the burden of heart disease increased. In the past several years, cardiovascular diseases accounted for ~30% of death worldwide and for nearly 50% of deaths in the industrial world [2]. The majority of cardiovascular deaths are related to coronary heart disease (Fig. 1.1). It is predicted that by the year 2020 coronary heart disease will exceed infectious disease as the world's leading cause of death and morbidity [3]. While nutritional standards and control of infectious illnesses has markedly improved, cardiovascular diseases and associated mortality continue to increase. These diseases have been gradually replaced by chronic diseases such as coronary heart disease and cancer. The trend of replacing infection and malnutrition with ischemic heart disease and malignancies initially appeared in developed countries, but also has been observed to gradually extend to developing countries. In parallel, behavioral changes have only directly contributed to the incidence of coronary heart disease; the transition to sedentary lifestyle and decreased daily caloric expenditure coupled with increased caloric intake enriched with saturated fat result in increased body weight, hypertension, diabetes, and other risk factors related to cardiovascular disease.

Heart disease has been the leading cause of death in the USA in the past 50 years. In the recent years, increased access to improved medical therapy and the adoption of healthier life style, contributed to a decline in cardiovascular death in the USA (Fig. 1.2).

G.W. Barsness and D.R. Holmes Jr. (eds.), *Coronary Artery Disease*,
DOI 10.1007/978-1-84628-712-1_1, © Springer-Verlag London Limited 2012

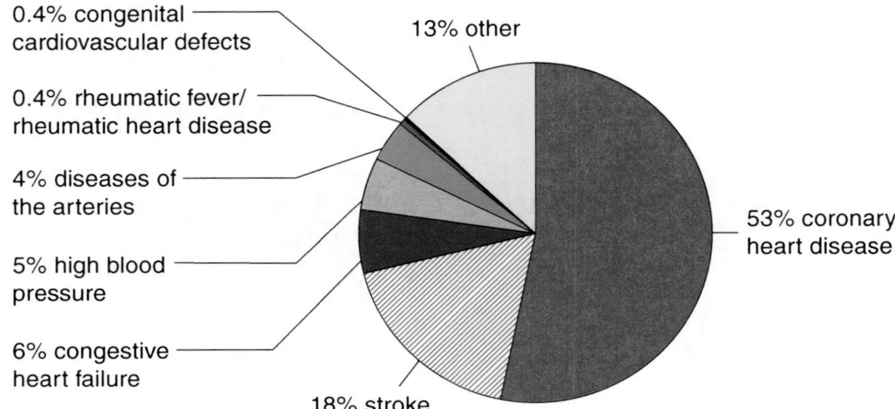

Fig. 1.1 Breakdown of death from cardiovascular disease. Unites States 2002 (Source: AHA, with permission)

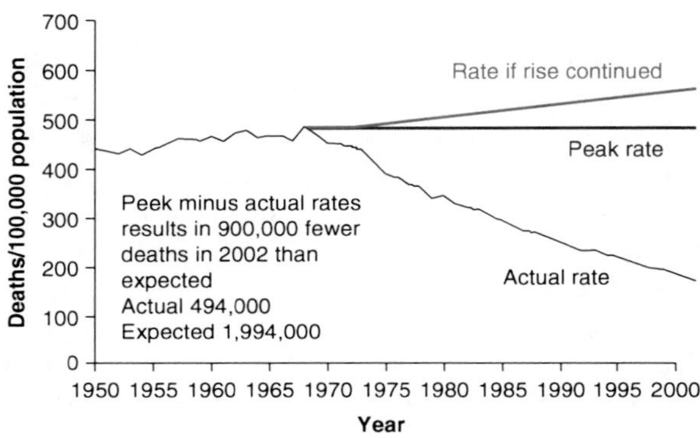

Fig. 1.2 Age-adjusted death rates for coronary heart disease, actual and expected, United States, 1950–2002 (Source: NIH, with permission)

The reduction can be seen in both coronary heart disease and stroke [4]. The data indicates a decline in cardiovascular mortality without a significant change in the incidence of myocardial infarction. Among men, age adjusted mortality from coronary heart disease declined from 2.2 per 1,000 in 1987 to 2.2 per 1,000 in 1991 with a steady mortality rate afterward during surveillance until 1994. Among women, coronary heart disease mortality decreased in the same years from 1.1 per 1,000 to 0.9 per 1,000 [5].

The Minnesota Heart Survey examined trends in mortality and morbidity due to coronary heart disease in the second half of the 1980s, among 30–74 year-old residents in a large metropolitan area: Minneapolis–St. Paul, Minnesota, and the surrounding suburbs. According to this survey, the age-adjusted rate of mortality due to coronary heart disease declined by approximately 25% in both sexes from 1985 to 1990. Decline in death rates were observed in both in-hospital and out of hospital coronary heart disease death. The decline in mortality rates from ischemic heart disease in the Minneapolis–St. Paul area during the 1970s and 1980s reflect national trends during these time periods. The decline in mortality was about 3.5% annually during the 1960s and reached a 25% reduction between the years 1985 and 1990. It is estimated that the decline in death due to coronary heart disease in the Twin Cities area in the latter half of the 1980s can be explained by both improved survival of patients hospitalized with myocardial infarction and reduced incidence of acute myocardial infarction in this population [6].

Data from the Framingham Heart Study and the offspring's cohorts reveal even a larger decrease in coronary heart disease death of 59% from 1950–1969 to 1990–1999 [7]. Despite the decrease in the mortality from heart disease in developed countries, heart disease remains the leading cause of death in these countries.

The decline in mortality from heart disease in developed countries may be attributed to both primary and secondary prevention strategies. Decreased rate of out-of-hospital death from coronary heart disease probably reflects primary prevention successes while the decline in hospital mortality in patients with acute coronary syndrome represents improved medical care [6]. Overall, the decline in cardiovascular mortality leads eventually to increase in the prevalence of chronic heart disease in developed countries.

It should be noted that in contrast to data from the USA, it is predicted that cardiovascular mortality will increase in developing countries as a consequence of social and economic factors and especially adoption of Western diet [8]. In a global viewpoint, mortality from cardiovascular causes is expected to increase.

Trends in Cardiovascular Risk Factors

Changes in risk factors status have a direct effect on trends in cardiovascular disease in broad populations. As the population ages and the tendency for a sedentary life style increases, the prevalence of many risk factors increases. Here we will provide a short summary of the trends in cardiac risk factors.

Hypertension: There is a continuous, consistent, and independent relationship between blood pressure levels and the risk of cardiovascular events. Hypertension affects approximately one billion individuals worldwide. More than 60% of the adult population in the USA has above normal blood pressure values, including 30% with hypertension, and another 31% who have prehypertension, defined as systolic blood pressure between 120 and 139 mmHg or diastolic blood pressure between 80 and 89 mmHg. It is estimated that the prevalence of hypertension will increase even further as the population ages as the lifetime risk for developing hypertension in normotensive subjects at 55 years of age is 90%. Reduction in blood pressure by 12–13 mmHg can reduce myocardial infarctions by 21%, and cardiovascular deaths by 25% [1, 9, 10]. Thus, improvement in blood pressure control has a significant potential for reduction in cardiovascular event rate.

Cholesterol: Many prospective trials revealed the relationship between high levels of low density lipoprotein (LDL) cholesterol and coronary heart disease. Hypercholesterolemia has a major effect on public health as about 50% of the population has cholesterol levels above 200 mg/dL [11]. A 10% decrease in total blood cholesterol levels may reduce the incidence of coronary heart disease by as much as 30% [11]. However, less than half of those who qualify receive lipid reduction therapy and more than 80% of people with high blood cholesterol do not have their lipid levels and blood pressure adequately controlled [1, 11, 12].

Diabetes mellitus: The prevalence of diabetes worldwide was estimated to be 2.8% in year 2000 and is projected to increase to 4.4% in 2030, particularly among individuals >65 years of age. It is estimated that the number of people with diabetes will more than double as a consequence of aging of the population and urbanization.

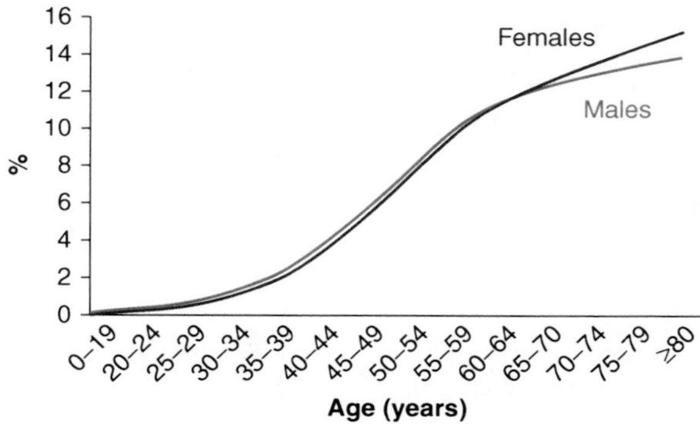

Fig. 1.3 Global diabetes prevalence by age and sex for 2000 (Source: Diabetes Care, with permission)

A further increase in diabetes prevalence is related to the enormous increase in obesity [13]. Coronary heart disease mortality is estimated to be 4.3-fold higher in patients with diabetes compared to nondiabetics [14]. Despite the decrease in cardiovascular death in the overall population in the industrial world, mortality attributable to diabetes is increasing, principally due to cardiovascular disease [14] (Figs. 1.3 and 1.4).

Smoking: The decrease in the coronary heart disease mortality is partially attributed to the steady decline in smoking, especially among males, from 1965 to 1990 [12]. The prevalence of current smokers among adults aged 18 years and over in the USA declined from 24.7% in 1997 to 20.9% in 2004 [15].

Obesity: Over the past 25 years, there has been a marked increase in the body mass index among individuals in the USA, with the prevalence of obesity among adults aged 20–74 years rising from 13% to 31% [16]. According to The Third Report of the National Cholesterol Education Program Expert Panel on Detection, Evaluation, and Treatment of High Blood Cholesterol in Adults definition, approximately 22% of American adults have metabolic syndrome [17]. Currently, 122 million adults are considered overweight or obese, a condition that further contributes to the rise in blood pressure levels [9].

Acute Coronary Syndrome Incidence

In the year 2002, an acute coronary syndrome was the primary diagnosis for in-patient hospitalization in nearly one million admissions in the USA. It is estimated that approximately 1.6 million patients

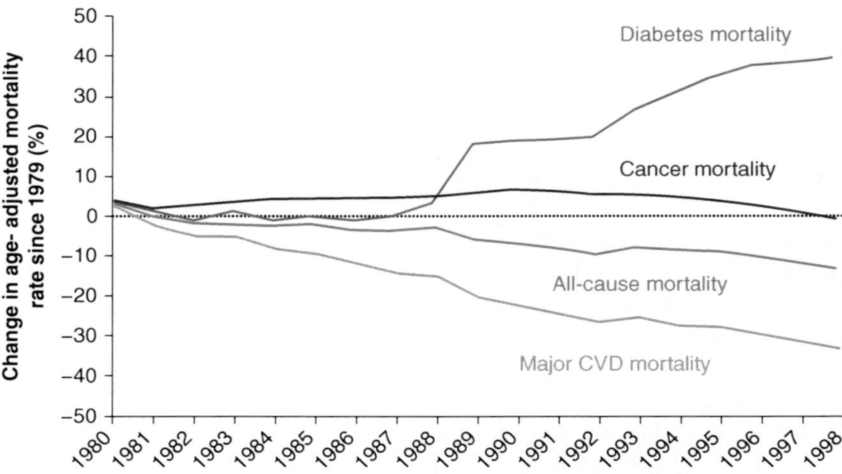

Fig. 1.4 Change in age-adjusted mortality rates since the year 1979 in the USA by cause of mortality (Centers for Disease Control and Prevention Mortality Database) (Source: Circulation, with permission)

with an acute coronary syndrome were hospitalized annually [12].

The hospitalization rates for acute myocardial infarction in the Minnesota Heart Survey show a moderate decline between 1985 and 1990. The main reduction was in the rate of first-time acute myocardial infarction and mirrored the favorable trend in the risk-factor profile of the general population [6]. In contrast to previous studies, this study showed increase in the discharge rate of patients with a diagnosis of acute coronary heart disease. Partial explanation is the introduction in the late 1980s of the ICD-9-CM code and the effects of reimbursement according to diagnosis-related groups. Both potentially could increase artifactually the diagnosis of acute coronary heart disease at discharge [6]. In a later report, the incidence of hospitalization due to myocardial infarction remained stable and even slightly increased. Therefore, the decrease in mortality from coronary heart disease during these years in this survey is mainly attributed to improvements in therapy and not decrease in the occurrence of new events [5].

Stable Angina Pectoris: Prevalence and Outcome

For epidemiologic studies, it has been long recognized that the reported incidence of myocardial infarction (MI) and sudden death may not accurately represent the prevalence of ischemic heart disease. Despite these limitations, however, because these events are routinely reported, they have been often adopted as surrogates for coronary artery disease. A report from the Mayo Clinic observed temporal trends in the incidence of hospitalized myocardial infarction and sudden death in Olmsted County, Minnesota [18]. In this report, the incidence of sudden death and MI declined by 17% between 1979 and 1998. During the second decade of the study period (1988–1998), when utilization of angiography had stabilized, coronary disease trends paralleled the trends observed in MI and in the combined incidence of MI and sudden death combined. Therefore, it was concluded that these events may be suitable indicators of trends in coronary disease prevalence [18].

Population surveys from the USA reveal that more than 60 million patients have cardiovascular disease, including more that 13 million with ischemic heart disease [12]. Cardiovascular disease is emerging as a leading chronic disease in the industrial world. As described previously, it may be difficult to estimate accurately the prevalence of angina pectoris. Nevertheless, the number of patients with angina pectoris can be extrapolated from the incidence of myocardial infarction. It is estimated that there are about 30 patients with angina for each patient with myocardial infarction who is hospitalized [19]. Accordingly, there are approximately 16,500,000 patients with stable angina in the USA [19].

Often significant ischemia exists with minimal or no symptoms. Silent myocardial ischemia was found in 11.4% of middle-aged and elderly subjects with no apparent heart disease [20]. Silent ischemia may account for up to 75% of all ischemic episodes in patients with angina pectoris [21]. These events are often recognized by electrocardiographic changes using an ambulatory electrocardiographic recorder or retrospectively after prior MI has been diagnosed by ECG or echocardiography. Therefore, national surveys likely underestimate the true prevalence of coronary heart disease.

According to the Framingham Study, 5 year death rate in middle-aged men with angina but with no evidence of previous infarction is 15–20%. Infarction rate during 1 year is 4–5% in these patients. More recent data, obtained in the setting of contemporary standards of care with aspirin, beta blockers, and statins reveal a reduced infarction rate of 1.7% in uncomplicated angina and 10 year mortality of 19% [22]. Also, there is a an association between the duration of chest pain and outcome. Patients with persistent angina have more indicators of severe disease and are more likely to experience subsequent cardiac events. In a study of 7,109 men with established coronary artery disease, those who reported anginal symptoms, both at the beginning of the study and after 5 years, had a twofold event risk compared with those who had ischemic symptoms only in the beginning of the follow-up [23].

Coronary Artery Bypass Grafting and Percutaneous Coronary Interventions

Percutaneous or surgical coronary revascularization is usually recommended to alleviate symptoms related to myocardial ischemia, and to reduce future risks. There is a steady increase in the number of cardiac catheterizations and revascularizations (Fig. 1.5). By the year 2000, more than 1,202,000 percutaneous coronary interventions (PCIs) and 519,000 surgical revascularization procedures were being performed annually in the USA [24].

Generally, two groups of patients may benefit from revascularization as opposed to medical therapy alone: Patients with significant angina despite medical therapy and patients who have significant coronary diseases accompanied by reduced left ventricular function. The recommendations for revascularization in stable angina pectoris are based primarily on dated clinical trials that compared medical therapy with coronary bypass surgery. Overall, bypass surgery extended the survival of surgical patients compared with medically treated patients by 4.3 months at 10 years of follow-up [25]. In these trials, coronary artery bypass surgery proved to be superior to medical therapy in patients with multivessel coronary artery disease or left main coronary artery disease, especially in the presence of left ventricular dysfunction.

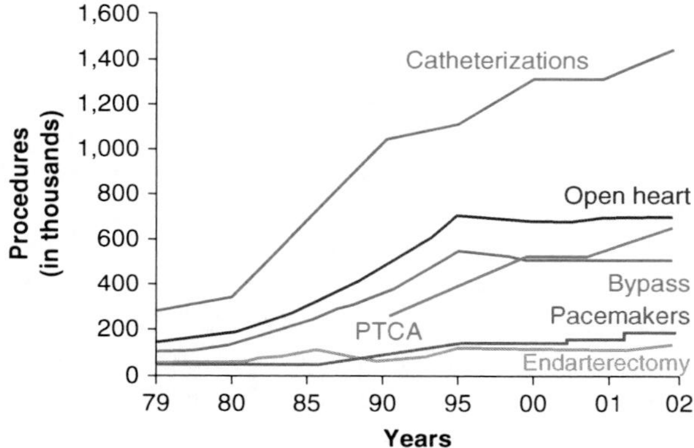

Fig. 1.5 Trends in cardiovascular operations and procedures. United States: 1979–2002 (Source AHA, with permission)

Information about the long-term outcome of patients who are not revascularized can be obtained from clinical trials that compared invasive treatment to medical therapy, as well as from longitudinal studies in which patients were mainly treated conservatively. Studies of patients with acute coronary syndromes generally involved early versus late interventions and not medical therapy alone and will not be discussed here.

Several studies compared PCI to medical therapy alone. In the Randomized Intervention Treatment of Angina (RITA)-2 trial, 1,018 patients, who were at a relatively low risk were treated by either medical therapy or percutaneous transluminal coronary intervention (PTCA). The mortality rate at 7 years was 8.5% in the medical therapy group and similar to that in the PTCA group. PTCA did improve symptoms compared to medical treatment alone [26]. It is noteworthy to mention that the current practice has changed considerably, with the liberal use of stents, drug eluting stents, and antiplatelet therapy. However, at the same time, there was also progress in medical therapy and intensive medical regimens including high-dose statins, blood pressure reduction, and routine antiplatelet therapy are now employed more often.

The Trial of Invasive versus Medical therapy in Elderly patients with chronic angina (TIME) compared an optimized medical strategy to an invasive strategy in patients 75 years of age. In this trial, patients were selected according to clinical presentation and not according to angiographic results. Class III or IV angina was present in 82% of patients. The rate of crossover was relatively large: 46% of the medical assigned patients were revascularized and 28% of the invasive assigned patients did not undergo revascularization, including 13% who were not suitable for revascularization. 4 year mortality was 28% and similar in both groups [27].

The Medicine, Angioplasty, or Surgery Study (MASS-II) was a controlled clinical trial that compared three treatment options: Surgery, PCI, and medical therapy in nonacute coronary syndrome patients with angiographically documented proximal multivessel disease. Medical therapy was assigned to 203 patients. Cardiac death rate in the medical arm at 1 year follow-up was 1.5%. Five percent had uncomplicated infarction and 8% were referred for revascularization. Cardiac death and myocardial infarction rates were similar to the surgical and PCI groups [28].

In a meta-analysis of six trials comparing PTCA to medical therapy in stable coronary artery disease patients, three trials included patients with multivessel disease. There was a greater relief of 30% in angina in the PTCA group, but with no significant difference in term of fatal and nonfatal infarctions [29].

We can conclude from the mentioned randomized trials that the outcome of patients with stable angina pectoris treated by medical therapy is generally benign in terms of death and myocardial infarction. However, the patients that were included in those trials were suitable for revascularization.

Medical Treatment Only Studies

The Angina Prognosis Study in Stockholm was a single center study that evaluated long-term use of anti-anginal medications, verapamil or metoprolol in patients with stable angina pectoris. The patient's outcomes were similar in both groups. Recently, an extended follow-up of 809 patients was reported and compared to matched individuals in a reference population. Objective signs of ischemia or previous manifestations of ischemic heart disease were present in 69% of patients at baseline. Expected requirement for revascularization during the first month was an exclusion criterion. During follow-up for a median of 9.1 years, 5% died from MI and additional 4% died from other cardiovascular causes. Total mortality and fatal MI among males were 19% and 6.6% respectively, and among females 6% and 1.6%, respectively.

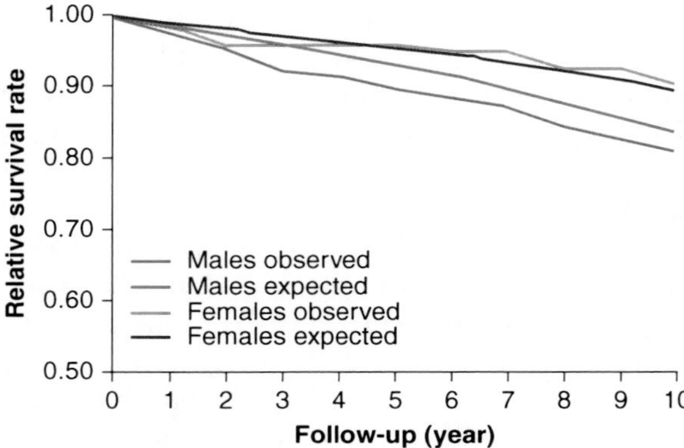

Fig. 1.6 Cumulative survival rates among male and female patients with stable angina pectoris (observed), and age-matched male and female subjects in a reference population from the same area (expected) (Source: Heart, with permission)

Most patients in this study had moderate angina (68%). Mild angina was present in 26% and class III angina in only ~5%. No association was found between angina type and event rate. Overall, these patients had a good prognosis. Female patients and the reference cohort had similar mortality rates throughout the study period. Male patients had slightly increase mortality in the first years, and thereafter survival curves paralleled those of the control cohort (Fig. 1.6). It can be concluded from this study that most patients with stable angina treated by medical therapy have favorable prognosis. It should be emphasized that revascularization was performed in 12% of patients during the initial 3.4 years of follow-up. Although this is a relatively low proportion, revascularization was used mainly for patients who were not controlled by medical therapy alone [30].

In another large prospective study, an initial approach based on intensive medical therapy, and strict criteria for coronary intervention was evaluated. A total of 693 patients with proved CAD were followed for 4.6 years. Long-term outcomes were excellent with an annual incidence of nonfatal MI, cardiac mortality, and total mortality of 2.2%, 0.8%, and 1.4%, respectively. Revascularization was performed in 24% of subjects [31].

Refractory Angina Pectoris

In order to define refractory angina, several criteria should be met: presence of angina for more than 3 months, objective evidence of reversible ischemia, and exhaustion of ordinary means for treating angina including medical therapy, angioplasty, and coronary bypass surgery [32]. It is noteworthy to mention, that sometimes a patient who is labeled as "not suitable candidate for revascularization" might undergo revascularization by another operator. Therefore, the potential for revascularization should be evaluated by other operators before putting the patient in the refractory angina category [33].

Surgical and catheter-based interventions are the mainstay treatment of angina pectoris in high risk patients and in those patients whose symptoms are not controlled by medical therapy. A large number of patients with ischemic heart disease have diffuse coronary disease that is not amenable to surgical or percutaneous revascularization. This results in an increasing number of patients with ischemic symptoms that are not controlled by conventional means.

Some of these patients underwent revascularization in the past, including multiple PCIs as well as surgical revascularization, and therefore sometimes they are not candidates for additional procedures. Others have comorbidities that preclude surgical or percutaneous intervention. Quite a few have small distal vessel disease or unfavorable morphologic characteristics such as severely degenerated vein grafts or chronic total occlusion that disqualifies them from revascularization. Patients who had previous bypass surgery may not have any more available conduits for repeat surgical procedures.

It is estimated that the amount of patients who are ineligible for revascularization will grow. Life expectancy increases gradually and constantly and reached 75.5 years at birth at 1991 [34]. As the population gets older and life expectancy increases, many patients who have anginal symptoms acquire more comorbidities that may disqualify them from undergoing invasive procedures. More patients survive after coronary events, the number of patients who undergoes repeat revascularization procedures increases and eventually they might get to a point in which repeat revascularization will not be appropriate for them anymore.

There is limited data concerning the long-term outcome of patients who are not suitable for revascularization. Clinical trials that compared medical to surgical or percutaneous revascularization were done on patients that were good candidates for both arms of the study. Those who did not were excluded from these trials.

The Mediators of Social Support Study (MOSS) was a nonrandomized longitudinal observational study, performed at Duke University Medical Center that evaluated prospectively outcomes of patients with significant CAD who underwent cardiac catheterization. Of 1,189 patients with advanced coronary artery disease and reduced left ventricular function or severe angina, 487 (41%) patients were not treated by revascularization. The remaining of the cohort with similar coronary disease severity that underwent revascularization by surgery or PCI represented a reference group for study end points. After median follow-up of 2.2 years, mortality for patients who were not treated by revascularization was 38% compared with 15% among patients who were treated by angioplasty and 19% for the bypass surgery group (Fig. 1.7). However, measures of functional status and quality of life were similar in both groups [35]. Long-term follow-up of patients from the Coronary Artery Surgery Study (CASS) registry show that surgery prolonged the life of patients with >60% left main coronary artery disease and abnormal LV systolic function [36]. In a small study that included 51 patients who had indication for CABG but were not referred to surgery because of distal coronary artery disease, a high mortality and morbidity rates were reported. It should be mentioned that patients with normal LV function had favorable prognosis [37]. We can conclude from these studies that the outcome of patients with refractory angina and/or left ventricular dysfunction is poor in the absence of revascularization.

It is unknown how many patients are not suitable for revascularization. In a study from the Cleveland Clinic that comprised 500 patients with symptomatic documented ischemia, 59 patients (12%) were considered unsuitable for coronary artery bypass grafting or PCI. The major cause of disqualification for revascularization in this study was at least one coronary artery with chronic total occlusion (64%). Mortality rate in these patients was 16.9% and the rate of myocardial infarction was 25.5%. Based on 12% of patients not entitled for revascularization, it can be estimated that about 200,000 patients who are referred for cardiac catheterization each year in the USA, may not be eligible for revascularization [38, 39]. We should emphasize that with current practice more patients having chronic total occlusions are referred for PCIs; therefore, this estimate might be above the actual figures.

There is some information on the outcome of patients with severe coronary artery disease who are treated by medicine alone, from clinical trials that compared novel approaches such as percutaneous transmyocardial laser revascularization (TMR) to

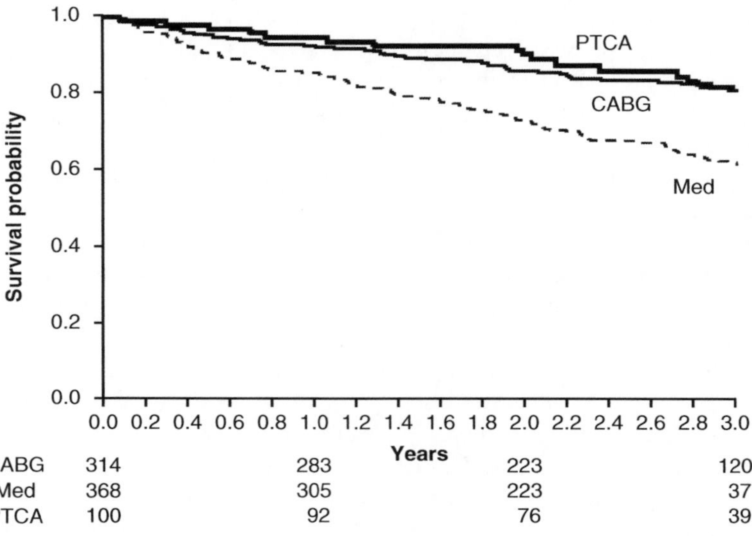

Fig. 1.7 Kaplan–Meier curves from the MOSS study demonstrating mortality among treatment groups beginning 30 days after diagnostic catheterization (MED, advanced coronary disease cohort; PTCA, angioplasty cohort; CABG, bypass surgery cohort) (Source: Am Heart J, with permission)

conventional medical therapy. These studies were usually relatively small and the follow-up period was not long. Surgical TMR is often performed as adjunct to coronary artery bypass grafting and less often as TMR alone. There is a large variability in patient's outcome in the different studies related to the extent of coronary disease, degree of ischemia and comorbidities.

In a study that compared TMR to maximal medical therapy, 141 patients with class III or IV angina, and failed PCI due to chronic total occlusion were included. Six-month death rates were 8.8% in the medical therapy group (not different from the TMR group) [40]. In another study that compared TMR to medical therapy in patients that could not be treated with percutaneous or surgical revascularization, 32% of patients in the medical group had improvement in angina at 12 months [41].

In a meta-analysis of randomized trials that evaluated the effect of TMR as a sole revascularization therapy, 1 year mortality in the medical treated groups ranged from 0% to 21% [42].

Cost

The economic expenditure due to cardiovascular disease is substantial and it grows as the population ages. In 2003, the cost of heart disease and stroke was projected to be $351 billion: $209 billion for health care expenditures and $142 billion for lost productivity from death and disability [1]. Direct costs of hospitalization due to stable angina are more than $ 15 billion. Indirect costs related to reduced productivity, medications, and workday lost are estimated to be as great as direct costs [19]. Although the initial hospital costs of patients with advanced coronary disease who are treated by medical therapy alone is substantially less than that of patients undergoing angioplasty and surgery, over time hospital costs exceeds those of patients undergoing revascularization [35]. It is estimated that the cost per patient is considerably higher in patients who are not suitable for revascularization, mainly due to indirect costs.

References

1. Preventing heart disease and stroke addressing the Nation's leading killers 2005. Centers for Disease Control, 2005. http://www.cdc.gov/nccdphp/aag/aag_cvd.htm. Accessed 29 Apr 2005.
2. World Health Organization. World health report 2004: changing history. Geneva: World Health Organization; 2004.
3. Gaziano JM. Global burden of cardiovascular disease. In: Zipes, editor. Braunwald's heart disease: a textbook of cardiovascular medicine, 7th ed. Philadelphia, PA: W.B. Saunders; 2005.
4. Ergin A, Muntner P, Sherwin R, He J. Secular trends in cardiovascular disease mortality, incidence, and case fatality rates in adults in the United States. Am J Med. 2004;117(4):219–27.
5. Rosamond WD, Chambless LE, Folsom AR, et al. Trends in the incidence of myocardial infarction and in mortality due to coronary heart disease, 1987–1994. N Engl J Med. 1998; 339(13):861–7.

6. McGovern PG, Pankow JS, Shahar E, et al. Recent trends in acute coronary heart disease – mortality, morbidity, medical care, and risk factors. N Engl J Med. 1996;334(14):884–90.
7. Fox CS, Evans JC, Larson MG, Kannel WB, Levy D. Temporal trends in coronary heart disease mortality and sudden cardiac death from 1950–1999: the Framingham heart study. Circulation. 2004;110(5):522–7.
8. Critchley J, Liu J, Zhao D, Wei W, Capewell S. Explaining the increase in coronary heart disease mortality in Beijing between 1984 and 1999. Circulation. 2004;110(10):1236–44.
9. Chobanian AV, Bakris GL, Black HR, et al. The seventh report of the Joint National Committee on prevention, detection, evaluation, and treatment of high blood pressure: the JNC 7 report. JAMA. 2003;289(19):2560–71.
10. Vasan RS, Beiser A, Seshadri S, et al. Residual lifetime risk for developing hypertension in middle-aged women and men: the Framingham heart study. JAMA. 2002;287(8): 1003–10.
11. American Heart Association. Heart disease and stroke statistics – 2005 update. Dallas: American Heart Association; 2005.
12. National Institutes of Health. Morbidity and mortality: 2004 chart book on cardiovascular, lung, and blood diseases. Bethesda: National Heart, Lung, and Blood Institute; 2004.
13. Wild SMB, Roglic G, Green AM, Sicree RM, King HM. Global prevalence of diabetes: estimates for the year 2000 and projections for 2030. Diabetes Care. 2004;27(5): 1047–53.
14. Sobel BE, Frye R, Detre KM. Burgeoning dilemmas in the management of diabetes and cardiovascular disease: rationale for the Bypass Angioplasty Revascularization Investigation 2 Diabetes (BARI 2D) Trial. Circulation. 2003;107(4):636–42.
15. National Center for Health Statistics, 2005. http://www.cdc.gov/nchs/nhis.htm. Accessed 29 Apr 2005.
16. Gregg EW, Cheng YJ, Cadwell BL, et al. Secular trends in cardiovascular disease risk factors according to body mass index in US adults. JAMA. 2005;293(15):1868–74.
17. Ford ES, Giles WH, Dietz WH. Prevalence of the metabolic syndrome among US adults: findings from the third National Health and Nutrition Examination survey. JAMA. 2002; 287(3):356–9.
18. Arciero TJ, Jacobsen SJ, Reeder GS, et al. Temporal trends in the incidence of coronary disease. Am J Med. 2004; 117(4):228–33.
19. ACC/AHA guideline update for the management of patients with chronic stable angina: a report of the American College of Cardiology/American Heart Association Task Force on practice guidelines (Committee to update the 1999 guidelines for the management of patients with chronic stable angina). 2002. Accessed at: http://www.acc.org/clinical/guidelines/stable/stable.pdf.
20. Sajadieh A, Nielsen OW, Rasmussen V, Hein HO, Hansen JF. Prevalence and prognostic significance of daily-life silent myocardial ischaemia in middle-aged and elderly subjects with no apparent heart disease. Eur Heart J. 2005;26(14): 1402–9.
21. Cohn PF, Fox KM, Daly C. Silent myocardial ischemia. Circulation. 2003;108(10):1263–77.
22. Lampe FC, Whincup PH, Wannamethee SG, Shaper AG, Walker M, Ebrahim S. The natural history of prevalent ischaemic heart disease in middle-aged men. Eur Heart J. 2000;21(13):1052–62.
23. Lampe FC, Whincup PH, Shaper AG, Wannamethee SG, Walker M, Ebrahim S. Variability of angina symptoms and the risk of major ischemic heart disease events. Am J Epidemiol. 2001;153(12):1173–82.
24. Rihal CS, Raco DL, Gersh BJ, Yusuf S. Indications for coronary artery bypass surgery and percutaneous coronary intervention in chronic stable angina: review of the evidence and methodological considerations. Circulation. 2003;108(20): 2439–45.
25. Eagle KA, Guyton RA, Davidoff R, et al. ACC/AHA guidelines for coronary artery bypass graft surgery: executive summary and recommendations: a report of the American College of Cardiology/American Heart Association Task Force on practice guidelines (Committee to revise the 1991 guidelines for coronary artery bypass graft surgery). Circulation. 1999;100(13):1464–80.
26. Henderson RA, Pocock SJ, Clayton TC, et al. Seven-year outcome in the RITA-2 trial: coronary angioplasty versus medical therapy. J Am Coll Cardiol. 2003;42(7):1161–70.
27. Pfisterer M, Trial of invasive versus Medical therapy in Elderly patients Investigators. Long-term outcome in elderly patients with chronic angina managed invasively versus by optimized medical therapy: four-year follow-up of the randomized Trial of Invasive Versus Medical Therapy in Elderly Patients (TIME). Circulation. 2004;110(10): 1213–8.
28. Hueb W, Soares PR, Gersh BJ, et al. The medicine, angioplasty, or surgery study (MASS-II): a randomized, controlled clinical trial of three therapeutic strategies for multivessel coronary artery disease: one-year results. J Am Coll Cardiol. 2004;43(10):1743–51.
29. Bucher HC, Hengstler P, Schindler C, Guyatt GH. Percutaneous transluminal coronary angioplasty versus medical treatment for non-acute coronary heart disease: meta-analysis of randomised controlled trials. BMJ. 2000;321(7253):73–7.
30. Hjemdahl P, Eriksson SV, Held C, Forslund L, Nasman P, Rehnqvist N. Favourable long-term prognosis in stable angina pectoris: an extended follow-up of the Angina Prognosis Study in Stockholm (APSIS). Heart. 2005;92(2): 177–82. doi:hrt.2004.057703.
31. Jabbour S, Young-Xu Y, Graboys TB, et al. Long-term outcomes of optimized medical management of outpatients with stable coronary artery disease. Am J Cardiol. 2004;93(3):294–9.
32. Mannheimer C, Camici P, Chester MR, et al. The problem of chronic refractory angina. Report from the ESC Joint Study Group on the treatment of refractory angina. Eur Heart J. 2002;23(5):355–70.
33. Kim MC, Kini A, Sharma SK. Refractory angina pectoris: mechanism and therapeutic options. J Am Coll Cardiol. 2002;39(6):923–34.
34. Life expectancy at birth, 65 and 85 years of age, by sex and race: United States, selected years 1900–2002. Center for Disease Control. http://209.217.72.34/aging/TableViewer/tableView.aspx. Accessed 29 Apr 2005.
35. Kandzari DE, Lam LC, Eisenstein EL, et al. Advanced coronary artery disease: appropriate end points for trials of novel therapies. Am Heart J. 2001;142(5):843–51.

36. Caracciolo EA, Davis KB, Sopko G, et al. Comparison of surgical and medical group survival in patients with left main coronary artery disease: long-term CASS experience. Circulation. 1995;91(9):2325–34.
37. da Rocha CAS, Rodrigues Dassa NP, Monassa Pittella FJ, et al. High mortality associated with precluded coronary artery bypass surgery caused by severe distal coronary artery disease. Circulation. 2005;112(9 suppl):I-328–31.
38. Mukherjee D, Bhatt DL, Roe MT, Patel V, Ellis SG. Direct myocardial revascularization and angiogenesis – how many patients might be eligible? Am J Cardiol. 1999;84(5):598–600.
39. Mukherjee D, Comella K, Bhatt DL, Roe MT, Patel V, Ellis SG. Clinical outcome of a cohort of patients eligible for therapeutic angiogenesis or transmyocardial revascularization. Am Heart J. 2001;142(1):72–4.
40. Stone GW, Teirstein PS, Rubenstein R, et al. A prospective, multicenter, randomized trial of percutaneous transmyocardial laser revascularization in patients with nonrecanalizable chronic total occlusions. J Am Coll Cardiol. 2002;39(10):1581–7.
41. Allen KB, Dowling RD, Fudge TL, et al. Comparison of transmyocardial revascularization with medical therapy in patients with refractory angina. N Engl J Med. 1999; 341(14):1029–36.
42. Liao L, Sarria-Santamera A, Matchar DB, et al. Meta-analysis of survival and relief of angina pectoris after transmyocardial revascularization. Am J Cardiol. 2005;95(10):1243–5.

Basic Science Concepts

2

Brendan Doyle and Noel Caplice

Introduction

Therapeutic options for atherosclerosis have expanded enormously over the past three decades. In particular, the development of surgical and percutaneous revascularization strategies for treating focal coronary lesions has effectively reduced morbidity and (to a lesser extent) mortality for a large number of patients. Greater attention is now being focused on a significant minority of patients with coronary arteriosclerosis who have significant but diffuse disease which is not amenable to mechanical revascularization. Even with optimal medical treatment, morbidity, mortality, and associated costs in this group remain high. Considerable hope has been vested in strategies which seek to augment the endogenous neovascularization response to ischemia. Although early clinical trials of a number of agents have been disappointing, continuing advances in our understanding of the mechanisms and key molecular pathways involved suggest we can remain optimistic that this approach will ultimately be successful.

The process of new blood vessel growth is frequently referred to as angiogenesis. More recently, this term has come to denote a specific biological process that does not encompass the entire spectrum of events that can result in new blood vessel development. The term angiogenesis is used here only in this narrow sense, and blood vessel growth is referred to in general as neovascularization. As currently understood, neovascularization may be achieved through three conceptually distinct mechanisms: angiogenesis, arteriogenesis, and possibly vasculogenesis [1]. Each is discussed here in turn, highlighting some of the most promising new avenues for therapeutic targeting. Other aspects of pro-angiogenic therapy are discussed in greater detail in Chap. 7 (Fig. 2.1).

Angiogenesis and Arteriogenesis

Angiogenesis is defined as the extension of an existing vascular bed by sprouting of new capillaries from post-capillary venules. Proteolytic degradation of the extracellular matrix is followed by chemotactic migration and proliferation of endothelial cells, formation of a lumen, and functional maturation of the newly formed capillary by tightening of inter-endothelial cell junctions. In contrast, arteriogenesis refers to a process of maturation (or perhaps de novo growth) of larger caliber collateral conduits which are invested with a smooth muscle cell coat, and are frequently of sufficient size to be visualized angiographically. The initial triggers of arteriogenesis are physical forces, most notably intravascular pressure gradients and fluid shear stress. Subsequent collateral vessel growth is linked to attraction and invasion of circulating blood cells, proliferation of vascular endothelial and smooth muscle cells, and remodeling processes which include digestion and rearrangement of the extracellular matrix and elastic lamina. Both angiogenesis and arteriogenesis are appropriate targets for therapy; proximal arterioles provide bulk flow to tissue while distal capillaries

B. Doyle (✉) • N. Caplice
Division of Cardiovascular Diseases, Department of Internal Medicine, Mater Private Hospital, Cork, Ireland
e-mail: drbdoyle2@materprivate.ie

G.W. Barsness and D.R. Holmes Jr. (eds.), *Coronary Artery Disease*,
DOI 10.1007/978-1-84628-712-1_2, © Springer-Verlag London Limited 2012

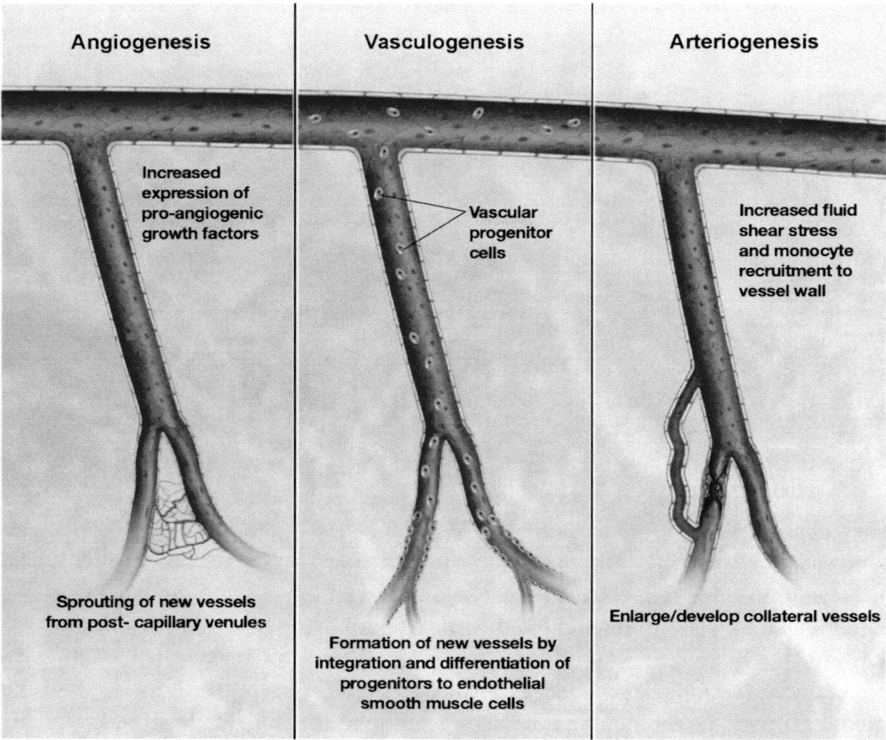

Fig. 2.1 Neovascularization, the process of new blood vessel growth, may be achieved through three conceptually distinct mechanisms: angiogenesis, arteriogenesis, and or vasculogenesis

distribute this flow. Although there is some degree of overlap, current understanding of the differences between initiating stimuli and molecular regulators of angiogenesis and arteriogenesis suggest that therapy directed at enhancing both will probably need to be multifaceted.

Oxygen Sensing, the HIF System, and Angiogenesis

The first experimental indication that angiogenesis must be subject to some form of metabolic regulation was provided by the striking correlation between muscle capillary density and the metabolic rate of different species in studies by Krogh almost a century ago [2]. Further insights were gained from pathophysiological studies of vascular and neoplastic disease, but it is only in recent years that the central role of a transcriptional complex called hypoxia inducible factor 1 (HIF-1) in oxygen sensing and the regulation of angiogenic growth factor gene expression has finally been elucidated [3].

HIF-1 is an $\alpha\beta$-heterodimer composed of HIF-α and HIF-β subunits, both of which can directly bind to DNA. HIF-1β subunits are constitutive nuclear proteins and their concentration remains stable under most conditions. HIF-α subunits are inducible by hypoxia. Among many genes induced by HIF-1α, those directly involved in angiogenesis include most prominently the VEGF family of genes, angiopoietins, and the inducible form of nitric oxide synthase (iNOS) [1]. The interface between the HIF system and tissue oxygen levels is efficiently direct. Oxygen-mediated hydroxylation of HIF-α results in the extremely rapid targeting of this molecule for proteasomal destruction [4–7], which in adequately perfused tissues provides a mechanism of HIF inactivation and inhibition of pro-angiogenic growth factor gene transcription, efficiently coupling metabolic demand to angiogenic activity.

Immunohistochemical staining of tissues for levels of HIF-α have advanced our understanding of the activity of this system in vivo. Such studies have confirmed that HIF-α levels are generally low in normoxic tissues, and may be undetectable even in physiologically hypoxic regions such as the renal medulla [8]. Levels are substantially increased after systemic hypoxia or tissue ischemia, although the extent and time course of induction varies between tissues [9–11]. Furthermore, HIF-α induction is often cell-type-specific within a particular region, suggesting that cellular thresholds for activation of the response may differ [8, 10, 11]. The fundamental role of tissue hypoxia and HIF system interfacing in the regulation of angiogenesis was recently reviewed in-depth by Pugh and Ratcliffe [3].

Pro-angiogenic Growth Factors and Angiogenesis

The existence of angiogenic growth factors was initially proposed on the basis of the strong neovascular response induced by transplanted tumors. Similar pro-angiogenic activity was subsequently demonstrated by non-neoplastic tissues. Many molecules have since been identified as positive regulators of angiogenesis including members of the VEGF gene family, platelet-derived growth factor (PDGF), fibroblast growth factors (FGFs), transforming growth factor (TGF)-α, TGF-β, hepatocyte growth factor (HGF), tumor necrosis factor-α, interleukin (Il)-8, and the angiopoietins [12, 13]. Among these, VEGF and PDGF appear to play a central role in neovascularization and their biology has been subject to the greatest scrutiny thus far.

The human VEGF gene is organized as eight exons separated by seven introns [14]. Alternative exon splicing was initially shown to result in the generation of four different isoforms having 121, 165, 189, and 206 amino acids, after signal sequence cleavage. As amino acid number increases, diffusion of the different isoforms through tissues decreases. Thus, VEGF189 and VEGF206 are both essentially sequestered in the extracellular matrix, VEGF121 is freely diffusible, and VEGF165 exhibits intermediate diffusion. VEGF isoforms have variable heparin-binding affinity, a property which has been shown to significantly influence mitogenic activity of the isoform. Overall, it appears that VEGF165 has optimal characteristics of bioavailability and biological potency with regard to the induction of angiogenesis. VEGF gene expression is regulated by oxygen tension (discussed above) and by several major growth factors, inflammatory cytokines, and by certain oncogenic mutations. The biological effects of VEGF are mediated by two receptor tyrosine kinases (RTK), VEGFR-1 and VEGFR-2, which differ considerably in signaling properties. Although VEGFR-1 was the first RTK to be identified as a VEGF receptor more than a decade ago [15] the precise function of this molecule is still debated. Both pro- and antiangiogenic effects have been demonstrated. Recent evidence indicates that the conflicting reports may be due, at least in part, to the fact that the functions and signaling properties of this receptor can differ depending on the developmental stage of the animal and the cell type (for instance, endothelial cells versus bone marrow cells). VEGFR-2, in contrast, has unequivocally emerged as the key mediator of the mitogenic, angiogenic, and permeability-enhancing effects of VEGF [14].

Platelet-derived growth factor is structurally related to VEGF [16] and was one of the first growth factors shown to regulate vessel maturation. Four members of this family have since been identified, PDGF-A, PDGF-B, PDGF-C, and PGDF-D. These must form dimers (AA, BB, etc.) to be physiologically active. PDGF-BB has an essential role in the maturation of nascent blood vessels recruiting smooth muscle cells and pericytes to the vessel wall but the therapeutic potential of this agent to augment blood supply to ischemic tissue appears limited, achieving significant neovascularization only when coadministered with other angiogenic growth factors [17]. PDGF-CC has emerged as arguably the more attractive candidate for use in the clinic, demonstrating revascularization of ischemic tissues through mechanisms which include mobilization and enhanced differentiation of bone marrow-derived endothelial progenitor cells [18].

New capillary development requires a coordinated interplay between VEGF, PDGF, and several other pro-angiogenic growth factors in a multi-step process which results in mature neovessel formation [19]. The initial step in angiogenesis involves nitric oxide-mediated vasodilation. Vascular permeability subsequently increases in response to VEGF, allowing extravasation of plasma proteins that lay down a provisional scaffold for migrating endothelial cells. For endothelial cells to emigrate from their resident site at the luminal surface of the vessel wall they need to loosen interendothelial cell contacts and to relieve periendothelial cell support; that is, mature vessels need to become destabilized. Angiopoietin 2 (Ang2) may be involved in detaching smooth muscle cells and loosening the matrix. Proteinases further degrade the extracellular matrix and may activate or liberate further pro-angiogenic growth factors sequestered within the matrix. Once a path has been cleared, proliferating endothelial cells migrate to distant sites under the influence of a number of pro-angiogenic growth factors (mainly those of the VEGF family). Endothelial cells may assemble as solid cords that subsequently acquire a lumen, the latter process promoted by VEGF and angiopoietin 1 (Ang1). Even after incorporation within new patent vessels, survival of endothelial cells remains dependent for some time on pro-angiogenic growth factor signaling. Endothelial apoptosis may arise following deprivation of these survival signals as occurs, for instance, in premature babies exposed to hyperoxia resulting in downregulation of VEGF and regression of retinal vessels.

Shear Stress, Monocytes, and Arteriogenesis

Unlike angiogenesis, the regulation of arteriogenesis does not appear dependent on local tissue hypoxia but upon the growth and remodeling of preexisting collateral anastomoses [20]. The potential for arteriogenesis to increase blood flow to ischemic tissue is considerably greater than that of angiogenesis and as such is regarded as an extremely attractive therapeutic target.

Following occlusion of an artery, the pressure in its distal stump falls to very low levels. When a vascular connection exists between the high-pressure region proximal to the occlusion and the distal low-pressure region, a steep pressure gradient develops which increases blood flow through these connections. Distension of the vessel wall by increased intravascular pressure increases circumferential wall stress, which in turn may activate smooth muscle cell proliferation [21]. Furthermore, increased blood flow through these nascent collateral vessels also augments fluid shear stress, or the viscous drag that flowing blood exerts on the endothelial lining. Fluid shear stress (FSS) is a relatively weak force but its role in arteriogenesis is still significant. Endothelium lining the collateral conduit exposed to fluid shear stresses becomes activated, recruiting circulating cells to the vessel wall. How the endothelial cell senses changes in FSS and transforms this signal into a change in gene expression is not yet understood. An elegant explanation has been proposed whereby tight coupling of the cell membrane with the cytoskeleton forms a "tensegrity" architecture so that the entire cell, when deformed by FSS, acts as a sensor [22–24]. Before this structure is deformed, FSS may also be detected by sensitive structures such as integrins, tyrosine kinase receptors, caveolae, and several ion channels within the endothelial cell membrane [25–27]. An intermediary role for the actin filaments of the cytoskeleton has been suggested, wherein the endothelial cytoskeleton is at least indirectly connected to all shear receptors [28, 29] which signal to several endothelial compartments including the nucleus [30, 31]. More than 40 genes have been reported to contain shear stress responsive elements within their promoter [20].

The biomechanical stimulus described above leads to marked alterations in the expression of numerous genes [32–35], including several which code for chemoattractant or activating cytokines (including growth factors), and for adhesion molecules [36–40]. This leads to the recruitment of circulating cells to the collateral vessel wall. Monocytes in particular appear to play a critical role in subsequent collateral enlargement and maturation, stimulating vascular smooth muscle and endothelial cell proliferation. This process is initiated as early as 24 h after experimental occlusion of the femoral artery in a rabbit model and peaks at days 3–7. Endothelial cell mitosis precedes that of smooth muscle cells by a few hours [41]. Increased smooth muscle cell mitosis coincides with a morphological change in these cells: the appearance of a prominent rough endoplasmic reticulum and many free ribosomes indicating that smooth muscle cells have been transformed from a contractile to a proliferative/synthetic phenotype [42]. During this phase, a neointima composed of smooth muscle cells is formed and increased matrix metalloproteinase activity (most likely derived from monocytes/macrophages) can be observed in the perivascular space of growing collaterals. It is possible that the latter may play a role in tissue digestion around the enlarging vessel, facilitating positive remodeling and maximizing final lumen size. As collateral vessel diameter gradually increases, fluid shear stress falls. This normalization of fluid shear stress may be a signal for maturation, downregulating endothelial cell activation and completing the transformation of a small microvascular resistance vessel into a large conductance artery [20].

Vasculogenesis

Until recently, concepts of endogenous neovascularization in the adult were limited in scope to the proliferation of existing terminally differentiated cells within vascular tissue and remodeling of preexisting collateral conduits as outlined above. The discovery of progenitor cells in peripheral blood that can differentiate into endothelial and smooth muscle cells has led to the reevaluation of these beliefs, with paradigms of vascular regeneration and repair now extended to include the possibility of postnatal vasculogenesis.

Vasculogenesis is defined as the formation of new blood vessels by the differentiation of precursor cells in situ and is the preeminent mechanism of new vessel formation in the embryo. Accumulating evidence now supports a role for circulating and vessel wall-derived progenitor cells in adult vascular biology. The first description of circulating adult endothelial progenitor cells (EPCs) published by Asahara et al. in 1997 [43] demonstrated that peripheral blood cells enriched for CD34 positivity could differentiate into endothelial-like cells in vitro, expressing a range of proteins characteristic of this cell type and exhibiting functional characteristics consistent with endothelial cells. Intravenous infusion of fluorescently labeled CD34 positive peripheral blood mononuclear cells (PBMCs) into murine and rabbit models of hindlimb ischemia resulted in neovascularization with vascular incorporation of these cells. VEGF-receptor2 positive enriched PBMCs also exhibited this capacity for postnatal vasculogenesis. Subsequent studies affirmed these findings by demonstrating endothelial cell differentiation capacity by a number of hematopoietic stem cell starting populations, including human CD133 positive cells [44]. Furthermore, single cell marrow reconstitution by a fluorescent labeled hemangioblast in a murine model demonstrated progenitor cell incorporation within a neovascularized region of the retina [45]. In addition to endothelial progenitors, circulating adult smooth muscle progenitors have also been identified in humans [46]. Evidence supporting bone marrow origin of vascular smooth muscle cells has been provided by a study demonstrating the presence of smooth muscle cells of donor origin in atherosclerotic lesions of patients receiving gender-mismatched bone marrow transplants [47].

These findings, although unexpected before the initial discovery by Asahara et al., were not counterintuitive given the common origins of vascular and hematopoietic stem cells in embryogenesis. What has been more intriguing has been the variety of cell types that have since been shown to reserve endothelial and smooth muscle cell differentiation capability. Vascular progenitors have been identified from a number of bone marrow and peripheral blood cell populations, and also from organs such as the heart, liver, spleen, and gut [48]. Indeed, a hierarchy of progenitors has recently been characterized within the vessel wall itself [49]. In hematopoiesis, the most proliferative progenitor that can be cultured in the absence of a stromal cell monolayer is termed the high-proliferative potential colony-forming cell [50]. Using a novel single-cell deposition clonogenic assay, Ingram et al. [49] demonstrated the presence of both low-proliferative and high-proliferative potential endothelial progenitors within the vessel wall, providing a new framework for the classification of cells supporting endopoiesis akin to that already established for the hematopoietic system [49].

Notwithstanding the exciting new perspectives these discoveries have brought to vascular biology, the true significance of the role of vascular progenitors in health and disease has yet to be fully elucidated. In particular, the contribution of vascular progenitor biology to endogenous neovascularization following ischemia is unclear. Improvements in tissue perfusion following infusion of ex vivo-expanded EPCs and autologous bone marrow mononuclear cells have been demonstrated in both animal [51–54] and human [55] peripheral vascular insufficiency. Measurements of tissue perfusion and myocardial contractile function have also improved in association with progenitor cell therapy in animal models of ischemic heart disease [54, 56, 57]. The precise mechanism underlying the apparent involvement of these cells in tissue perfusion remains to be defined, but may involve promotion of one (or more) of the three distinct neovascularization processes already discussed – vasculogenesis, angiogenesis, and arteriogenesis.

One might expect that amelioration of tissue ischemia by cells with the capacity for vascular cell differentiation would come about as a result of new vessel formation through vasculogenesis. In reality it appears that direct progenitor incorporation occurs at rates that are lower than might have been anticipated, although there is substantial variation depending on the model studied. In normal mice without injury, basal vascular incorporation of endothelial progenitors is extremely low at no more than 1.4% [58], rising to about 10% in the setting of significant vascular perturbation [59]. Mature adult endothelial cells have a half-life of approximately 3 years and retain the capacity to proliferate in response to minor injury, consistent with these relative rates of incorporation. In keeping with a putative evolutionary role of progenitor cells in vascular repair that would be sufficient to confer a survival advantage, models that employ substantial vascular injury such as allogenic cardiac/vascular transplantation without immunosuppression [60, 61] and wire-induced injury sufficient to cause medial necrosis [62] have been associated with the highest percentage of direct incorporation with rates of up to 80%.

However, the improvements in tissue perfusion do not uniformly correlate as expected with the observed level of progenitor cell integration in the neovasculature. Indeed, some groups have demonstrated important contributions to angiogenesis and arteriogenesis in the absence of direct incorporation of progenitors [63, 64]. The secretion of pro-angiogenic and survival factors by vascular progenitors is a potential supportive mechanism which may be relevant in these circumstances. A range of blood-borne, bone marrow-derived, and other tissue-derived vascular progenitors have been shown to produce cytokines and growth factors such as VEGF and HGF, which may be released and impact neighboring cells in a paracrine manner [65]. The biologic role of these factors may be revealed not only in the potentiation of the ischemic tissues instrinsic angiogenic and arteriogenic response, but also (by modulating processes such as apoptosis) in survival of target tissue cells, such as cardiomyocytes. In addition, mobilization and recruitment of endogenous vascular progenitors from remote sources to ischemic tissue in response to these factors may provide a means of maintaining and augmenting these beneficial effects [66]. How this might be harnessed in the treatment of vascular insufficiency is discussed below.

Failure of the Endogenous Response to Ischemia

Despite the potential for endogenous mechanisms of neovascularization to maintain myocardial perfusion and function even in the setting of critical coronary artery disease, the response is more frequently inadequate. In fact, atherosclerosis is associated with severe impairment of angiogenesis and arteriogenesis [67] although the reasons for this are still not entirely clear. The development of coronary collateral vessels can be predicted to a certain extent by a number of factors such as the duration, location, and severity of disease, and the level of physical activity of the patient. Nonetheless, much of the differences observed between patients in clinical practice remain unexplained [68, 69].

The ability of the vasculature to respond to pro-angiogenic growth factor stimulation may be a key factor in this context. Although we know relatively little about what regulates vascular responsiveness it is apparent that this diminishes with age [1] and a number of disease states. The mechanisms underlying this are now being examined. For instance, in a recent study of patients with coronary artery disease, those with diabetes were found to have increased VEGF expression within ischemic myocardial tissue when compared to normal controls and to nondiabetic patients [70]. Interestingly, diabetics were also found to have decreased expression of VEGF receptors and down-regulation of VEGF signal transduction [70]. Further evidence supporting the concept of vascular resistance to pro-angiogenic stimuli has been provided by studies of monocyte function in diabetics, which revealed impairment of the ability of these cells to migrate toward a gradient of VEGF-A. This deficiency appears to arise as a result of a signal transduction defect within the monocyte [71]. Other aspects of monocyte function may also be important, such as the ability of these cells to respond to hypoxia by increasing HIF-1α, a function which was demonstrated to correlate with the extent of collateral development. Greater understanding of these and other post-receptor defects in neovascularization may be critically important to the success of future attempts to develop effective treatments. Most work to date has focused almost exclusively on increasing expression of pro-angiogenic growth factors within ischemic tissue, an approach which may have significant limitations when considered within this conceptual framework.

An exclusive focus on pro-angiogenic factors may also have other limitations. Increased expression and availability of such factors may not, in isolation, be sufficient to induce angiogenesis due to the countervailing influence of angiogenesis inhibitors. These include the thrombospondins [72, 73], platelet factor 4 [74, 75], endostatin [76], and kallistatin [77] among a growing list of recognized endogenous agents. The competitive balance between these agonists and inhibitors has been the subject of intense study in tumor biology and therapeutics. Less in known at present about their role in vascular disease, although emerging data suggests this may indeed be significant. For instance, single-nucleotide polymorphisms of thrombospondin 1, 2 and 4 are associated with increased risk of premature myocardial infarction [78]. Furthermore, experimental animal models support a role for endogenous systems of angiogenesis inhibition as an important mechanism in the regulation of plaque growth. Evidence is now emerging to support an inhibitory role for endogenous angiogenesis inhibitors in collateral vessel formation, higher pericardial endostatin levels having been associated with the absence of collateral coronary vessel growth [79]. Endostatin is a potent inhibitor of angiogenesis, limiting proliferation and migration of endothelial cells in addition to inducing endothelial cell apoptosis [80, 81]. Further studies will be needed to more clearly define the role of this and similar agents in the regulation of endogenous neovascularization following ischemia.

Translation: Basic Science Concepts, New Treatments

During the past decade, attempts to translate encouraging preclinical data to effective therapies in the clinic have on the whole been disappointing. Nonetheless, greater understanding of the fundamental mechanisms and regulatory elements of endogenous neovascularization are now allowing us to approach the development of new therapies in a more focused manner. In particular, new blood vessel growth is now recognized as a complex, multigene event and it appears likely that multiple growth factors acting over a prolonged period of time will be required if clinically meaningful and sustained neovascularization is to be induced. Several strategies have been proposed to achieve this goal.

Gene transfer is one such method, used as a gain-of-function strategy to replace or augment defective or under-compensating genes that are involved in the endogenous response to ischemia. The therapeutic potential of gene transfer has been demonstrated in several animal models of cardiovascular disease using a wide range of therapeutic targets [82]. The major hindrance to the development of effective gene therapies for vascular disease has been the lack of efficient vectors and delivery tools for the genetic manipulation of blood vessels. Most of the current vectors lack tissue specificity and express transgenes over a relatively brief timeframe [83, 84]. Recombinant viruses which deliver genetic material with higher efficiency than nonviral vectors are now preferred for cardiovascular gene transfer. Some of these, such as lentivirus and adeno-associated virus, are capable of sustained expression of the therapeutic gene although this too may be attenuated by immune reaction to viral proteins. Of course, prolonged and unregulated expression of an angiogenic agent may also have unwanted effects. In order to tailor angiogenic therapy to tissue requirements, future vectors should ideally incorporate physiologically responsive promoter elements that are capable of adjusting therapeutic gene expression in response to changes in tissue milieu such as reduced oxygen tension. The possibility of multigene transfer allowing the simultaneous expression of multiple growth factors is now also emerging as a therapeutic option and several studies are underway to assess efficacy of this approach for inducing neovascularization.

Another approach to sustained delivery of multiple angiogenic growth factors in ischemic vascular beds is cell therapy. As discussed above, various vascular progenitor cell types have been shown to enhance neovascularization by enhancing angiogenesis, arteriogenesis, and vasculogenesis. Most of these studies have employed cells which have been expanded ex vivo before use in treatment. Clearly, such an approach in the clinic would be cumbersome and would likely restrict availability to highly specialized cell therapy centers. From a practical standpoint, strategies directed at enhancing the endogenous progenitor response using pharmacologic means would be preferable. The mechanisms underlying progenitor cell mobilization, target tissue homing and integration, and the functional capabilities of these cells are now being elucidated [48] and may eventually facilitate such an approach.

Key to the successful evolution of these novel treatments will be improvements in our ability to monitor efficacy, and in particular, our ability to image the microcirculation in vivo. Molecular imaging of angiogenesis by targeting various "angiogenic" endothelial cell-specific antigens such as $\alpha v\beta 3$ integrin [85] and VEGF receptors [86] has demonstrated early evidence of feasibility. Other technological advances which should complement direct visualization of the microvasculature include improved methodologies for assessing the effects of enhanced neovascularization, such as increased tissue perfusion, oxygenation, or function. MRI and PET offer high spatial resolution and sensitivity which are now being effectively applied in this context, although experience with both in large clinical trials is limited.

Conclusions

Insight into the fundamental mechanisms regulating endogenous neovascularization has progressed rapidly in recent years, as has our understanding of the reasons why previous attempts to augment this response have failed. Exciting advances in cardiovascular and molecular imaging should accelerate further still developments in this field. In this setting, the concept that pro-angiogenic therapies may soon offer a viable therapeutic option for patients with refractory angina now appears increasingly reasonable. What form these therapies may ultimately take is explored more fully in Chap. 8.

References

1. Simons M. Angiogenesis: where do we stand now? Circulation. 2005;111:1556–66.
2. Krogh A. The number and distribution of capillaries in muscles with calculations of the oxygen pressure head necessary for supplying the tissue. J Physiol. 1919;52:409–15.
3. Pugh CW, Ratcliffe PJ. Regulation of angiogenesis by hypoxia: role of the HIF system. Nat Med. 2003;9: 677–84.
4. Ivan M, Kondo K, Yang H, Kim W, Valiando J, Ohh M, et al. HIFalpha targeted for VHL-mediated destruction by proline hydroxylation: implications for O_2 sensing. Science. 2001;292:464–8.
5. Jaakkola P, Mole DR, Tian YM, Wilson MI, Gielbert J, Gaskell SJ, et al. Targeting of HIF-alpha to the von Hippel-Lindau ubiquitylation complex by O_2-regulated prolyl hydroxylation. Science. 2001;292:468–72.
6. Yu F, White SB, Zhao Q, Lee FS. HIF-1alpha binding to VHL is regulated by stimulus-sensitive proline hydroxylation. Proc Natl Acad Sci USA. 2001;98:9630–5.
7. Masson N, Willam C, Maxwell PH, Pugh CW, Ratcliffe PJ. Independent function of two destruction domains in hypoxia-inducible factor-alpha chains activated by prolyl hydroxylation. EMBO J. 2001;20:5197–206.
8. Rosenberger C, Mandriota S, Jurgensen JS, Wiesener MS, Horstrup JH, Frei U, et al. Expression of hypoxia-inducible factor-1alpha and -2alpha in hypoxic and ischemic rat kidneys. J Am Soc Nephrol. 2002;13:1721–32.
9. Lee SH, Wolf PL, Escudero R, Deutsch R, Jamieson SW, Thistlethwaite PA. Early expression of angiogenesis factors in acute myocardial ischemia and infarction. N Engl J Med. 2000;342:626–33.
10. Stroka DM, Burkhardt T, Desbaillets I, Wenger RH, Neil DA, Bauer C, et al. HIF-1 is expressed in normoxic tissue and displays an organ-specific regulation under systemic hypoxia. FASEB J. 2001;15:2445–53.
11. Wiesener MS, Jurgensen JS, Rosenberger C, Scholze CK, Horstrup JH, Warnecke C, et al. Widespread hypoxia-inducible expression of HIF-2alpha in distinct cell populations of different organs. FASEB J. 2003;17:271–3.
12. Folkman J, Shing Y. Angiogenesis. J Biol Chem. 1992;267:10931–4.
13. Yancopoulos GD, Davis S, Gale NW, Rudge JS, Wiegand SJ, Holash J. Vascular-specific growth factors and blood vessel formation. Nature. 2000;407:242–8.
14. Ferrara N, Gerber HP, LeCouter J. The biology of VEGF and its receptors. Nat Med. 2003;9:669–76.
15. de Vries C, Escobedo JA, Ueno H, Houck K, Ferrara N, Williams LT. The fms-like tyrosine kinase, a receptor for vascular endothelial growth factor. Science. 1992;255: 989–91.
16. Bergsten E, Uutela M, Li X, Pietras K, Ostman A, Heldin CH, et al. PDGF-D is a specific, protease-activated ligand for the PDGF beta-receptor. Nat Cell Biol. 2001;3:512–6.
17. Dimmeler S. Platelet-derived growth factor CC – a clinically useful angiogenic factor at last? N Engl J Med. 2005;352:1815–6.
18. Li X, Tjwa M, Moons L, Fons P, Noel A, Ny A, et al. Revascularization of ischemic tissues by PDGF-CC via effects on endothelial cells and their progenitors. J Clin Invest. 2005;115:118–27.
19. Carmeliet P. Angiogenesis in health and disease. Nat Med. 2003;9:653–60.
20. Heil M, Schaper W. Influence of mechanical, cellular, and molecular factors on collateral artery growth (arteriogenesis). Circ Res. 2004;95:449–58.
21. Scheel K. The possible role of mechanical stresses on coronary collateral development during gradual coronary occlusion. In: Schaper W, editor. The pathophysiology of myocardial perfusion. Amsterdam: Elsevier/North Holland; 1979. p. 489–518.
22. Ingber DE, Tensegrity I. Cell structure and hierarchical systems biology. J Cell Sci. 2003;116:1157–73.
23. Ingber DE, Tensegrity II. How structural networks influence cellular information processing networks. J Cell Sci. 2003;116:1397–408.
24. Ingber DE. Mechanical signaling and the cellular response to extracellular matrix in angiogenesis and cardiovascular physiology. Circ Res. 2002;91:877–87.
25. Resnick N, Yahav H, Shay-Salit A, Shushy M, Schubert S, Zilberman LC, et al. Fluid shear stress and the vascular endothelium: for better and for worse. Prog Biophys Mol Biol. 2003;81:177–99.
26. Topper JN, Gimbrone Jr MA. Blood flow and vascular gene expression: fluid shear stress as a modulator of endothelial phenotype. Mol Med Today. 1999;5:40–6.
27. Davies PF, Barbee KA, Volin MV, Robotewskyj A, Chen J, Joseph L, et al. Spatial relationships in early signaling events of flow-mediated endothelial mechanotransduction. Annu Rev Physiol. 1997;59:527–49.
28. Barbee KA. Changes in surface topography in endothelial monolayers with time at confluence: influence on subcellular shear stress distribution due to flow. Biochem Cell Biol. 1995;73:501–5.
29. Helmke BP, Davies PF. The cytoskeleton under external fluid mechanical forces: hemodynamic forces acting on the endothelium. Ann Biomed Eng. 2002;30:284–96.
30. Bojanowski K, Maniotis AJ, Plisov S, Larsen AK, Ingber DE. DNA topoisomerase II can drive changes in higher order chromosome architecture without enzymatically modifying DNA. J Cell Biochem. 1998;69:127–42.

31. Ingber D. In search of cellular control: signal transduction in context. J Cell Biochem Suppl. 1998;30–31:232–7.
32. Gimbrone Jr MA, Topper JN, Nagel T, Anderson KR, Garcia-Cardena G. Endothelial dysfunction, hemodynamic forces, and atherogenesis. Ann N Y Acad Sci. 2000;902: 230–9, discussion 239–40.
33. Shyy JY, Li YS, Lin MC, Chen W, Yuan S, Usami S, et al. Multiple cis-elements mediate shear stress-induced gene expression. J Biomech. 1995;28:1451–7.
34. Shyy JY, Lin MC, Han J, Lu Y, Petrime M, Chien S. The cis-acting phorbol ester "12-O-tetradecanoylphorbol 13-acetate"-responsive element is involved in shear stress-induced monocyte chemotactic protein 1 gene expression. Proc Natl Acad Sci USA. 1995;92:8069–73.
35. Resnick N, Collins T, Atkinson W, Bonthron DT, Dewey Jr CF, Gimbrone Jr MA. Platelet-derived growth factor B chain promoter contains a cis-acting fluid shear-stress-responsive element. Proc Natl Acad Sci USA. 1993;90:4591–5.
36. Scholz D, Ziegelhoeffer T, Helisch A, Wagner S, Friedrich C, Podzuweit T, et al. Contribution of arteriogenesis and angiogenesis to postocclusive hindlimb perfusion in mice. J Mol Cell Cardiol. 2002;34:775–87.
37. Hoefer IE, van Royen N, Rectenwald JE, Bray EJ, Abouhamze Z, Moldawer LL, et al. Direct evidence for tumor necrosis factor-alpha signaling in arteriogenesis. Circulation. 2002;105:1639–41.
38. Fernandez B, Buehler A, Wolfram S, Kostin S, Espanion G, Franz WM, et al. Transgenic myocardial overexpression of fibroblast growth factor-1 increases coronary artery density and branching. Circ Res. 2000;87:207–13.
39. Liu ZJ, Shirakawa T, Li Y, Soma A, Oka M, Dotto GP, et al. Regulation of Notch1 and Dll4 by vascular endothelial growth factor in arterial endothelial cells: implications for modulating arteriogenesis and angiogenesis. Mol Cell Biol. 2003;23:14–25.
40. Lee CW, Stabile E, Kinnaird T, Shou M, Devaney JM, Epstein SE, et al. Temporal patterns of gene expression after acute hindlimb ischemia in mice: insights into the genomic program for collateral vessel development. J Am Coll Cardiol. 2004;43:474–82.
41. Arras M, Ito WD, Scholz D, Winkler B, Schaper J, Schaper W. Monocyte activation in angiogenesis and collateral growth in the rabbit hindlimb. J Clin Invest. 1998;101:40–50.
42. Scholz D, Ito W, Fleming I, Deindl E, Sauer A, Wiesnet M, et al. Ultrastructure and molecular histology of rabbit hindlimb collateral artery growth (arteriogenesis). Virchows Arch. 2000;436:257–70.
43. Asahara T, Murohara T, Sullivan A, Silver M, van der Zee R, Li T, et al. Isolation of putative progenitor endothelial cells for angiogenesis. Science. 1997;275:964–7.
44. Gehling UM, Ergun S, Schumacher U, Wagener C, Pantel K, Otte M, et al. In vitro differentiation of endothelial cells from AC133-positive progenitor cells. Blood. 2000;95: 3106–12.
45. Grant MB, May WS, Caballero S, Brown GA, Guthrie SM, Mames RN, et al. Adult hematopoietic stem cells provide functional hemangioblast activity during retinal neovascularization. Nat Med. 2002;8:607–12.
46. Simper D, Stalboerger PG, Panetta CJ, Wang S, Caplice NM. Smooth muscle progenitor cells in human blood. Circulation. 2002;106:1199–204.
47. Caplice NM, Bunch TJ, Stalboerger PG, Wang S, Simper D, Miller DV, et al. Smooth muscle cells in human coronary atherosclerosis can originate from cells administered at marrow transplantation. Proc Natl Acad Sci USA. 2003; 100:4754–9.
48. Caplice NM, Doyle B. Vascular progenitor cells: origins, and mechanisms of mobilization, differentiation, integration and vasculogenesis. Stem Cells Dev. 2005;14(2):122–39.
49. Ingram DA, Mead LE, Moore DB, Woodard W, Fenoglio A, Yoder MC. Vessel wall-derived endothelial cells rapidly proliferate because they contain a complete hierarchy of endothelial progenitor cells. Blood. 2005;105:2783–6.
50. McNiece IK, Stewart FM, Deacon DM, Temeles DS, Zsebo KM, Clark SC, et al. Detection of a human CFC with a high proliferative potential. Blood. 1989;74:609–12.
51. Urbich C, Heeschen C, Aicher A, Dernbach E, Zeiher AM, Dimmeler S. Relevance of monocytic features for neovascularization capacity of circulating endothelial progenitor cells. Circulation. 2003;108:2511–6.
52. Kalka C, Masuda H, Takahashi T, Kalka-Moll WM, Silver M, Kearney M, et al. Transplantation of ex vivo expanded endothelial progenitor cells for therapeutic neovascularization. Proc Natl Acad Sci USA. 2000;97:3422–7.
53. Murohara T, Ikeda H, Duan J, Shintani S, Sasaki K, Eguchi H, et al. Transplanted cord blood-derived endothelial precursor cells augment postnatal neovascularization. J Clin Invest. 2000;105:1527–36.
54. Kawamoto A, Gwon HC, Iwaguro H, Yamaguchi JI, Uchida S, Masuda H, et al. Therapeutic potential of ex vivo expanded endothelial progenitor cells for myocardial ischemia. Circulation. 2001;103:634–7.
55. Tateishi-Yuyama E, Matsubara H, Murohara T, Ikeda U, Shintani S, Masaki H, et al. Therapeutic angiogenesis for patients with limb ischaemia by autologous transplantation of bone-marrow cells: a pilot study and a randomised controlled trial. Lancet. 2002;360:427–35.
56. Kocher AA, Schuster MD, Szabolcs MJ, Takuma S, Burkhoff D, Wang J, et al. Neovascularization of ischemic myocardium by human bone-marrow-derived angioblasts prevents cardiomyocyte apoptosis, reduces remodeling and improves cardiac function. Nat Med. 2001;7:430–6.
57. Askari AT, Unzek S, Popovic ZB, Goldman CK, Forudi F, Kiedrowski M, et al. Effect of stromal-cell-derived factor 1 on stem-cell homing and tissue regeneration in ischaemic cardiomyopathy. Lancet. 2003;362:697–703.
58. Crosby JR, Kaminski WE, Schatteman G, Martin PJ, Raines EW, Seifert RA, et al. Endothelial cells of hematopoietic origin make a significant contribution to adult blood vessel formation. Circ Res. 2000;87:728–30.
59. Urbich C, Dimmeler S. Endothelial progenitor cells: characterization and role in vascular biology. Circ Res. 2004;95: 343–53.
60. Shimizu K, Sugiyama S, Aikawa M, Fukumoto Y, Rabkin E, Libby P, et al. Host bone-marrow cells are a source of donor intimal smooth-muscle-like cells in murine aortic transplant arteriopathy. Nat Med. 2001;7:738–41.
61. Religa P, Bojakowski K, Maksymowicz M, Bojakowska M, Sirsjo A, Gaciong Z, et al. Smooth-muscle progenitor cells of bone marrow origin contribute to the development of neointimal thickenings in rat aortic allografts and injured rat carotid arteries. Transplantation. 2002;74:1310–5.

62. Sata M, Saiura A, Kunisato A, Tojo A, Okada S, Tokuhisa T, et al. Hematopoietic stem cells differentiate into vascular cells that participate in the pathogenesis of atherosclerosis. Nat Med. 2002;8:403–9.
63. De Palma M, Venneri MA, Roca C, Naldini L. Targeting exogenous genes to tumor angiogenesis by transplantation of genetically modified hematopoietic stem cells. Nat Med. 2003;9:789–95.
64. Ziegelhoeffer T, Fernandez B, Kostin S, Heil M, Voswinckel R, Helisch A, et al. Bone marrow-derived cells do not incorporate into the adult growing vasculature. Circ Res. 2004; 94:230–8.
65. Rehman J, Li J, Orschell CM, March KL. Peripheral blood "endothelial progenitor cells" are derived from monocyte/macrophages and secrete angiogenic growth factors. Circulation. 2003;107:1164–9.
66. Hattori K, Dias S, Heissig B, Hackett NR, Lyden D, Tateno M, et al. Vascular endothelial growth factor and angiopoietin-1 stimulate postnatal hematopoiesis by recruitment of vasculogenic and hematopoietic stem cells. J Exp Med. 2001;193:1005–14.
67. Kornowski R. Collateral formation and clinical variables in obstructive coronary artery disease: the influence of hypercholesterolemia and diabetes mellitus. Coron Artery Dis. 2003;14:61–4.
68. Koerselman J, van der Graaf Y, de Jaegere PP, Grobbee DE. Coronary collaterals: an important and underexposed aspect of coronary artery disease. Circulation. 2003;107: 2507–11.
69. Fujita M, Nakae I, Kihara Y, Hasegawa K, Nohara R, Ueda K, et al. Determinants of collateral development in patients with acute myocardial infarction. Clin Cardiol. 1999;22:595–9.
70. Sasso FC, Torella D, Carbonara O, Ellison GM, Torella M, Scardone M, et al. Increased vascular endothelial growth factor expression but impaired vascular endothelial growth factor receptor signaling in the myocardium of type 2 diabetic patients with chronic coronary heart disease. J Am Coll Cardiol. 2005;46:827–34.
71. Waltenberger J, Lange J, Kranz A. Vascular endothelial growth factor-A-induced chemotaxis of monocytes is attenuated in patients with diabetes mellitus: a potential predictor for the individual capacity to develop collaterals. Circulation. 2000;102:185–90.
72. Dameron KM, Volpert OV, Tainsky MA, Bouck N. Control of angiogenesis in fibroblasts by p53 regulation of thrombospondin-1. Science. 1994;265:1582–4.
73. Gupta K, Gupta P, Wild R, Ramakrishnan S, Hebbel RP. Binding and displacement of vascular endothelial growth factor (VEGF) by thrombospondin: effect on human microvascular endothelial cell proliferation and angiogenesis. Angiogenesis. 1999;3:147–58.
74. Sulpice E, Contreres JO, Lacour J, Bryckaert M, Tobelem G. Platelet factor 4 disrupts the intracellular signalling cascade induced by vascular endothelial growth factor by both KDR dependent and independent mechanisms. Eur J Biochem. 2004;271:3310–8.
75. Gupta SK, Hassel T, Singh JP. A potent inhibitor of endothelial cell proliferation is generated by proteolytic cleavage of the chemokine platelet factor 4. Proc Natl Acad Sci USA. 1995;92:7799–803.
76. Miosge N, Sasaki T, Timpl R. Angiogenesis inhibitor endostatin is a distinct component of elastic fibers in vessel walls. FASEB J. 1999;13:1743–50.
77. Miao RQ, Agata J, Chao L, Chao J. Kallistatin is a new inhibitor of angiogenesis and tumor growth. Blood. 2002;100:3245–52.
78. Topol EJ, McCarthy J, Gabriel S, Moliterno DJ, Rogers WJ, Newby LK, et al. Single nucleotide polymorphisms in multiple novel thrombospondin genes may be associated with familial premature myocardial infarction. Circulation. 2001;104:2641–4.
79. Panchal VR, Rehman J, Nguyen AT, Brown JW, Turrentine MW, Mahomed Y, et al. Reduced pericardial levels of endostatin correlate with collateral development in patients with ischemic heart disease. J Am Coll Cardiol. 2004;43:1383–7.
80. O'Reilly MS, Boehm T, Shing Y, Fukai N, Vasios G, Lane WS, et al. Endostatin: an endogenous inhibitor of angiogenesis and tumor growth. Cell. 1997;88:277–85.
81. Dixelius J, Larsson H, Sasaki T, Holmqvist K, Lu L, Engstrom A, et al. Endostatin-induced tyrosine kinase signaling through the Shb adaptor protein regulates endothelial cell apoptosis. Blood. 2000;95:3403–11.
82. Melo LG, Pachori AS, Gnecchi M, Dzau VJ. Genetic therapies for cardiovascular diseases. Trends Mol Med. 2005;11:240–50.
83. Mah C, Byrne BJ, Flotte TR. Virus-based gene delivery systems. Clin Pharmacokinet. 2002;41:901–11.
84. Niidome T, Huang L. Gene therapy progress and prospects: nonviral vectors. Gene Ther. 2002;9:1647–52.
85. Meoli DF, Sadeghi MM, Krassilnikova S, Bourke BN, Giordano FJ, Dione DP, et al. Noninvasive imaging of myocardial angiogenesis following experimental myocardial infarction. J Clin Invest. 2004;113:1684–91.
86. Lu E, Wagner WR, Schellenberger U, Abraham JA, Klibanov AL, Woulfe SR, et al. Targeted in vivo labeling of receptors for vascular endothelial growth factor: approach to identification of ischemic tissue. Circulation. 2003; 108:97–103.

Coronary Artery Disease: Development and Progression

3

Joerg Herrmann and Amir Lerman

Over the past decades the term "Coronary Artery Disease" (CAD) epitomized the involvement of the epicardial coronary circulation in the atherosclerotic disease process, classically in conjunction with the visualization of luminal narrowing by angiography. However, a disease state of the coronary arteries can develop independently from the systemic atherosclerotic disease process, for instance, as part of a vasculitis syndrome such as Kawasaki disease or systemic diseases such as amyloidosis. Moreover, CAD functionally involves the entire coronary circulation, including the myocardial microvasculature. This chapter will review CAD as part of the atherosclerotic cardiovascular disease (ASCVD) process. Specifically, it will focus on current concepts of its pathophysiology as it underlies clinical presentation and therapy.

Atherogenesis: The Pathophysiology of CAD

CAD was first recognized as part of a "degeneration to bones" by Fallopius in the sixteenth century, leading to the terminology of "arteriosclerosis" (derived from the Greek words for airpipe, i.e., "arteria," and hard, i.e., "scleros") by Lobstein in the nineteenth century. This term was modified to "atherosclerosis" (based on the Greek word for gruel, i.e., "atheroma") to reflect the experimental discovery by Anitschow in 1914 that arteries not only harden but accumulate cholesterol. Ever since, a number of theories have been forwarded to explain the development of atherosclerosis, including the monoclonal theory, the clonal senescence theory, the degenerative theory, the encrustation or thrombogenic theory, the platelet aggregation theory, the intima-filtration or response-to-retention theory, the iron theory, the oxidative stress theory, the inflammatory theory, and the response-to-injury theory.

The currently prevailing and integrative response-to-injury theory was sparked by Russell Ross and John Glomset in 1973 with subsequent modifications over the following decades [23–25]. In essence, it suggests that atherosclerosis develops as an inflammatory-proliferative response to repetitive injury of the inner lining of an artery, that is, the endothelium. This view focuses mainly on the endothelial monolayer of the intima but it has to be taken into consideration that an endothelial monolayer is the essence of the vasa vasorum in the adventitia as well. Hence, the response-to-injury theory should not be mistaken as an "inside-out-theory" but considers the entire vascular wall. Furthermore, the outcome of the injury ultimately depends on the quantity and quality of the repair mechanisms (Fig. 3.1).

Even though physical forces can be some of the injuring factors, the main mode of injury is biochemical in nature [11]. Hypercholesterolemia, hypertension, diabetes mellitus, smoking, and age, all cardinal risk factors for the development of ASCVD, lead to increased vascular oxidative stress (Fig. 3.2a) [4]. This is the consequence of an increase in the generation of reactive oxygen species (ROS), especially superoxide anions, over antioxidant capabilities, resulting in

J. Herrmann (✉) • A. Lerman
Department of Internal Medicine, Mayo Clinic Rochester, Rochester, MN, USA
e-mail: herrmann.joerg@mayo.edu

G.W. Barsness and D.R. Holmes Jr. (eds.), *Coronary Artery Disease*,
DOI 10.1007/978-1-84628-712-1_3, © Springer-Verlag London Limited 2012

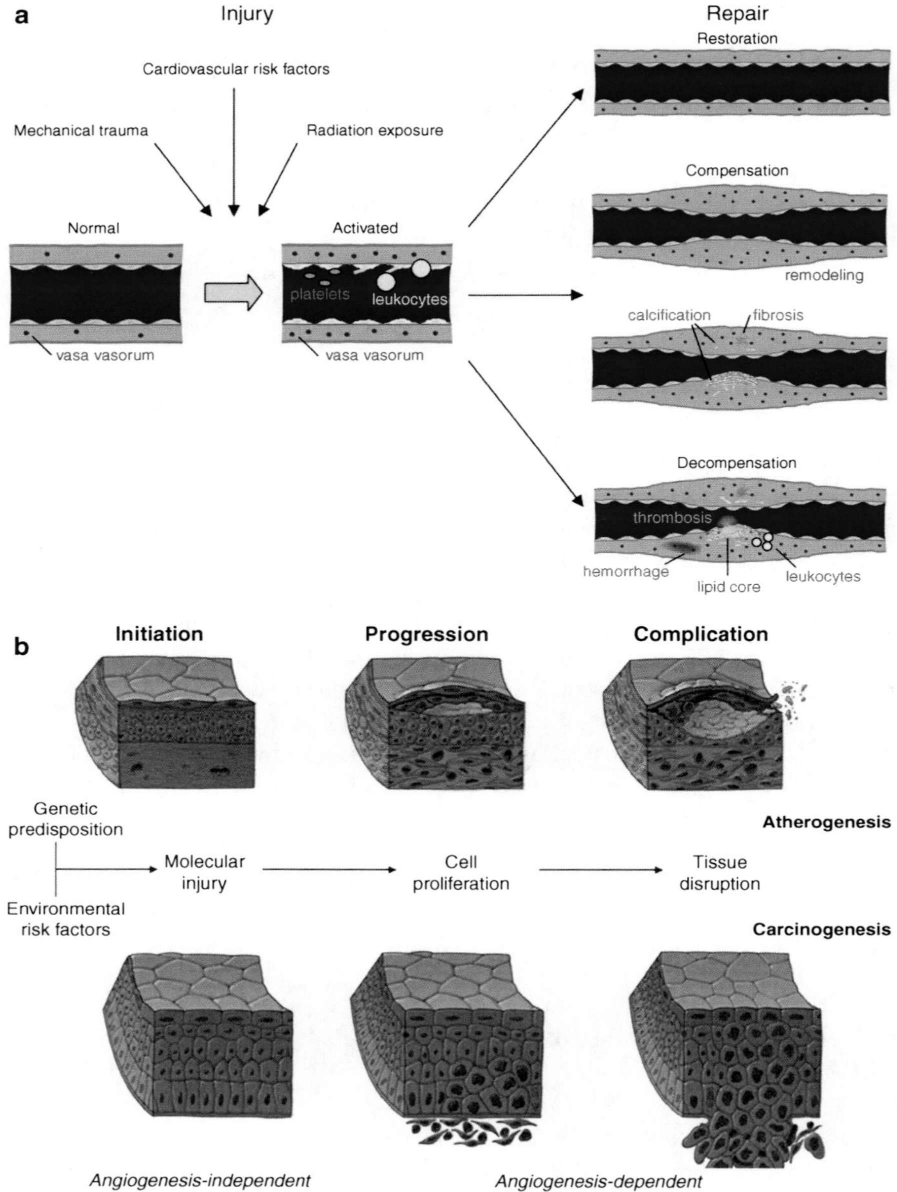

Fig. 3.1 Illustration of the response-to-injury theory of atherosclerosis, which entails the activation of the endothelial monolayer of the intima and of the adventitia with vasa vasorum neovascularization as well as transformation to a pro-thrombotic, pro-inflammatory, and pro-vasoconstrincting state (**a**). The outcome is determined by the repair mechanisms, allowing full restoration (*upper panel*), compensation with stable remodeling, including fibrosis and calcification (*middle panel*), or decompensation with unstable remodeling, including inflammation, neovascularization, and thrombosis (**a**). In pathoanatomical terms, the distinction between an initiation, a progression, and a complication stage of atherosclerosis can be made similar to cancer. Just like carcinogenesis, further growth of an atherosclerotic plaque seems to be dependent on angiogenesis following an initial angiogenesis-independent disease stage (**b**) (Image reproduced with permission of the American Heart Association [12])

the structural and functional modification of proteins, lipids, and DNA. For instance, superoxide rapidly reacts with nitric oxide (NO), generating the highly cytotoxic product peroxynitrite and reducing the bioavailability of NO, which constitutes the central endogenous antiatherogenic factor. In addition, modifications of signaling pathways lead to the stimulation of the local renin-angiotensin system (RAS) and the endogenous endothelin system as well as the alteration of the activity and expression of transcription factors such as nuclear factor kappa B (NFκB) [6].

These molecular processes lead to the attraction and binding of inflammatory cells to the endothelial monolayer and their infiltration into the subendothelial space where monocytes turn into macrophages and macrophages into foam cells by intracellular accumulation of lipids [16]. Lipids, especially low-density lipoproteins, cross the endothelium, which is impaired in barrier

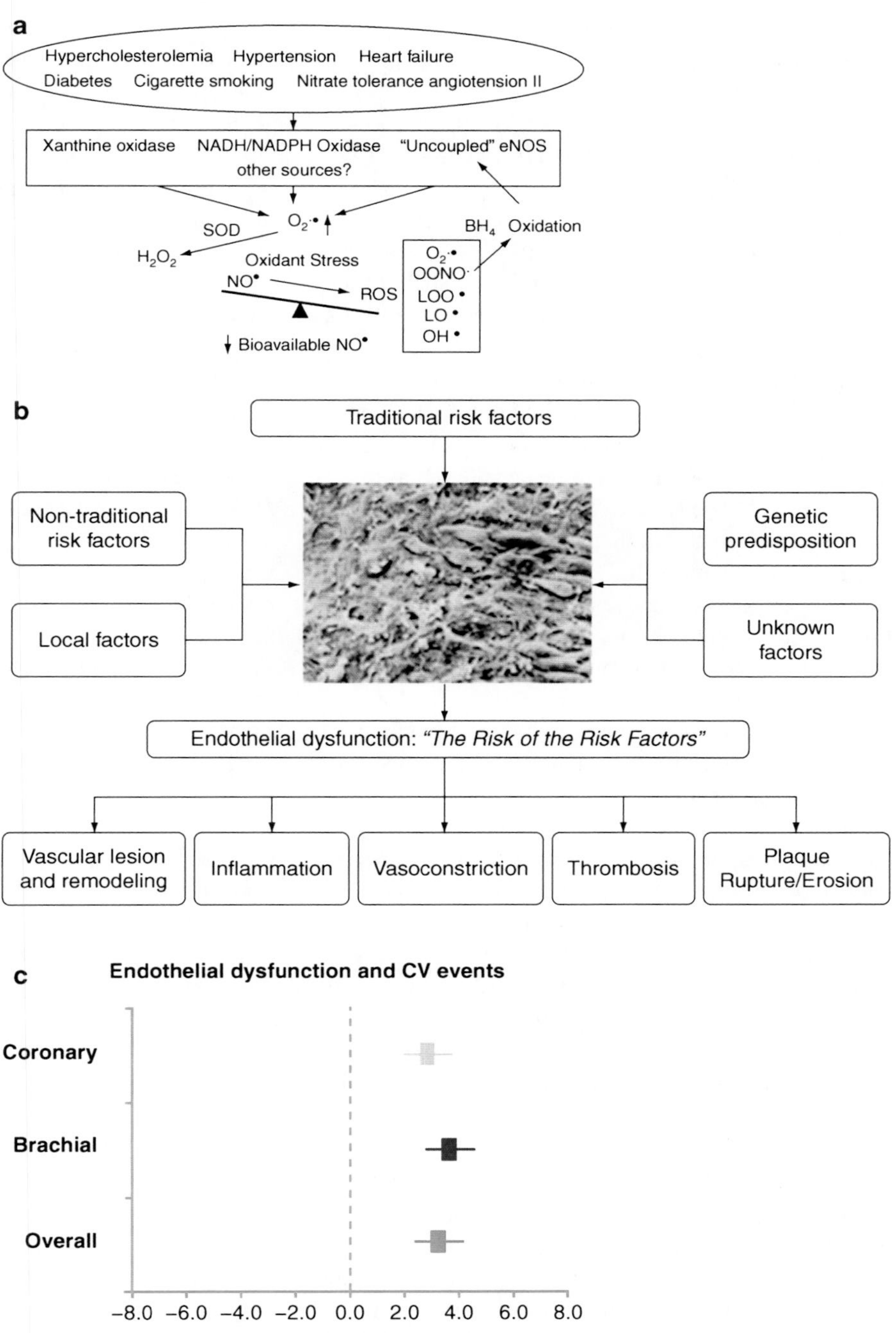

Fig. 3.2 Overview of the syndrome of endothelial dysfunction. Cardiovascular risk factors stimulate the production of reactive oxygen species, which reduce the bioavailability of NO (**a**). This impairs the antiatherosclerotic function of the endothelium. Within the outlined spectrum of effects, endothelial dysfunction represents a syndrome, "translating" the exposure to environmental factors, along with other variables, into clinical, cardiovascular risk (**b**). This is underscored by a multivariate analysis showing an approximately threefold higher risk of cardiovascular events in the presence of endothelial dysfunction, as assessed by coronary or brachial endothelium-dependent vasoreactivity testing (**c**) (Images reproduced with permission of the American Heart Association [3, 4, 15])

function, and accumulate in the intima. Media vascular smooth muscle cells (VSMCs) transform from a contractile to a proliferating, metabolic phenotype, which invades the subendothelial space and contributes to extracellular matrix formation. The extracellular matrix favors retention and oxidation of lipid particles. Eventually, a fibrous cap develops over an enlarging lipid core. Ulceration and erosion of the fibrous cap with subsequent thrombus formation lead to acute narrowing of the coronary artery lumen [18]. Thus, following initiation, coronary atherogenesis progresses to a complicated disease stage (Fig. 3.1b).

Endothelial Dysfunction: The Initiation Stage of CAD

Over the recent two decades, both experimental and clinical trials outlined impairment in endothelial function as the first manifestation of a diseased vascular wall and its presence and contribution throughout all stages of the atherosclerotic disease process. Given the numerous functions of the endothelium, the consequences of its dysfunctional state are quite diverse and endothelial dysfunction has to be considered as a syndrome (Fig. 3.2b) [3].

The one manifestation most classically linked to impairment in endothelial function is impairment in endothelium-dependent vasorelaxation. Along these lines, a reduction of coronary artery diameter and coronary blood flow in response to intracoronary infusion of acetylcholine has become the gold standard for the diagnosis of coronary endothelial dysfunction on epicardial and microvascular level. Patients diagnosed with coronary endothelial dysfunction by these means are also characterized by an increased level of circulating apoptotic endothelial microparticles, underscoring ongoing endothelial cell injury. Two main mechanisms of repair have been recognized: (1) regeneration by local endothelial cells and (2) regeneration by circulating endothelial progenitor cells. The overall outcome is therefore determined by the balance between injury and repair processes, and a reduction in NO bioavailability has a double negative impact on this balance [7].

In addition to impaired endothelium-dependent vasorelaxation, the injured endothelial monolayer is furthermore characterized by increased expression of pro-inflammatory, pro-thrombotic, and procoagulant molecules. These molecules have been studied as surrogate markers of endothelial cell injury. Tissue plasminogen activator, plasminogen activator inhibitor-1, thrombomodulin, and von-Willebrand factor were among the first molecules analyzed in this respect. Soluble forms of endothelial markers of activation like VCAM-1, ICAM-1, E-selectin, and P-selectin subsequently gained increasing attention. However, no marker is superior and the relationship between these markers and endothelial dysfunction as assessed by vasoreactive testing is not well characterized [11]. These vasofunctional tests rather than serum biomarkers have been found to be of prognostic significance in a number of different patient populations (Figs. 3.2c, d) [15].

In summary, dysfunction (activation) of the endothelium marks the initiation stage of the CAD. It is the consequence of an imbalance in endothelial injury and repair. Impairment in endothelium-dependent vasorelaxation serves as the diagnostic hallmark, and linked to atherosclerosis, as an important prognostic indicator.

Prinzmetal and Microvascular Angina: Variant Presentations of CAD

Apart from structural changes, functional narrowing of the coronary arteries, as it can occur with endothelial dysfunction, can lead to an acute decrease in myocardial blood flow and myocardial ischemia with alterations in potassium metabolism that account for both, the acute visceral chest pain sensation and acute ST segment elevation. The stimulus for this functional narrowing does not have to be physical exercise but can include mental stress with and without hyperventilation, hormonal changes such as low-estradiol menstrual cycle phase, and environmental factors such as tobacco smoke. Characteristically, these chest pain episodes occur during the night time hours, and the combination of these clinical elements characterizes the entity of variant angina. Prinzmetal initially thought it would relate to sudden increases in vascular tone in the proximity of higher-grade stenoses [22]. Subsequent work, however, highlighted that structural atherosclerotic burden is not a necessity for these vasofunctional episodes to occur. Indeed, abnormal coronary vasoconstriction in response to ergonovine and acetylcholine has been reported in patients without morphologic alteration of the vessel wall as assessed by either coronary angiography or intravascular ultrasound. Hyperventilation and cold pressor testing are two other maneuvers, used to provoke the reproduction of signs and symptoms of variant angina whereas exercise testing may or may not be useful. Of prognostic significance, various degrees of myocardial injury and cardiac arrhythmias can occur depending on the coronary arteries involved.

In some patients with angina and otherwise no concomitant disease, altered vasomotion of the resistance vessels seems to be of even greater significance. The combination of angina, positive cardiac stress test, namely, ischemic ECG changes, and a coronary angiogram negative for significant luminal narrowing has been termed cardiac syndrome X [5]. Atypical features suggestive of this presentation include a lack of response to nitroglycerine, prolonged persistence of angina (i.e., >15 min), and variations in the character of true visceral chest pain. These atypical features relate to the current concept of the underlying pathophysiology, which is impairment of myocardial microvascular function, myocardial ischemia, and increased pain sensitivity ("microvascular angina" or "sensitive heart syndrome"). The traditional view of the excellent prognosis of patients with cardiac syndrome X has recently been challenged as have been the diagnostic criteria for this syndrome [14].

Thus, relating to abnormal endothelial cell or smooth muscle cell function, constrictive dyscontrol of the epicardial coronary arteries and the myocardial microcirculation can lead to angina with atypical features. Overall prognosis is fair, bearing in mind that some patients with variant angina can experience acute cardiac events and patients with cardiac syndrome X can be debilitated by the chest pain episodes.

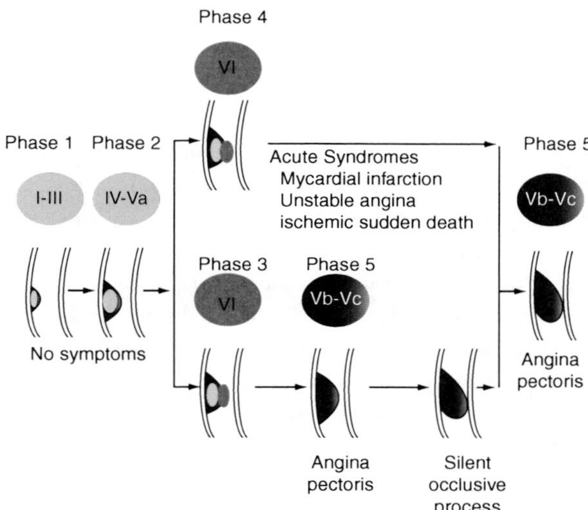

Fig. 3.3 Clinical-histological classification of atherosclerotic lesions. Phase 1 represents the early, asymptomatic stage of atherosclerosis with three different lesion types: macrophage/foam cell predominance with intracellular lipid droplets (type I), macrophages and smooth muscle cells and mild extracellular lipid droplets (type II), and smooth muscle cells with connective tissue and lipids deposits (type III). Phase 2 represents the advanced stage of atherosclerosis with two main lesion variants: cellular lesions with confluence of extracellular lipid (type IV) or fully developed fibrous cap overlying an established lipid core (type Va). Phase 3 represents the complication stage of atherosclerosis with plaque rupture or erosion, leading to mural, non-obstructing thrombosis (type VI), which remains clinically silent in most cases. On the contrary, Phase 4 represents acute complicated type VI lesions with fixed or repetitive occlusive, which leads to the presentation of acute coronary syndrome in most cases. Phase 5 represents the chronic stable stage of atherosclerosis with calcified (type Vb) or fibrotic (type Vc) lesions, which may cause chronic angina (Images reproduced with permission by the American College of Cardiology [8])

Chronic Stable Angina: The Progression Stage of CAD

Following the initial functional changes, coronary arteries undergo active structural modifications, which have been summarized under the term "remodeling" and individualized by three main classification systems, one of which is highlighted in Fig. 3.3 [8, 26, 27].

The initial structural changes include intimal thickening and adventitial vasa vasorum neovascularization. As they progress, they eventually join together in the formation of plaque neovessels [12]. Experimental data support an active contribution of these neovessels to plaque growth by maintaining oxygen and nutrient supply, even stimulated by hypoxia, increased metabolism, and oxidative stress. Furthermore, they may be both cause and consequence of vessel wall inflammation. Finally, given their fragile nature, they may contribute to the extravasation of red blood cells (RBCs). As RBC membranes possess the highest cholesterol content in the entire human organisms, this process has the potential to tremendously contribute to plaque growth [28]. Furthermore, frank intraplaque hemorrhage may bestow sudden, rapid plaque growth. Indeed, the progression of coronary atherosclerotic plaques can occur in acute, sudden spurs as well as a chronic, gradual process [30]. Moreover, the growth of atherosclerotic lesions is discontinuous and more prominent in the proximal segments of coronary arteries as well as at certain "hot spots" such as flow dividers. This phenomenon has been explained in part but not completely by rheological factors.

Importantly, the adventitial vasa vasorum contribute not only to the neovessels within but also around the plaque. This leads to collateral formation as the growing plaque encroaches into the lumen, finally to completely obstruct it. Due to this "endogenous bypass formation," even a complete obstruction of a coronary artery can remain clinically silent. Similarly, a growing plaque may not lead to clinical symptoms. One reason is that myocardial perfusion reserve remains unimpaired until luminal dimensions are reduced by 70–75% [10]. Starting at that point, coronary flow reserve is used to meet baseline demand and becomes less available for stress situations, leading to myocardial ischemia and the presentation of typical, exertional angina [29]. In addition to physical exercise, mental stress can trigger angina. In fact, ambulatory monitoring of hemodynamic and electrocardiographic parameters in patients with CAD has shown that most and even silent ischemic periods are preceded by sympathetic arousal [20]. Increased sympathetic activity renders especially the diseased vessel more sensitive to vasoconstriction and increases myocardial workload by positive chronotropic, dromotropic, and inotropic effects.

These pathophysiological processes underlie the classical presentation and testing of patients with chronic stable angina. In patients selected by these means, substantial lesions may stand out on coronary angiography but they may not be the highest risk substrate for acute clinical deterioration. Upon adjunctive coronary imaging, these prominent coronary artery lesions frequently display a high fibrous cap-to-lipid core ratio and deep calcification, that is, features associated with a low risk of surface disintegration.

Hence, chronic stable angina reflects the gradual progression type of CAD. While associated with the classical symptoms of CAD, obstructing lesions on coronary angiogram likely present only the tip of the iceberg of ASCVD.

Acute Coronary Syndrome (ACS): The Complication Stage of CAD

Another reason for the long symptomatic latency period is the phenomenon of positive remodeling, also called Glagov effect [9]. This entails the growth of the plaque to the abluminal side, which preserves luminal dimensions. Interestingly, it is this eccentric plaque growth that is associated with acute presentations. Other characteristics of the "vulnerable" plaque are a low fibrous cap-to-lipid core ratio ("thin-capped fibroatheroma") and inflammatory cell accumulation, particularly in the shoulder regions, which are also rich in neovessels [8]. In recent years, there has also been the realization that in addition to the culprit lesion, patients who present with an acute coronary syndrome harbor vulnerable plaques elsewhere in the coronary circulation and even in other vascular regions [17]. This has led to the concept of the vulnerable patient rather than the single vulnerable plaque. Identification of these patients by novel diagnostic techniques remains a challenge and subject to active research [19].

The eccentric anatomy predisposes to focal exaggeration of shear stress in plaque areas already weakened by the production of matrix degrading enzymes during the inflammatory and angiogenic processes. Intraplaque hemorrhage may contribute not only to sudden plaque growth but may acutely impair overall plaque integrity. Rupture of the fibrous cap, mainly in shoulder areas, exposes the highly thrombogenic plaque content to the blood stream [8]. One important component is tissue factor, which is produced in great amounts in macrophage-rich areas and initiates the extrinsic clotting cascade. Furthermore, exposure of von-Willebrand factor and collagen activates platelets, thereby contributing to acute coronary thrombosis. Activated platelets also favor coronary vasoconstriction by the release of substances such as serotonin and thromboxane-A_2. In addition, counteracting mechanisms are weakened by the dysfunctional state of the surrounding endothelium. While plaque rupture accounts for the majority of acute coronary events, still up to 40% of the cases of coronary thrombosis occur at sites at which plaque rupture cannot be identified. Superficial erosions are the pathoanatomic substrate under these circumstances and stand out in premenopausal women with ACS presentation.

In the setting of acute coronary occlusion, there is no collateral formation to sustain a minor level of coronary blood flow. Hence, myocardial perfusion sustains a sudden decrease. Depending on the localization of the plaque rupture, the extent of the thrombotic process, the baseline condition of the myocardium and the myocardial microvasculature, as well as other interfering factors, the clinical consequences vary from unstable angina to non-ST-segment elevation myocardial infarction to ST-segment elevation myocardial infarction and sudden cardiac death.

Thus, ACS develops in the vulnerable patient as the consequence of atherosclerotic plaque rupture or erosion. The pre-disposing anatomic substrate of the vulnerable plaque remains a diagnostic and therapeutic challenge.

Coronary Artery Restenosis: The Intervention Stage of CAD

Revascularization procedures allow the reopening or bypassing of significant coronary artery stenoses but themselves trigger a response-to-injury, leading to restenosis. Negative remodeling, including elastic recoil, is an important element for restenosis with percutanenous transluminal balloon angioplasty (PTCA) as is neointima formation for in-stent restenosis. As yet another distinction from primary atherosclerosis, the restenotic lesions after PTCA and stenting are rich in extracellular matrix (collagen and matrix proteoglycans) rather than cells [2]. Hence, restenotic lesions have been considered as largely fibrotic and stable. However, this view has changed with the ACS presentation and identification of in-stent restenosis as the culprit [1]. Very recently, the delayed healing response with first-generation drug-eluting stents has highlighted the overall vulnerable potential of these interventions [13].

Thrombosis accounts for early restenosis (i.e., within 1 month) after coronary artery bypass grafting (CABG) [21]. Subsequently, stenoses in arterial coronary bypasses are mainly observed at the anastomosis site and due to neointimal hyperplasia. On the contrary, accelerated atherosclerosis accounts for the development of stenoses with saphenous vein grafts (SVGs). SVG atherosclerosis is characterized by diffuse involvement of the entire bypass segment, the development of thin-capped lesions, and the absence of outward remodeling. This predisposes to late graft thrombosis and acute clinical presentations. Given the friable atherosclerotic plaque burden, percutaneous intervention of these lesions also remains a challenge with a higher risk of complications.

Hence, revascularization procedures are intended to preserve myocardial perfusion but can be complicated by further disease development. In addition to the ongoing disease process in the native coronary circulation, SVG-CABG is complicated by the development of accelerated atherosclerosis with the development of high-risk lesions in a relatively short period of time.

Summary

CAD as part of ASCVD is currently viewed as an inflammatory-proliferative disease in response to sustained injury to the endothelial monolayer, mainly by increase in endogenous oxidative stress secondary to cardiovascular risk exposure and genetic predisposition. Dysfunction or activation of the endothelium marks the first, functional, and reversible initiation stage of atherosclerosis. Intimal thickening and adventitial vasa vasorum neovascularization are the first structural changes of the coronary artery wall. Subsequent growth of the atherosclerotic plaque can be inward (negative remodeling) or outward (positive remodeling). The significantly lumen-obstructing coronary artery plaque leads to the typical presentation of angina and positive cardiac stress testing but in most cases not to acute presentations. On the contrary, the "vulnerable plaque," which underlies the entity of the acute coronary syndrome, can forgo detection by standard means. The current management strategies of CAD are based on risk stratification and clinical presentation as it relates to the outlined pathophysiology.

References

1. Assali AR, Moustapha A, et al. Acute coronary syndrome may occur within-stent restenosis and is associated with adverse outcomes (the PRESTO trial). Am J Cardiol. 2006;98(6):729–33.
2. Bennett MR. In-stent stenosis: pathology and implications for the development of drug eluting stents. Heart. 2003;89(2):218–24.
3. Bonetti PO, Lerman LO, et al. Endothelial dysfunction: a marker of atherosclerotic risk. Arterioscler Thromb Vasc Biol. 2003;23(2):168–75.
4. Cai H, Harrison DG. Endothelial dysfunction in cardiovascular diseases: the role of oxidant stress. Circ Res. 2000;87(10):840–4.
5. Crea F, Lanza GA. Angina pectoris and normal coronary arteries: cardiac syndrome X. Heart. 2004;90(4):457–63.
6. De Nigris F, Lerman LO, et al. Oxidation-sensitive transcription factors and molecular mechanisms in the arterial wall. Antioxid Redox Signal. 2001;3(6):1119–30.
7. Deanfield JE, Halcox JP, et al. Endothelial function and dysfunction: testing and clinical relevance. Circulation. 2007;115(10):1285–95.
8. Fuster V, Moreno PR, et al. Atherothrombosis and high-risk plaque: part I: evolving concepts. J Am Coll Cardiol. 2005;46(6):937–54.
9. Glagov S, Weisenberg E, et al. Compensatory enlargement of human atherosclerotic coronary arteries. N Engl J Med. 1987;316(22):1371–5.

10. Goldstein RA, Kirkeeide RL, et al. Relation between geometric dimensions of coronary artery stenoses and myocardial perfusion reserve in man. J Clin Invest. 1987;79(5): 1473–8.
11. Herrmann J, Lerman A. The endothelium: dysfunction and beyond. J Nucl Cardiol. 2001;8(2):197–206.
12. Herrmann J, Lerman LO, et al. Angiogenesis in atherogenesis. Arterioscler Thromb Vasc Biol. 2006;26(9):1948–57.
13. Joner M, Finn AV, et al. Pathology of drug-eluting stents in humans: delayed healing and late thrombotic risk. J Am Coll Cardiol. 2006;48(1):193–202.
14. Lanza GA. Cardiac syndrome X: a critical overview and future perspectives. Heart. 2007;93(2):159–66.
15. Lerman A, Zeiher AM. Endothelial function: cardiac events. Circulation. 2005;111(3):363–8.
16. Libby P. Current concepts of the pathogenesis of the acute coronary syndromes. Circulation. 2001;104(3):365–72.
17. Libby P. Atherosclerosis: disease biology affecting the coronary vasculature. Am J Cardiol. 2006;98(12A):3Q–9.
18. Libby P, Theroux P. Pathophysiology of coronary artery disease. Circulation. 2005;111(25):3481–8.
19. MacNeill BD, Lowe HC, et al. Intravascular modalities for detection of vulnerable plaque: current status. Arterioscler Thromb Vasc Biol. 2003;23(8):1333–42.
20. Moskowitz RM, Chatterjee K, et al. Silent myocardial ischemia: an update. Med Clin North Am. 1988;72(5):1033–54.
21. Motwani JG, Topol EJ. Aortocoronary saphenous vein graft disease: pathogenesis, predisposition, and prevention. Circulation. 1998;97(9):916–31.
22. Prinzmetal M, Kennamer R, et al. Angina pectoris. I. A variant form of angina pectoris; preliminary report. Am J Med. 1959;27:375–88.
23. Ross R. Atherosclerosis – an inflammatory disease. N Engl J Med. 1999;340(2):115–26.
24. Ross R, Glomset JA. Atherosclerosis and the arterial smooth muscle cell: proliferation of smooth muscle is a key event in the genesis of the lesions of atherosclerosis. Science. 1973;180(93):1332–9.
25. Ross R, Glomset J, et al. Response to injury and atherogenesis. Am J Pathol. 1977;86(3):675–84.
26. Stary HC. Natural history of calcium deposits in atherosclerosis progression and regression. Z Kardiol. 2000;89 Suppl 2:28–35.
27. Virmani R, Kolodgie FD, et al. Lessons from sudden coronary death: a comprehensive morphological classification scheme for atherosclerotic lesions. Arterioscler Thromb Vasc Biol. 2000;20(5):1262–75.
28. Virmani R, Kolodgie FD, et al. Atherosclerotic plaque progression and vulnerability to rupture: angiogenesis as a source of intraplaque hemorrhage. Arterioscler Thromb Vasc Biol. 2005;25(10):2054–61.
29. Wilson RF. Assessing the severity of coronary-artery stenoses. N Engl J Med. 1996;334(26):1735–7.
30. Yokoya K, Takatsu H, et al. Process of progression of coronary artery lesions from mild or moderate stenosis to moderate or severe stenosis: a study based on four serial coronary arteriograms per year. Circulation. 1999;100(9): 903–9.

Therapeutic Goals in Patients with Refractory Angina

4

Mauricio G. Cohen and E. Magnus Ohman

Introduction

Refractory angina is a major clinical challenge in contemporary cardiovascular medicine. As therapeutic strategies evolve, there is increased life expectancy for ischemic heart disease with more patients reaching advanced stages. Due to a better understanding of the disease process and technological advances, coronary revascularization, by means of coronary by-pass grafting (CABG) and percutaneous coronary interventions (PCI), is now offered to a wide spectrum of high-risk patients. The inception of drug eluting stents in routine clinical practice has reduced the restenosis rates to single digits [1, 2], extending the indications of PCI to poor operative candidates with unprotected left main stenosis or diabetics with diffuse small vessel disease. In a similar fashion, more generalized use of major surgical revascularization breakthroughs, such as off-pump CABG and arterial grafts, have resulted in significant improvements in surgical outcomes [3]. Despite these advances, a significant proportion of patients with preserved left ventricular fraction and no life-threatening arrhythmias remain symptomatic with severe debilitating angina due to progression of native atherosclerotic disease associated with failure or unfeasibility of revascularization. In a prospective observational study, Hemingway et al. showed that at 1-year follow-up angina persists in 52% of patients treated with PCI and 40% of those treated with CABG [4]. Similar findings were observed in the multicenter international ARTS randomized trial, in which only 19% of PCI patients and 38% of CABG patients were free of angina and antianginal therapy at 1-year follow-up [5]. Moreover, in a meta-analysis of 11 randomized trials comparing PCI with medical therapy in stable patients with chronic coronary artery disease, PCI offered no survival benefit [6].

The ESC Joint Study Group has defined refractory angina as a *chronic condition (>3 months) characterized by the presence of angina caused by coronary insufficiency in the presence of coronary artery disease which cannot be controlled by a combination of medical therapy, angioplasty, and coronary by-pass surgery. The presence of reversible myocardial ischemia should be clinically established to be the cause of the symptoms* [7]. Multiple clinical studies have shown that the 1-year mortality risk of this group of patients is relatively low at approximately 5% or less [8, 9]. For example, the sample size estimation in the Impact of Nicorandil in Angina (IONA) trial that enrolled high-risk patients with chronic stable angina was based in the assumption of a 13% event rate after an average of 21 months of follow-up in the combined end point of coronary heart disease death, nonfatal myocardial infarction, or unplanned hospital admission for chest pain and 8% for the composite of coronary heart disease death or nonfatal MI [10]. The actual all-cause mortality rate at mean follow-up of 1.6 years in the

M.G. Cohen (✉)
Cardiovascular Division, Department of Medicine, University of Miami Miller School of Medicine, Miami, FL, USA

Cardiac Catheterization Laboratory, University of North Carolina at Chapel Hill, Chapel Hill, NC, USA
e-mail: mgcohen@med.miami.edu

E.M. Ohman
Division of Cardiology, Department of Medicine, Duke University Medical Center, Durham, NC, USA

G.W. Barsness and D.R. Holmes Jr. (eds.), *Coronary Artery Disease*,
DOI 10.1007/978-1-84628-712-1_4, © Springer-Verlag London Limited 2012

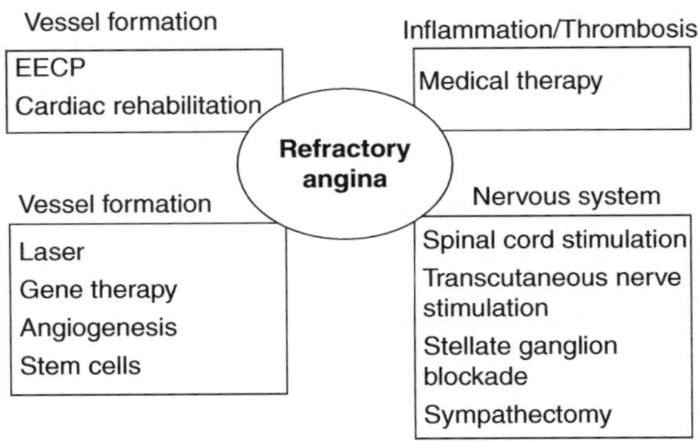

Fig. 4.1 Therapeutic opportunities in refractory angina (From DeJongste et al. [12].)

IONA trial was 4.3% in the Nicorandil group and 5% in the placebo group [11]. Therefore, the low-event rates in this population suggest that the goal of therapy should be mostly directed at improving quality of life, provided that the patients are already on optimal medical therapy. As depicted in Fig. 4.1, despite the lack of revascularization options in these patients, there are multiple therapeutic opportunities.

General Goals of Therapy: Improve Adherence to Evidence-Based Therapies

Similar to other patients with atherosclerotic coronary artery disease, the major determinants of survival in patients with refractory angina include older age, male gender, low ejection fraction, extent of coronary disease, previous MI, and diabetes mellitus [8]. Therefore, medical treatments for this patient population should be divided in two groups with separate goals, therapies that stabilize atherosclerosis and prevent disease progression, recurrent coronary events, preserve left ventricular function, and improve overall survival and therapies that reduce the anginal threshold by decreasing oxygen demand or by improving hemodynamics to increase myocardial oxygen supply. The first set of goals can be accomplished using appropriate evidence-based medical therapies and aggressive risk factor modification [13, 14] (see Table 4.1). Recommended pharmacological treatments include aspirin, clopidogrel (for patients with aspirin allergy or post-PCI), beta-blockers, non-dihydropyridine calcium channel blockers, lipid lowering agents, and ACE-inhibitors. Statin therapy appears to play a crucial role in the management of patients with chronic angina, not only due to its effects in decreasing lipid levels but to the so-called pleiotropic effects, which encompasses improvements in endothelial dysfunction, increased nitric oxide bioavailability, antioxidant properties, inhibition of inflammatory responses, and stabilization of atherosclerotic plaques [15]. In the REVERSAL trial,

Table 4.1 General measures for the treatment of refractory angina

Measure	Recommendation	Level of evidence
Pharmacologic		
Aspirin	I	A
Clopidogrel (if aspirin is contraindicated)	IIb	B
Beta-blockers	I	A
Calcium channel blockers (when beta-blockers are contraindicated)	I	B
Long-acting nitrates	I	B
Lipid lowering therapy	I	A
ACE-inhibitors (in the presence of CHF or EF≤40%)	I	A
Low-intensity oral anticoagulation	IIb	B
Risk factor modification		
Hypertension control (<130/85 mmHg)	I	A
Smoking cessation therapy	I	B
Physical activity (Cardiac rehabilitation)	I	B
Diabetes management	I	B
Dietary counseling and modification (Weight loss for obese patients with hypertension, diabetes, or hyperlipidemia)	I	B
Other measures		
Assessment and correction of Anemia	I	C
Thyroid function	–	–
Stress management (anxiety or depression)	–	–
Control heart rate in case of atrial fibrillation	–	–
Hypoxemia	–	–
Assessment of valvular heart disease	–	–

intensive lipid lowering with 80 mg of atorvastatin during 18 months was associated with a significant reduction in progression of atheromatous plaque volume as measured by intravascular ultrasound compared with a moderate regimen consisting of 40 mg of pravastatin. The apparent effects observed on plaque stabilization translated into significant clinical benefits in the large multicenter PROVE-IT trial. This study randomized 4,162 patients with acute coronary syndromes to the same lipid lowering regimens used in the REVERSAL trial. At a mean follow-up of 24 months, the LDL-cholesterol levels in the atorvastatin and pravastatin groups were 62 and 92 mg/dL, respectively. This difference was associated with a 16% relative risk reduction in the study primary endpoint (death, myocardial infarction, rehospitalization for unstable angina, revascularization procedures, and stroke) in the group receiving intensive therapy [16]. The results of these trials prompted a change in the recommended goal of lipid lowering therapy to LDL-cholesterol levels of less than 70 mg/dL for high-risk patients [17].

Despite the wide availability of clinical management guidelines [13], a number of registries in different settings have shown that proven therapies for ideal candidates are underutilized in real-world clinical practice. The recently published Euro Heart Survey showed that the use of secondary prevention and antianginal agents is far from ideal in Europe. This multinational registry enrolled a total 3,779 patients with stable angina. Even though all patients in this registry had been evaluated by a cardiologist, the use of aspirin was 78%, statins 48%, beta-blockers 67%, nitrates 61%, calcium channel blockers 27%, and ACE-inhibitors 40% [18]. A major reason for not prescribing beta blockers has been attributed to possible side effects. However, there is clear evidence that the general belief that blocker therapy is associated with substantial risks of depressive symptoms, fatigue, and sexual dysfunction is not supported by data from clinical trials [19].

In the USA, the Cardiovascular Hospitalization Atherosclerosis Management Program (CHAMP) aimed at initiating evidence-based therapies such as aspirin, lipid-lowering agents (LDL goal ≤ 100 mg/dL), beta-blockers, and ACE inhibitors in conjunction with dietary and exercise counseling in patients with established coronary artery disease before hospital discharge. The program was implemented in 1994 and utilized a number of tools designed to facilitate initiation of therapy throughout hospital stay in patients without contraindications. At 1 year follow-up, patients enrolled in CHAMP showed a substantially higher use of evidence-based medicines, such as aspirin, beta-blockers, statins, and ACE-inhibitors, compared to patients treated in a period prior to the implementation of the program. Most importantly, as depicted in Fig. 4.2, adherence to recommended

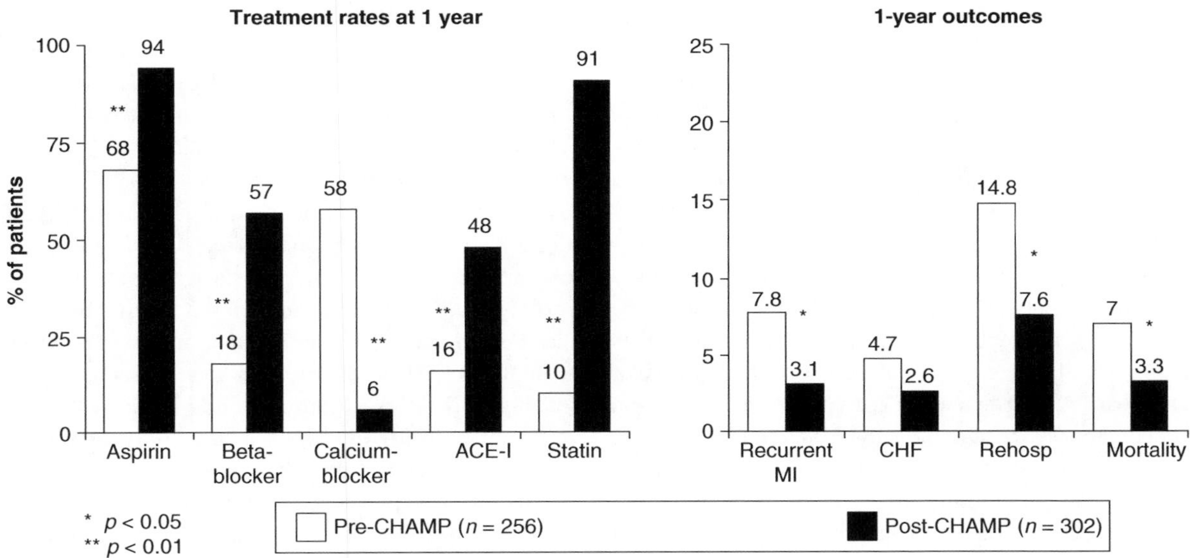

Fig. 4.2 Adherence to recommended therapies result in improved outcomes. Result from CHAMP

Table 4.2 Conventional medical therapies for chronic stable angina

Beta blockers	First-line therapy
	Heart rate reduction
	Reduction of myocardial contractility
Calcium channel blockers	
Non-dihydropyridine	Heart rate reduction
Hydropiridine	Blood pressure reduction
	Dilation of coronary vessels
Nitrates	Preload reduction
	Afterload reduction
	Dilation of coronary vessels

therapies resulted in a significant reduction of recurrent ischemic events, heart failure, rehospitalization, and death at year [20].

In a more acute setting, the CRUSADE (Can Rapid Risk Stratification of Unstable Angina Patients Suppress Adverse Outcomes with Early Implementation of the ACC/AHA Guidelines?) registry, with more than 150,000 patients enrolled, showed that use of evidence-based recommendations continues to be suboptimal resulting in increased in-hospital morbidity and mortality [21].

Other general therapeutic goals that should not be overlooked include the assessment and correction of anemia, hyperthyroidism, hypoxemia, psychological stress, and tachyarrhythmias (Table 4.2). Over the past few years, anemia has emerged as an independent risk factor for adverse cardiovascular outcomes. In the population-based Atherosclerosis Risk in Communities (ARIC) study, the presence of anemia, as defined by a hemoglobin value ≤12 g/dL in women and ≤13 g/dL in men, was associated with a 40% increase in cardiovascular outcomes defined as definite or probable myocardial infarction, coronary angioplasty, CABG or definite cardiovascular death in 14,410 individuals [22].

In addition to these general measures, the coronary anatomy of patients with refractory angina should be revisited periodically by interventional cardiologists and cardiothoracic surgeons with different levels of expertise. A significant underuse of revascularization procedures has been demonstrated in clinical practice. A multicenter study in Britain showed that 34% and 26% of patients initially treated with medicines were appropriate candidates for revascularization with PCI and CABG, respectively, according to a nine-point scale for specific clinical indications. Over 2.5 years of follow-up, these medically treated patients had higher mortality and a higher prevalence of angina than patients who underwent revascularization. Appropriate candidates for PCI who received medical treatment were more likely to have angina at follow-up (OR 95%CI, 1.97; 1.29–3.00). Likewise, patients classified as appropriate candidates for CABG but were treated with medical therapy were more likely to have angina at follow-up (OR 95% CI: 3.03, 2.08–4.42). Moreover, these medically treated CABG-eligible patients were more likely to die or have a nonfatal myocardial infarction during follow-up with a hazard ratio (95% CI) of 4.08 (2.82–5.93) [4].

Specific Goals of Therapy for Patients with Refractory Angina

Quality of Life

By definition, patients diagnosed with refractory angina are those who have failed all standard therapies recommended for the management of chronic stable angina and have coronary anatomy not suitable for revascularization as assessed by a cardiothoracic surgeon and an interventional cardiologist. Therefore, treatments in this situation should be aimed at improving the patient's quality of life without compromising quantity of life. The extent of quality of life compromise in patients with established coronary artery disease has been well defined in the Randomized Intervention Treatment of Angina (RITA) trial that compared PCI versus CABG in 1,011 patients. This study showed that angina persists in approximately 15–20% of all patients 3 years after a revascularization procedure. In this group of patients, the presence and severity of angina has a marked impact in quality of life, affecting all aspects of self-perceived health status, including level of energy, sleep, emotional reactions, social isolation, and physical mobility. In addition, angina has an unfavorable impact in employment status [23]. Similar results were observed in the ensuing trial RITA-2 that compared medical therapy versus PCI in 1,018 patients. In this study, quality of life was affected not only by the presence of angina, but also by the presence of shortness of breath and decreased exercise capacity [24].

Even though there is no specific data linking quality of life and mortality in patients with refractory angina, it has been demonstrated that quality of life determines prognosis in patients with a wide variety of cardiac conditions. In the Studies of Left Ventricular Dysfunction (SOLVD), that enrolled 5,025 patient with left ventricular systolic dysfunction, the baseline assessment of quality of life, more specifically in the domains of activities of daily living and self-reported general health of the short form health survery-36 (SF-36), independently predicted mortality and rehospitalization in asymptomatic and symptomatic patients [25]. A substudy from the Eplerenone Post-Acute Myocardial Infarction Heart Failure Efficacy and Survival (EPHESUS) study showed that health status, as assessed with a disease-specific instrument during the first outpatient visit, was strongly associated with subsequent 1-year hospitalization and death rates in 1,516 patients with heart failure post-MI [26]. Rumsfeld et al. looked at the same question in 2,480 post-CABG patients in 14 Veteran Affairs Hospitals. A multivariable model showed that the domains of activities of daily living and general health were independently associated with all-cause mortality at 36 months [27]. In a cohort of 945 patients treated at Australian public hospitals for unstable angina, MI, chronic ischemic heart disease, and heart failure, Dixon et al. found that subjects with low quality of life were two times more likely to experience an adverse outcome (death or emergent rehospitalization) at 8 months follow-up, even after adjusting for other prognostic clinical variables, compared with subjects with high scores of quality of life [28]. In the large IONA trial, which enrolled 5,126 patients with chronic stable angina, no specific instruments for the assessment of quality of life were used. However, the multivariable analysis showed that the strongest predictor of cardiac death and/or nonfatal MI was baseline angina class, one of the most important determinants of quality of life. The adjusted hazard ratio (95%CI) for cardiac death and/or nonfatal MI was 2.17 (1.44–3.25) for angina class III–IV compared with class I, greater than the hazard ratios for other classic prognostic factors such as age and left ventricular hypertrophy [29].

Quality of life can be further improved by just implementing standardized management strategies. In addition, there is a placebo effect associated with various treatments or procedures, an effect previously demonstrated by Benson and McCallie [30]. More contemporary evidence supporting this notion comes from the RITA-2 trial in which a significant proportion of patients randomized to the medical arm experienced a significant improvement in ratings of physical role functioning , emotional role functioning, social functioning, pain, and mental health at 3-year follow-up [24]. This "placebo" effect was further demonstrated in the DMR In Regeneration of Endomyocardial Channels Trial (DIRECT), which randomized 298 patients with severe refractory angina to low- or high-dose direct myocardial revascularization with laser, or a sham procedure in a blinded fashion. Patients undergoing the sham procedure experienced significant improvements at 6 and 12 months in quality of life, exercise duration, time to 1 mm ST-segment depression, and angina severity [31].

On the other hand, it has to be kept in mind that the severity of angina, degree of disability, and treatment satisfaction may not directly correlate with the severity and extent of coronary artery disease. Increased levels of anxiety, depression, and psychological stress play a major role in patients with refractory angina. A number of studies have shown that response to therapy depends more on psychological features such as anxiety, depression, neuroticism, and hypochondriasis rather than the extent and degree of coronary disease. Misconceptions about the nature of anginal episodes may further contribute to the increased levels of stress in this patient population [32–36]. Therefore, education, coaching, optimal implementation of secondary prevention therapies, and exercise programs are key elements in the management of refractory angina patients. The implementation of a dedicated patient-centered multidisciplinary program for the management of refractory angina in the UK was associated with significant improvements in quality of life. This program involves extensive education, optimization of medical therapies, rehabilitation, and other specific therapies. Patients, relatives, and physicians were able to define realistic goals and tailor therapies accordingly, based on full knowledge of all available and relevant therapeutic options. The 1-year results of this program were evaluated in a cohort of 66 patients using three instruments including the abbreviated short form health survey (SF-12), the Seattle angina questionnaire, and the hospital and depression scale. All patients received outpatient counseling, cardiac rehabilitation, and cognitive behavior therapy, 64% received transcutaneous nerve stimulation, and 14% temporary sympathectomy. At 1 year, patients enrolled in the program experienced clinically significant improvements in angina stability, angina frequency, treatment satisfaction, and quality of life. In addition, levels of anxiety and depression were reduced by 38%. Additional details on this comprehensive refractory angina program are available at www.angina.org [37].

Other strategies such as the wide implementation of nurse-led clinics to promote medical and lifestyle aspects of secondary prevention have also been tested in patients with established coronary artery disease. In northeast Scotland, a randomized clinical trial including 1,173 patients, 50% of them with chronic angina, showed significant improvement in functional status, as assessed with the SF-36 questionnaire, and less hospital admissions at 1 year, however angina, depression, and anxiety scores were marginally affected [38]. At 4 years, patients who attended the secondary prevention clinics not only achieved better control of their risk factors, but also obtained a significant survival benefit. Cumulative death rates were 14.5% for the intervention group and 18.9% for the control group ($P=0.038$), and the relative risk for total mortality was 0.78 (95% confidence interval 0.61–0.99). Attendance to the clinics was associated with better adherence to risk factor modification measures, including aspirin use, blood pressure control, lipid management, and exercise [39].

Quantifiable Goals of Therapy

Most clinical trials testing pharmacological agents or devices for refractory angina are designed on the basis of more quantifiable goals than quality of life. Common end points used in testing these therapies include frequency of angina attacks, use of short-acting nitrates, and exercise-testing parameters such as exercise duration, time to onset of angina, and time to 1-mm ST-depression. As depicted in Table 4.3, specific antianginal therapies including ranolazine, ivabradine, and nicorandil have been able to achieve improvements in most of these end points in moderate-sized clinical trials [9, 40–43]. Noninvasive methods such as enhanced external counterpulsation (EECP) and transcutaneous electrical nerve stimulation (TENS) have also shown similar results [44, 45]. Satisfactory results have also been obtained using neuromodulation through a more invasive approach such as spinal cord stimulation (SCS). With this approach, an electrical current is applied to the spinal cord with an electrode placed in the epidural space between C7 and T1, which is connected to a pulse generator located in a subcutaneous pocket in the anterior abdominal wall. An observational study using SCS in 517 refractory angina patients showed significant improvement in angina class [8]. SCS has been further tested in a randomized trial versus CABG, assessing frequency of angina attacks, use of short-acting nitrates, and time to ischemia in exercise testing. The results showed that CABG ($n=51$) and SCS ($n=53$) had similar efficacy in reducing nitrate consumption and frequency of angina attacks. However, CABG was associated with better exercise capacity and less ST-segment depression at maximum workload [46].

Table 4.3 Current limitations of antianginal therapies

Peripheral vascular disease
Chronic obstructive pulmonary disease
Asthma
Diabetes
Depression
Sexual dysfunction
Lethargy/fatigability
Hypotension
Gastrointestinal dysfunction
Headache
Acquired tolerance

In contrast, disappointing results were obtained with gene therapy and percutaneous myocardial revascularization (PMR). Despite promising preliminary data in small sample size trials, larger randomized studies showed no benefit associated with the use of these therapies [47, 48]. The AGENT-III trial testing two doses of an adenovirus-based intracoronary infusion of the human angiogenic FGF-4 gene (Ad5fgf-4) was stopped for futility after enrolling more than 400 patients. The 12-week results showed that patients in the placebo and treatment arms experimented a similar ~30% increase in mean exercise duration [49]. Similar results were observed with PMR in the DIRECT trial. At 6 months, the change in exercise duration of approximately 30 s was not different among those patients treated with a sham ($n=100$), low-dose laser ($n=98$), or high-dose laser ($n=98$) procedure [31].

Scintigraphic end points have also been used in clinical trials testing therapies for refractory angina but seem to be less consistent than exercise capacity or symptoms. Studies using scintigraphic end point are

Table 4.4 Treatment strategies and goals of therapy

Treatment	Time to ST depression	Exercise duration	Anginal class	Myocardial perfusion	FDA approved (Guidelines indication)
Pharmacological					
Ranolazine [9, 40]	↑	↑	↓	NA	Yes
Ivabradine [41, 42]	↑	↑	↓	NA	No
Nicorandil [11, 43, 52]	↑	↑	↓	↑	No
Noninvasive			↓		
EECP [44]	↑	↑	↓	↑	Yes (IIb)
TENS [45]	↑	↑	↓	NA	Yes
Invasive					
SCS [8, 46]	↑	↑	↓	↑	Yes (IIb)
TMR [50]	Unchanged	↑	↓	Unchanged	Yes (IIa)
PMR [31]	Unchanged	Unchanged	Unchanged	Unchanged	No
Gene therapy [49, 53]	↑	Unchanged	↓	↑	No

Adapted from: Yang et al. [54].
EECP enhanced external counterpulsation, *FDA* Food and Drug Administration, *NA* not available, *PMR* percutaneous myocardial revascularization, *SCS* spinal cord stimulation, *TENS* transcutaneous electrical nerve stimulation, *TMR* transmyocardial revascularization

usually smaller and provide preliminary data for larger studies using symptom and/or exercise end points. In general, myocardial perfusion is evaluated with a radionuclide scintigraphy at baseline and at different timepoints after starting a new therapy for refractory angina. Scintigraphic parameters include tracer uptake, magnitude of reversibility, average thickening fraction, and left ventricular ejection fraction. Even though multiple observational retrospective studies examining the effects of EECP have shown significant resolution of perfusion defects [50], a more recent prospective multicenter study did not show any improvements in scintigraphic parameters despite significant improvements in angina attacks and exercise capacity [51]. Similar observations were reported with other therapeutic modalities such as TMR, PMR, and medical therapies, suggesting that improvements in exercise capacity and symptom relief may not be directly related to enhanced myocardial perfusion.

Conclusions

Refractory angina is a debilitating condition and its treatment remains problematic. Due to advances in revascularization strategies and medical therapies, the survival of patients with atherosclerotic coronary artery disease has improved substantially over the past two decades. In fact, the 1-year survival rate of patients with refractory angina is approximately 95%. The goals of therapy need to be individualized in each case and expectations should be discussed with patients and their families. The coronary anatomy should be reviewed periodically by interventional cardiologists and cardiothoracic surgeons to confirm that revascularization is not an option. Assuring adherence to evidence-based therapies and correction of precipitating factors is crucial for the stabilization of atherosclerosis, which in turn may result in a survival benefit. Therapies that reduce the anginal threshold by decreasing oxygen demand or improving hemodynamics also play an important role. Management strategies aimed at improving quality of life are fundamental in the management of these patients and may also be associated with a survival benefit. These strategies include psychological support, education, and exercise programs (cardiac rehabilitation). More specific therapies such as EECP, TENS, and SCS also have an important place in the treatment of these patients, keeping in mind that there is a significant "placebo" effect with each one of these specific therapies (Table 4.4).

References

1. Stone GW, Ellis SG, Cox DA, Hermiller J, O'Shaughnessy C, Mann JT, et al. A polymer-based, paclitaxel-eluting stent in patients with coronary artery disease. N Engl J Med. 2004;350:221–31.

2. Moses JW, Leon MB, Popma JJ, Fitzgerald PJ, Holmes DR, O'Shaughnessy C, et al. Sirolimus-eluting stents versus standard stents in patients with stenosis in a native coronary artery. N Engl J Med. 2003;349:1315–23.
3. Pretre R, Turina MI. Choice of revascularization strategy for patients with coronary artery disease. JAMA. 2001;285: 992–4.
4. Hemingway H, Crook AM, Feder G, Banerjee S, Dawson JR, Magee P, et al. Underuse of coronary revascularization procedures in patients considered appropriate candidates for revascularization. N Engl J Med. 2001;344:645–54.
5. Serruys PW, Unger F, Sousa JE, Jatene A, Bonnier HJ, Schonberger JP, et al. Comparison of coronary-artery bypass surgery and stenting for the treatment of multivessel disease. N Engl J Med. 2001;344:1117–24.
6. Katritsis DG, Ioannidis JP. Percutaneous coronary intervention versus conservative therapy in nonacute coronary artery disease: a meta-analysis. Circulation. 2005;111:2906–12.
7. Mannheimer C, Camici P, Chester MR, Collins A, DeJongste M, Eliasson T, et al. The problem of chronic refractory angina; report from the ESC Joint Study Group on the Treatment of Refractory Angina. Eur Heart J. 2002;23: 355–70.
8. TenVaarwerk IA, Jessurun GA, DeJongste MJ, Andersen C, Mannheimer C, Eliasson T, et al. Clinical outcome of patients treated with spinal cord stimulation for therapeutically refractory angina pectoris. The Working Group on Neurocardiology. Heart. 1999;82:82–8.
9. Chaitman BR, Pepine CJ, Parker JO, Skopal J, Chumakova G, Kuch J, et al. Effects of ranolazine with atenolol, amlodipine, or diltiazem on exercise tolerance and angina frequency in patients with severe chronic angina: a randomized controlled trial. JAMA. 2004;291:309–16.
10. IONA Study Group. Trial to show the impact of nicorandil in angina (IONA): design, methodology, and management. Heart. 2001;85:E9.
11. The IONA Study Group. Effect of nicorandil on coronary events in patients with stable angina: the Impact Of Nicorandil in Angina (IONA) randomised trial. Lancet. 2002;359:1269–75.
12. DeJongste MJ, Tio RA, Foreman RD. Chronic therapeuti-S refractory angina pectoris. Heart. 2004;90:225–30.
13. Gibbons RJ, Chatterjee K, Daley J, Douglas JS, Fihn SD, Gardin JM, et al. ACC/AHA/ACP-ASIM guidelines for the management of patients with chronic stable angina: a report of the American College of Cardiology/American Heart Association Task Force on Practice Guidelines (Committee on Management of Patients With Chronic Stable Angina). J Am Coll Cardiol. 1999;33:2092–197.
14. King 3rd SB. Angioplasty is better than medical therapy for alleviating chronic angina pectoris. Arch Intern Med. 2005;165:2589–92.
15. Davignon J. Beneficial cardiovascular pleiotropic effects of statins. Circulation. 2004;109:III39–43.
16. Cannon CP, Braunwald E, McCabe CH, Rader DJ, Rouleau JL, Belder R, et al. Intensive versus moderate lipid lowering with statins after acute coronary syndromes. N Engl J Med. 2004;350:1495–504.
17. Grundy SM, Cleeman JI, Merz CN, Brewer Jr HB, Clark LT, Hunninghake DB, et al. Implications of recent clinical trials for the National Cholesterol Education Program Adult Treatment Panel III guidelines. Circulation. 2004;110: 227–39.
18. Daly CA, Clemens F, Sendon JL, Tavazzi L, Boersma E, Danchin N, et al. The clinical characteristics and investigations planned in patients with stable angina presenting to cardiologists in Europe: from the Euro Heart Survey of Stable Angina. Eur Heart J. 2005;26:996–1010.
19. Ko DT, Hebert PR, Coffey CS, Sedrakyan A, Curtis JP, Krumholz HM. Beta-blocker therapy and symptoms of depression, fatigue, and sexual dysfunction. JAMA. 2002;288:351–7.
20. Fonarow GC, Gawlinski A, Moughrabi S, Tillisch JH. Improved treatment of coronary heart disease by implementation of a Cardiac Hospitalization Atherosclerosis Management Program (CHAMP). Am J Cardiol. 2001;87: 819–22.
21. Peterson ED, Roe MT, Lytle BL, Newby LK, Fraulo ES, Gibler WB, et al. The association between care and outcomes in patients with acute coronary syndromes: national results from CRUSADE. J Am Coll Cardiol. 2004;43:406A.
22. Sarnak MJ, Tighiouart H, Manjunath G, MacLeod B, Griffith J, Salem D, et al. Anemia as a risk factor for cardiovascular disease in the Atherosclerosis Risk in Communities (ARIC) study. J Am Coll Cardiol. 2002;40:27–33.
23. Pocock SJ, Henderson RA, Seed P, Treasure T, Hampton JR. Quality of life, employment status, and anginal symptoms after coronary angioplasty or bypass surgery. 3-year follow-up in the Randomized Intervention Treatment of Angina (RITA) Trial. Circulation. 1996;94:135–42.
24. Pocock SJ, Henderson RA, Clayton T, Lyman GH, Chamberlain DA. Quality of life after coronary angioplasty or continued medical treatment for angina: three-year follow-up in the RITA-2 trial. Randomized Intervention Treatment of Angina. J Am Coll Cardiol. 2000;35: 907–14.
25. Konstam V, Salem D, Pouleur H, Kostis J, Gorkin L, Shumaker S, et al. Baseline quality of life as a predictor of mortality and hospitalization in 5,025 patients with congestive heart failure. SOLVD Investigations. Studies of Left Ventricular Dysfunction Investigators. Am J Cardiol. 1996;78:890–5.
26. Soto GE, Jones P, Weintraub WS, Krumholz HM, Spertus JA. Prognostic value of health status in patients with heart failure after acute myocardial infarction. Circulation. 2004;110:546–51.
27. Rumsfeld JS, MaWhinney S, McCarthy Jr M, Shroyer AL, VillaNueva CB, O'Brien M, et al. Health-related quality of life as a predictor of mortality following coronary artery bypass graft surgery. Participants of the Department of Veterans Affairs Cooperative Study Group on Processes, Structures, and Outcomes of Care in Cardiac Surgery. JAMA. 1999;281:1298–303.
28. Dixon T, Lim LL, Heller RF. Quality of life: an index for identifying high-risk cardiac patients. J Clin Epidemiol. 2001;54:952–60.
29. The IONA Study Group. Determinants of coronary events in patients with stable angina: results from the impact of nicorandil in angina study. Am Heart J. 2005;150:689.
30. Benson H, McCallie Jr DP. Angina pectoris and the placebo effect. N Engl J Med. 1979;300:1424–9.

31. Leon MB, Kornowski R, Downey WE, Weisz G, Baim DS, Bonow RO, et al. A blinded, randomized, placebo-controlled trial of percutaneous laser myocardial revascularization to improve angina symptoms in patients with severe coronary disease. J Am Coll Cardiol. 2005;46:1812–9.
32. Smith TW, Follick MJ, Korr KS. Anger, neuroticism, type A behaviour and the experience of angina. Br J Med Psychol. 1984;57(Pt 3):249–52.
33. Jenkins CD, Stanton BA, Klein MD, Savageau JA, Harken DE. Correlates of angina pectoris among men awaiting coronary by-pass surgery. Psychosom Med. 1983;45:141–53.
34. Hlatky MA, Haney T, Barefoot JC, Califf RM, Mark DB, Pryor DB, et al. Medical, psychological and social correlates of work disability among men with coronary artery disease. Am J Cardiol. 1986;58:911–5.
35. Channer KS, O'Connor S, Britton S, Walbridge D, Rees JR. Psychological factors influence the success of coronary artery surgery. J R Soc Med. 1988;81:629–32.
36. Lewin RJ. Improving quality of life in patients with angina. Heart. 1999;82:654–5.
37. Moore RK, Groves D, Bateson S, Barlow P, Hammond C, Leach AA, et al. Health related quality of life of patients with refractory angina before and one year after enrolment onto a refractory angina program. Eur J Pain. 2005;9: 305–10.
38. Campbell NC, Thain J, Deans HG, Ritchie LD, Rawles JM, Squair JL. Secondary prevention clinics for coronary heart disease: randomised trial of effect on health. BMJ. 1998;316:1434–7.
39. Murchie P, Campbell NC, Ritchie LD, Simpson JA, Thain J. Secondary prevention clinics for coronary heart disease: four year follow up of a randomised controlled trial in primary care. BMJ. 2003;326:84.
40. Chaitman BR, Skettino SL, Parker JO, Hanley P, Meluzin J, Kuch J, et al. Anti-ischemic effects and long-term survival during ranolazine monotherapy in patients with chronic severe angina. J Am Coll Cardiol. 2004;43:1375–82.
41. Borer JS, Fox K, Jaillon P, Lerebours G. Antianginal and antiischemic effects of ivabradine, an I(f) inhibitor, in stable angina: a randomized, double-blind, multicentered, placebo-controlled trial. Circulation. 2003;107:817–23.
42. Tardif JC, Ford I, Tendera M, Bourassa MG, Fox K. Efficacy of ivabradine, a new selective I(f) inhibitor, compared with atenolol in patients with chronic stable angina. Eur Heart J. 2005;26:2529–36.
43. Ciampricotti R, Schotborgh CE, de Kam PJ, van Herwaarden RH. A comparison of nicorandil with isosorbide mononitrate in elderly patients with stable coronary heart disease: the SNAPE study. Am Heart J. 2000;139:939–43.
44. Arora RR, Chou TM, Jain D, Fleishman B, Crawford L, McKiernan T, et al. The multicenter study of enhanced external counterpulsation (MUST-EECP): effect of EECP on exercise-induced myocardial ischemia and anginal episodes. J Am Coll Cardiol. 1999;33:1833–40.
45. Borjesson M, Eriksson P, Dellborg M, Eliasson T, Mannheimer C. Transcutaneous electrical nerve stimulation in unstable angina pectoris. Coron Artery Dis. 1997;8:543–50.
46. Mannheimer C, Eliasson T, Augustinsson LE, Blomstrand C, Emanuelsson H, Larsson S, et al. Electrical stimulation versus coronary artery bypass surgery in severe angina pectoris: the ESBY study. Circulation. 1998;97:1157–63.
47. Grines CL, Watkins MW, Mahmarian JJ, Iskandrian AE, Rade JJ, Marrott P, et al. A randomized, double-blind, placebo-controlled trial of Ad5FGF-4 gene therapy and its effect on myocardial perfusion in patients with stable angina. J Am Coll Cardiol. 2003;42:1339–47.
48. Kornowski R, Baim DS, Moses JW, Hong MK, Laham RJ, Fuchs S, et al. Short- and intermediate-term clinical outcomes from direct myocardial laser revascularization guided by biosense left ventricular electromechanical mapping. Circulation. 2000;102:1120–5.
49. Henry T. AGENT 3: A multicenter, randomized, double-blind, placebo controlled study to evaluate the efficacy and safety of Ad5FGF-4 in patients with stable angina. Presented at Late Breaking Clinical Trials Session of the Transcatheter Cardiovascular Therapeutics, Washington, DC, 2004. http://www.tctmd.com/csportal/appmanager/tctmd/main?_nfpb=true&_pageLabel=TCTMDContent&hdCon=847395. Accessed 23 Dec 2005.
50. Saririan M, Eisenberg MJ. Myocardial laser revascularization for the treatment of end-stage coronary artery disease. J Am Coll Cardiol. 2003;41:173–83.
51. Michaels AD, Raisinghani A, Soran O, de Lame PA, Lemaire ML, Kligfield P, et al. The effects of enhanced external counterpulsation on myocardial perfusion in patients with stable angina: a multicenter radionuclide study. Am Heart J. 2005;150:1066–73.
52. Yamazaki J, Iida M, Igarashi M, Hosoi H, Ishiguro S, Hou M, et al. Evaluation of the efficacy of nicorandil in patients with ischemic heart disease by exercise Tl-201 myocardial SPECT. Int J Clin Pharmacol Ther. 1994;32:183–91.
53. Grines C, Patel A, Zijlstra F, Weaver WD, Granger C, Simes RJ. Primary coronary angioplasty compared with intravenous thrombolytic therapy for acute myocardial infarction: six-month follow up and analysis of individual patient data from randomized trials. Am Heart J. 2003;145:47–57.
54. Yang EH et al. Current and future treatment strategies for refractory angina. Mayo Clin Proc. 2004;79(10):1284–92.

Medical Therapy for Chronic Refractory Angina

5

Gregory W. Barsness, Thomas J. Kiernan, and David R. Holmes Jr.

Medical therapy is the cornerstone of treatment for patients with chronic refractory angina, as it is across the entire spectrum of vascular disease. As part of a comprehensive risk modification program, including exercise, diet, and appropriate revascularization, optimal medical therapy offers significant benefit in reducing symptoms of ischemic heart disease and improving long-term prognosis. Indeed, current medical regimens, far superior to those offered only a decade ago, afford patients with refractory angina a marked survival benefit. Newer agents have demonstrated a marked symptomatic benefit, as well. This chapter will explore the importance of optimal medical therapy in improving prognosis, as well as details potential for imparting a much needed boost to quality of life and symptom amelioration.

Goals and Rationale of Optimal Medical Therapy

The impact of medical therapy has grown with the introduction of advanced antiplatelet therapy, statins, and angiotensin-converting enzyme and receptor inhibition, among other established and evolving therapies that provide important moderation of the inexorable progression of coronary disease. Indeed, appropriate application of evidence-based therapy has had important societal health implications, with a resultant measurable reduction in adverse cardiac events over the past several decades. While appropriate revascularization in patients with chronic angina contributed an estimated 5% to this observed reduction in coronary heart disease mortality between 1980 and 2002, a much larger 50% of the total reduction is attributed to improvement in the risk factor profiles of those populations in jeopardy, largely due to improved agents and greater application of this medical therapy [1].

In fact, the important prognostic benefit associated with optimal medical therapy has been clearly demonstrated, even in patients suitable for coronary revascularization. A prime example of this is the Clinical Outcomes Utilizing Revascularization and Aggressive Drug Evaluation (COURAGE) trial [2], the largest trial yet performed to evaluate the relative impact of PCI over optimal medical therapy alone. This trial randomized 2,287 patients to optimal medical therapy (OMT) or OMT with early percutaneous revascularization (PCI), utilizing predominantly bare metal stents. Optimal medical therapy was intended to include antiplatelet therapy, beta-blockade with metoprolol, ACE inhibition or ARB therapy, and anti-ischemic measures, including amlodipine and/or nitrate therapy. Diet, exercise, and smoking cessation were also encouraged. At a mean follow-up of 4.6 years, there was no significant difference in the primary end point of death or myocardial infarction between the PCI and medical treatment groups (OR 1.05, 95% CI 0.87–1.27, $p=0.62$), nor was there a

G.W. Barsness (✉) • D.R. Holmes Jr.
Mayo Clinic College of Medicine,
Rochester, MN, USA
e-mail: barsness.gregory@mayo.edu

T.J. Kiernan
Division of Cardiovascular Diseases, Mayo Clinic,
Rochester, MN, USA

G.W. Barsness and D.R. Holmes Jr. (eds.), *Coronary Artery Disease*,
DOI 10.1007/978-1-84628-712-1_5,

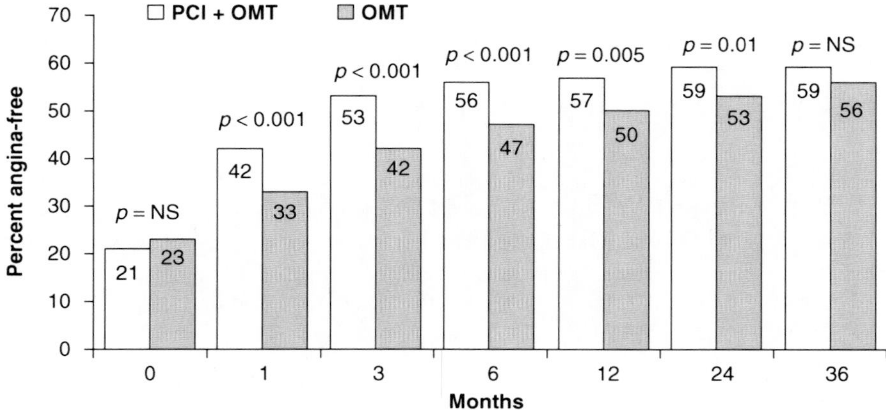

Fig. 5.1 Changes in the Angina-Frequency Scale of the Seattle Angina Questionnaire over time within the COURAGE trial cohorts of percutaneous revascularization with optimal medical therapy (*PCI + OMT*) and optimal medical therapy alone (*OMT*). The early anginal benefit demonstrated with PCI+OMT is reduced over time as patients within the OMT group experience progressively greater freedom from angina over the initial 3 years of follow-up (Modified with permission: Weintraub et al. [3])

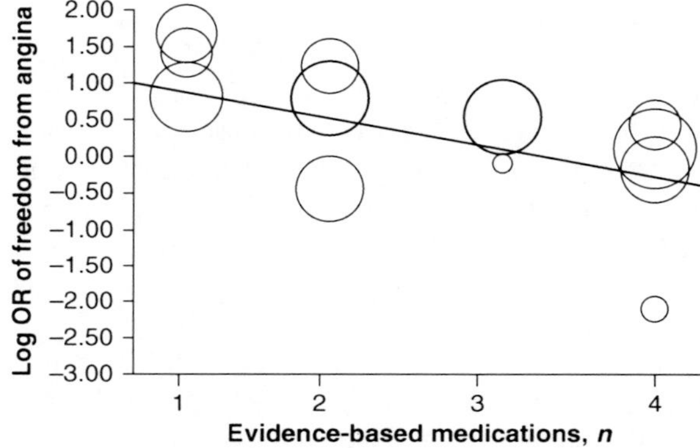

Fig. 5.2 Meta-regression demonstrating an inverse relationship between freedom from angina and adherence to optimal evidence-based medical regimens within individual trial components of the meta-analysis. In more contemporary trials, evidence-based medication was used more frequently and the measurable symptom relief benefit of PCI was diminished (Reproduced with permission: Wijeysundera et al. [4])

difference in overall mortality (7.6% vs 8.3%, $p=0.38$) or freedom from angina (74% vs 72%, $p=0.35$). However, in patients treated with PCI, in addition to medical therapy, freedom from angina was significantly greater up to 3 years, with the medical therapy cohort exhibiting a "catch-up" pattern only after the initial 2 years of follow-up (Fig. 5.1) [3]. These results support the widespread use of optimal medical therapy in patients with established coronary arterial disease and emphasize the tremendous potential impact of this therapeutic strategy in patients with refractory angina, both in terms of reduction in major cardiac events, and also in terms of symptom control (Fig. 5.2) [4].

Components of Optimal Medical Therapy

Angina is the result of myocardial ischemia that occurs when the supply of oxygen is unable to meet its demand. Treatment strategies focus on decreasing oxygen demand and or increasing its supply (Fig. 5.3). The standard treatment for symptomatic relief in chronic stable angina should include beta-blockers and or non-dihydropyridine calcium channel blockers titrated to the lowest heart rate and blood pressure tolerated. In addition, a long acting nitrate should be given utilizing an interrupted dosing schedule to prevent nitrate tolerance. Aggressive risk factor modification with smoking cessation, cholesterol modifying agents, and exercise training should also be offered to these patients.

Although offering important prognostic benefit and good antianginal efficacy, traditional anti-ischemic agents do not provide angina relief uniformly, and significant variations in individual response are well recognized. No recent comparative efficacy studies are available for currently available agents, although beta-blockers have been shown to provide better antianginal efficacy than calcium channel blockers (not including amlodipine or felodipine) in a large meta-analysis [5]. Combination therapy is similarly underexplored, although the combination of beta-blockade with nitrates

Fig. 5.3 Physiologic and hemodynamic effects of cardiac antianginal medications

	O_2 Supply	O_2 Demand			
Drug	Coronary blood	Heart	Arterial pressure	Venous return	Myocardial contractility
Beta blockers	—	↓	↓	—	↓
DHP calcium blockers	↓	↑	↓	—	↓
Non-DHP calcium blockers	↑	↓	↓	—	↓
Long-acting nitrates	↑	↑/ —	↓	↓	—

Table 5.1 Summary of mechanistic effects of novel pharmacologic therapies for refractory angina

Agent	Mechanism	Clearance	Half-life	Adverse reactions
Nicorandil	(1) Nitrate-like vasodilation, (2) K_{ATP} channel activation	Hepatic	45 min	Headache, GI distress
Ivabradine	Heart rate-lowering agent via I_f ion channel blockade	Hepatic	2 h	Visual disturbance, abdominal discomfort
L-arginine	Endothelium-dependent vasodilator as a substrate for nitric oxide (NO) synthase and increased nitric oxide	Hepatic	1.5–2 h	Hypotension, hyperkalemia
Ranolazine	Metabolic modulator inhibiting late sodium channels and preventing intracellular sodium overload	Hepatic	2 h	Constipation, dizzy, nausea, asthenia, QT interval prolongation
Trimetazidine	Metabolic modulator increasing myocardial glucose utilization and inhibiting oxidation of fats via 3-ketoacyl coenzyme A thiolase (3-KAT) inhibition	Renal	6 h	GI burning

Adapted with permission: Yang and Barsness [80]

Table 5.2 Summary of demonstrated effects of novel pharmacologic therapies for refractory angina

Treatment	Improvement in time to ST-depression	Improvement in total exercise time	Reduction in anginal class	Improvement in myocardial perfusion	FDA approved (AHA Class Indication)
Ranolazine	+	+	+	NA	+
Ivabradine	+	+	+	NA	–
Nicorandil	+	+	+	+	–
Trimetazidine	+	–	+	–	–
L-Arginine	+	+	NA	NA	+
Testosterone	+	–	NA	NA	+
Estrogen	+	+	+	NA	+

Adapted with permission: Yang and Barsness [80]
NA data not available, *AHA* American Heart Association, + = yes, – = no

and/or calcium channel blockade has theoretical benefits in reducing ischemic burden through both myocardial supply and demand pathways. Even with the combined use of all three classes of medications, a significant anginal burden may persist, with approximately 5–15% of patients refractory to these combinations [6, 7]. Those patients with ongoing anginal symptoms despite being on optimal standard therapy should be considered for the alternative treatment strategies described in the following sections (Tables 5.1 and 5.2).

Novel Antianginal Agents

L-Arginine

Nitric oxide is synthesized from the amino acid L-arginine by a family of enzymes through the L-arginine–nitric oxide pathway [8]. L-Arginine is the substrate for the production of nitric oxide synthase. It has been shown that L-arginine administration improves endothelium dependent vasodilation in patients with risk factors for atherosclerosis, such as hypercholesterolemia [9], smoking [10], aging [11], and hypertension [12] and in patients with coronary artery disease [13–15] (including dilatation of coronary stenoses) [16], microvascular angina pectoris [17], and peripheral arterial disease [18]. In animal models, L-arginine has improved endothelial dysfunction after coronary angioplasty [19] and protected against ischemia-reperfusion injury [20].

The clinical studies on oral L-arginine therapy as an antianginal are somewhat contradictory. Short-term administration of L-arginine improves coronary microvascular function in hypercholesterolemic subjects [21] and therefore might be expected to improve myocardial ischemia in patients with stable angina. Walker et al. observed no greater improvement in exercise tolerance than in the placebo group in a group of 40 men with stable angina receiving L-arginine 5 mg or placebo [22]. However, a single-center, double-blind, placebo-controlled trial involving 22 patients with stable angina showed that treatment with L-arginine resulted in an increase in exercise duration and maximum workload during stress testing as well as an increase in the time to onset of ST-segment depression (Fig. 5.4) [23]. L-arginine has been shown to improve the clinical symptoms in a selected group of patients with intractable angina pectoris [24]. The contradictory nature of these results may be related to the possibility that improvement with dietary L-arginine may depend upon the predominant mechanism underlying the endothelial dysfunction. Young patients with marked hypercholesterolemia or patients with nonobstructive CAD, for example, may benefit from oral L-arginine to a greater extent than older patients with symptomatic coronary atherosclerosis. L-arginine is currently licensed by the Food and Drug Administration for use in the USA.

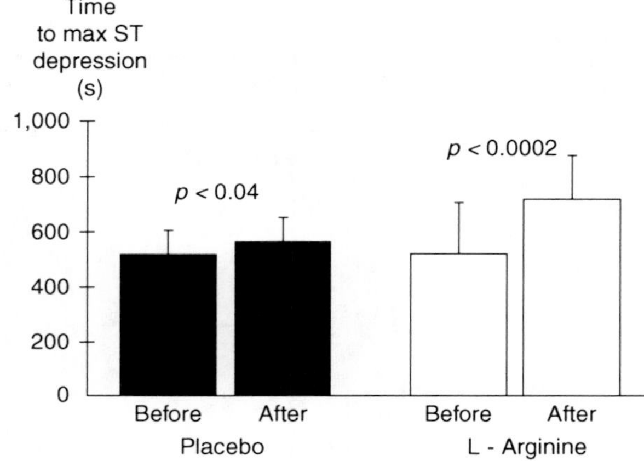

Fig. 5.4 Time to maximal ST-segment depression during exercise testing before and after oral L-arginine administration (2 g, three times each day for 3 days) or placebo (With permission: Ceremuzynski et al. [23])

Ranolazine

Ranolazine belongs to a new group of drugs known as metabolic modulators [25, 26]. Metabolic modulators are believed to exert their effect by increasing the energy available to cardiac cells (Fig. 5.5) and improving the metabolic use of cardiac substrates [26]. Ranolazine is a piperazine derivative that inhibits the late sodium channels, thereby protecting ischemic myocardial cells by lowering total inward sodium flux and subsequent intracellular calcium overload [27, 28].

CARISA (Combination Assessment of Ranolazine in Stable Angina) was a randomized, double-blind, placebo-controlled, three group parallel trial of 823 patients with symptomatic chronic angina [25]. Patients received placebo, 750 mg, or 1,000 mg of sustained-release ranolazine twice daily. Patients were included if they had coronary artery disease and a minimum 3-month history of exertional angina. Eligible subjects had ST segment depression of at least 1 mm; limited exercise capacity, defined as 3–9 min, on a modified Bruce protocol; and reproducible angina. In addition to placebo or ranolazine, participants received commonly prescribed agents for treatment of angina (atenolol 43%, amlodipine 31.1%, diltiazem 25.9%). The majority of patients were male, with a mean age of 77 years.

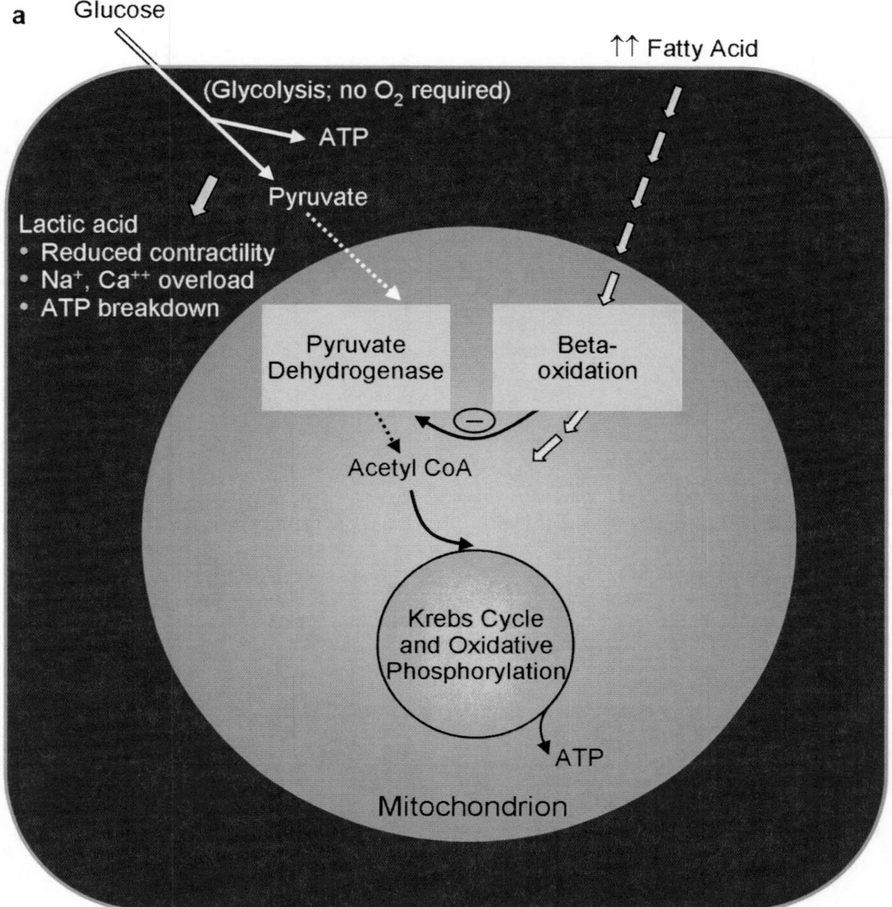

Fig. 5.5 Carbohydrate metabolism regulation by fatty acid oxidation and possible effects of ranolazine. Predominating pathways are represented by *open arrows*; inhibited pathways are represented by *dotted arrows*. (**a**) Pyruvate dehydrogenase is the enzyme mediating conversion of pyruvate to acetyl CoA, permitting its entry into the Krebs cycle. In the presence of elevated fatty acid levels, the end products of β-oxidation reduce pyruvate dehydrogenase activity. As a result, oxygen-wasting fatty acid oxidation predominates, pyruvate oxidation is inhibited, and lactate accumulates. (**b**) Inhibiting fatty acid oxidation with ranolazine may alter the inhibition of pyruvate dehydrogenase, promoting glucose and lactate oxidation, which phosphorylates ATP using less oxygen than the fatty acid oxidation pathway. In addition, lactate accumulation is diminished (With permission: Chaitman et al. [27])

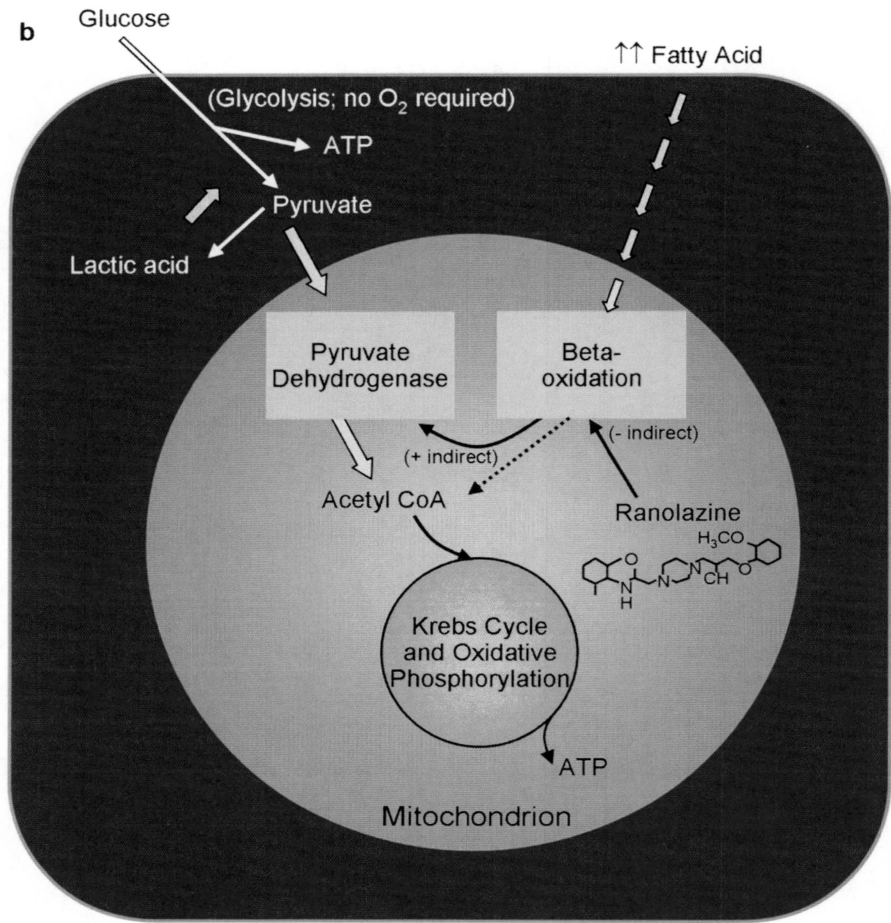

Fig. 5.5 (continued)

The main outcomes assessed in this trial included change in exercise duration, time to onset of ischemia, time to onset of angina, nitroglycerin use, and number of anginal attacks. The main efficacy parameter was change from baseline in exercise treadmill time at trough concentration. Ranolazine significantly improved ($p<0.01$) exercise duration, time to angina attacks, and electrocardiographic changes indicative of ischemia versus placebo. Ranolazine also significantly reduced ($p<0.02$) the mean weekly anginal attacks and nitroglycerin consumption. Ranolazine provided additional antianginal and anti-ischemic efficacy in patients with chronic angina who were symptomatic despite use of other commonly prescribed agents without affecting hemodynamic parameters.

MARISA (Monotherapy Assessment of Ranolazine in Stable Angina) was a randomized, double-blind, placebo-controlled, four period crossover study [27]. The goal was to assess the dose–response relationship of sustained-release ranolazine on symptom-limited exercise duration. Similar to the CARISA population, patients were included if they had coronary artery disease and a minimum 3 month history of exertional angina. All patients discontinued antianginal treatment, except sublingual nitroglycerin, during the trial. The majority of subjects were white males, and mean age was 64 years. Sustained-release ranolazine was administered twice daily for 1 week at 500, 1,000, or 1,500 mg. The brief treatment periods were employed to minimize the exposure of patients with severely limiting angina to placebo treatment. At the end of each period, exercise treadmill tests were performed 4 and 12 h after dosing at times approximating peak and trough ranolazine plasma concentrations. Compared with placebo, all three doses of ranolazine produced a longer time to 1 mm ST-segment depression, increased exercise duration, and lengthened time between anginal attacks.

Commonly reported adverse effects in clinical trials included dizziness, nausea, constipation, asthenia, and minor changes in Bazett's QTc interval; it appears that adverse effects are dose related [25, 27, 29].

Ranolazine is approved by the FDA for use in patients with angina. As the first agent approved for this indication in nearly 30 years, it provides a viable treatment option for patients with angina, although further research is needed to determine the impact of its multiple potential effects. In addition, more studies are required to fully elucidate its mechanism of action either supporting or refuting the current hypothesis regarding partial fatty acid oxidation inhibition and any prognostic benefit associated with this effect.

Nicorandil

Nicorandil, a nicotinamide-nitrate ester [*N*-(2-hydroxyethyl)-nicotinamide nitrate] is the only clinically available potassium channel opener with antianginal effects, and with comparable efficacy and tolerability to existing antianginal therapy. In addition to causing nitrate effects via cyclic guanosine monophosphate, it opens adenosine triphosphate-dependent potassium channels (K_{ATP} channels) [30–32]. Nicorandil thus causes vasodilation not only in epicardial coronary artery but also in small coronary vessels [33]. Through its K_{ATP} channel opening function, nicorandil is thought to reduce calcium influx into myocytes and to limit membrane depolarization, and consequently to attenuate ATP consumption during ischemia. Of note, the K+ ATP channel has been shown to be involved in the phenomenon of myocardial preconditioning, and studies in animal models of ischemia-reperfusion-induced myocardial stunning or infarction indicate that nicorandil has cardioprotective effects. Studies in patients undergoing percutaneous transluminal coronary angioplasty (PTCA) have shown that the administration of nicorandil reduces ST-segment elevation during ischemia.

The IONA (impact of nicorandil in angina) trial was carried out in the UK in which 5,126 high risk angina patients were randomly assigned to receive either placebo ($n=2{,}561$) or nicorandil 20 mg ($n=2{,}565$) twice daily in addition to full conventional treatment [34, 35]. Nicorandil reduced the risk of the primary composite end point (CHD death, nonfatal myocardial infarction (MI), or unplanned hospitalization with cardiac chest pain) by 17% ($p=0.014$) over a mean follow-up of 1.6 years [35]. Comparative and noncomparative studies support the use of nicorandil as monotherapy or in combination with other antianginal therapy for stable angina pectoris.

Nicorandil is not currently FDA approved in the USA but is licensed and used in Europe and also much used in Japan. There have been infrequent case reports of mouth ulcers in patients receiving nicorandil; causality has not been conclusively established, but product prescribing information indicates that an alternative treatment should be considered if persistent aphthous or severe mouth ulceration occurs. Infrequent case reports concerning a potential potassium-channel opening syndrome that can cause hyperkalemia and cardiovascular compromise has also been reported in the literature. In summary, nicorandil seems to be a well-tolerated antianginal with a good safety profile and proven efficacy in chronic stable angina.

Ivabradine

Angina is a symptom of myocardial ischemia, which occurs when insufficient oxygen is supplied to the heart muscle. Heart rate is a primary determinant of myocardial oxygen demand and may also affect myocardial perfusion. Lowering heart rate increases the duration of diastole relative to cardiac cycle length, allowing more time for effective left ventricular (LV) filling and coronary perfusion. Therefore, lowering the heart rate may improve both the aspects of myocardial oxygen balance.

Spontaneous pacemaker activity involves interplay between several ionic currents that influence spontaneous diastolic depolarization of the sinoatrial node, including the I_f current [36]. The "f" denotes "funny," so called because it had unusual properties compared with other current systems known at the time of its discovery. The I_f current is carried by both sodium and potassium ions across the sarcolemma; it is inward at voltages in the diastolic range, is activated on hyperpolarization (within the diastolic range of voltages regularly observed in cardiac pacemaker tissue) [37], and is characterized by unusually low single-channel conductance and slow activation kinetics. The I_f current is directly activated by intracellular cyclic adenosine monophosphate (cAMP), not linked to cAMP-dependent phosphorylation activity [38], and is carried by the hyperpolarization-activated cyclic nucleotide-gated family of ion channels [39].

More than three decades ago, the search began for pure heart rate-lowering agents that would prevent angina without the adverse effects of β-blockers. Currently, ivabradine is the only I_f current inhibitor in the late stage of clinical development. Ivabradine reduces the firing rate of the pacemaker cells in the sinoatrial node without affecting the duration of the action potential [36, 40], whilst acting at concentrations that have no effect on other ionic currents, making ivabradine a selective I_f inhibitor [41]. Ivabradine blocks I_f channels in a concentration-dependent manner by entering the channel pore from the intracellular side [41, 42]. Blockade is only possible when the I_f channel is open, and the magnitude of I_f inhibition is directly related to the frequency of channel opening. Unlike other heart rate-lowering mechanisms, direct I_f blockade depends on the current driving force, as block dramatically increases across the voltage interval, and on sodium concentration in the surrounding milieu [42]. Thus, ivabradine would be expected to be most effective at higher heart rates, where its clinical usefulness would also be greatest.

A randomized, placebo-controlled, double-blind, multicenter, multinational study in 360 patients with stable angina for at least 3 months and documented coronary artery disease evaluated ivabradine in a short dose-ranging phase and in longer-term use [43]. The reduction in heart rate during exercise was associated with a significant increase in time to 1-mm ST-segment depression during ETT in a dose-dependent manner, and there was a statistical trend to improvement in time to limiting angina after just 2 weeks, albeit that these were soft end points.

The results of the International Trial on the Treatment of angina with Ivabradine vs Atenolol (INITIATIVE) were published in 2005 [44]. This randomized, double-blind study compared ivabradine with atenolol over 4 months in 939 patients with stable angina pectoris and documented coronary artery disease. At 4 months, noninferiority of ivabradine 7.5 mg to atenolol was retained for all parameters except time to 1-mm ST-segment depression, again no hard end points were used in this study. The benefit and safety of Ivabradine has also been shown in combination with other antianginals such as beta blockers, nitrates, or calcium-channel blockers [45, 46].

Data from clinical trials demonstrated that visual symptoms were reported in less than 2% of patients receiving the 5 mg bid dosage of ivabradine. Ivabradine reduces heart rate without any observed effects on myocardial contractility and does not alter the cardiac conduction system [47, 48]. In conclusion, Ivabradine appears to be a safe antianginal agent as a monotherapy or in combination with conventional antianginals for the treatment of patients with refractory angina.

Trimetazidine

Trimetazidine, a metabolic antianginal agent that is similar to perhexiline, exerts no significant negative inotropic or vasodilatory properties at rest or during exercise [49, 50]. The actual mechanism of antianginal effect is debatable with some research demonstrating a reduction in the rate of FFA oxidation accompanied by an increase in glucose oxidation rate during low-flow ischemia thought to be due to the inhibition of a key enzyme in the β-oxidation pathway, including 3-ketoacyl coenzyme A thiolase (3-KAT) [50]. Conversely, other studies have not demonstrated this effect [51] (although the underlying mechanism of antianginal action is believed to be induction of a metabolic shift) [52]. Trimetazidine has been shown to be an inhibitor of CPT-I, although a much weaker inhibitor of CPT-I than perhexiline [53].

The benefit of trimetazidine in ischemic heart disease has been clearly demonstrated. The TRIMPOL II study, a large randomized controlled trial conducted in Poland involving 426 patients with stable angina pectoris randomized to receive either 20 mg three times per day trimetazidine or placebo in addition to 50 mg twice daily metoprolol reported favorable results of mean nitrate consumption, angina frequency, and improved time to ST segment depression during exercise testing [54]. A meta-analysis of 12 clinical trials of trimetazidine in stable angina found a significant reduction in anginal frequency [55].

In patients with chronic stable CAD, trimetazidine induced a significant reduction in the perfusion defect assessed by stress ^{201}TI scintigraphy together with an improvement in the ischemic threshold [49]. On the basis of this observation, authors suggested that trimetazidine may correct cell swelling and extravascular compression on coronary microcirculation during ischemia.

In a multicenter, double-blind, placebo-controlled study, Sellier and Broustet [56] confirmed the anti-ischemic

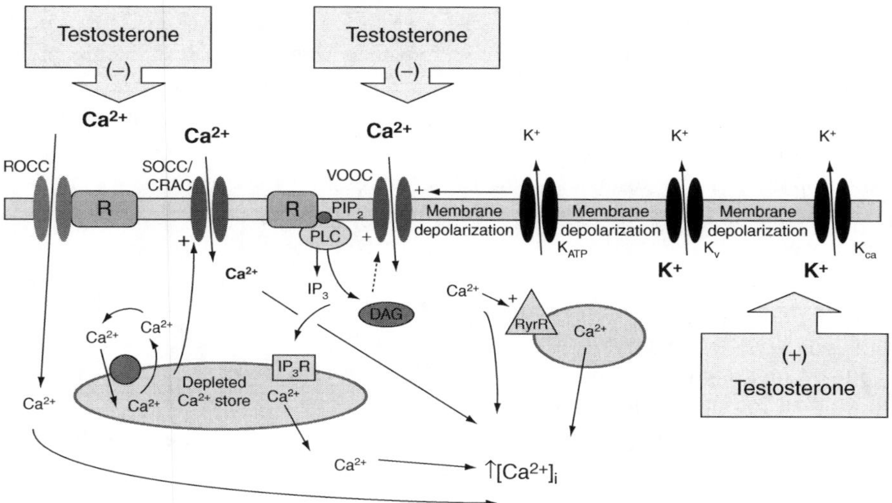

Fig. 5.6 Proposed sites of action to explain the vasodilatory activity of testosterone. $\uparrow[Ca]_i$ elevation in intracellular calcium, *DAG* diacyl glycerol, IP_3 inositol triphosphate, IP_3R inositol triphosphate receptor, K_{ATP} ATP-sensitive potassium channel, K_{Ca} calcium-sensitive potassium channel, *KCl* potassium chloride, K_V voltage-sensitive potassium channel, *NA* noradrenaline, *PLC* phospholipase C, $PGF_{2\alpha}$ prostaglandin $F_{2\alpha}$, PIP_2 phosphatidyl inositol biphosphate, *ROOC* receptor-operated calcium channel, *RyrR* ryanadine receptor, *SOCC* store operated calcium channel, *Thap* thapsigargin, *VOCC* voltage-operated calcium channel (With permission: Jones et al. [67])

and antianginal efficacy of the new formulation in patients with stable angina pectoris receiving atenolol 50 mg/daily; this new trimetazidine formulation was also well tolerated over 6 months.

Trimetazidine's efficacy in stable angina pectoris has been conclusively demonstrated [57]. Several double-blind, randomized studies have compared trimetazidine to placebo or to traditional agents including nifedipine or propranolol, as well as the combination of trimetazidine with nifedipine, β-blockers, or diltiazem. The effects of acute administration of trimetazidine were initially tested in patients with chronic stable effort angina during exercise. Trimetazidine administered from 4 weeks to 6 months improves exercise capacity and total workload of patients with effort angina [58, 59], and reduces the frequency of the anginal attacks and nitroglycerin consumption [60].

Etomoxir

Etomoxir, the least investigated of these "novel" metabolic antianginal agents was initially introduced into the clinical market as a potential diabetic agent [61] and has shown potential as an antianginal agent in ex vivo research but is yet to be investigated in a randomized controlled trial [52]. Similar to perhexiline, etomoxir is a potent CPT-I inhibitor [62]. One small, open-labeled clilnical trial examining the potential benefits of etomoxir in New York Heart Association Classes II-III heart failure found 3 months of 80 mg/day etomoxir improved left ventricular ejection fraction, cardiac output at peak exercise, and clinical status [63]. A planned larger study was stopped prematurely due to the recognition of increased liver transaminase levels in four patients randomized to active agent [64]. In a rat model, using palmitate-perfused ischemic rat hearts, a reduction in oxygen consumption during ischemic recovery and prevention of myocardial function depression was observed when treated with etomoxir [62].

Testosterone and Estrogen

Testosterone has been shown to result in coronary artery dilation and increased blood flow in humans. The mechanism appears to be endothelium independent and may involve the ion channels on vascular smooth muscle cells (Fig. 5.6) [65, 66], a mechanism demonstrated in both in vitro and in vivo studies [66–68]. Several groups have reported that testosterone therapy with intramuscular [69, 70], intravenous, [62] and transdermal preparations had a beneficial anti-ischemic effect in men with coronary disease [71]. The populations of men in these studies were randomly chosen and not selected on the basis of endogenous hormone concentrations. Given that testosterone therapy is of benefit to eugonadal men with coronary disease it would be expected that hormone replacement for hypogonadal men would be of even greater benefit. Since a large proportion of men with coronary disease are biochemically hypogonadal, this proof of concept was felt to be an important finding. In the past 30 years, at least six studies of various design have reported the effects of androgen therapy on coronary ischemia [69–74]; and all but one have reported a beneficial effect [74]. A randomized, double-blind, placebo-controlled trial involving 46 male patients with stable angina on medical therapy showed that treatment with transdermal testosterone resulted in an improvement in time to ST-segment depression during exercise testing and an improvement in quality of life. [71] Another study by Malkin and colleagues [75] looked exclusively at hypogonadal men and found an improvement in time to ischemic threshold to be greater than that among the randomly selected men reported by English and colleagues [71]. Although none of the patients experienced adverse prostatic or hematological effects, concern exists regarding possible health effects of long-term therapy with testosterone in the general male population.

Estrogen has also been investigated as an antianginal agent and has been shown to dilate coronary arteries and improve endothelial function [76]. A randomized, double-blind, placebo-controlled trial involving 74 female patients with stable angina showed that estradiol and norethindrone therapy improved exercise duration and the time to onset of ST-segment depression [77]. There was also a reduction in the number of ischemic events in the treatment group. However, concern was raised in the Women's Health Initiative study, which showed that overall health risks exceeded benefits from use of combined estrogen plus progestin for an average 5.2-year follow-up among healthy postmenopausal US women. All-cause mortality was not affected during the trial. The risk-benefit profile found in this trial was not consistent with the requirements for a viable intervention for primary prevention of chronic diseases and suggested that this regimen should not be initiated or continued for primary prevention of CHD [78]. These benefits, however, must be weighed against the potential for an initial increase in cardiac events caused by estrogen therapy in females with coronary artery disease [79]. In conclusion, the long-term use of either testosterone or estrogen for the treatment of refractory angina is fraught with potential concern in terms of side effects and therefore cannot be recommended as a routine therapeutic regiment.

Future Directions

Refractory angina is a difficult clinical dilemma that is growing in prevalence. As with the entire spectrum of coronary disease, optimal medical therapy and risk factor modification provides important prognostic and symptomatic benefit in these patients. However, when symptoms persist despite aggressive uptitration of standard therapies, a number of promising new pharmacological and nonpharmacological approaches are available. These new treatments; however, still need to undergo the scrutiny of large placebo-controlled randomized trials before we can state with confidence that they are effective. While new agents are currently in development, more complete utilization of currently available agents would provide significant symptomatic relief in the large patient cohort. It is also possible that combination therapy with multiple novel agents may provide additional benefit, although potential adverse effects associated with combination therapy has yet to be investigated.

References

1. Ford ES, Ajani UA, Croft JB, Critchley JA, Labarthe DR, Kottke TE, et al. Explaining the decrease in U.S. deaths from coronary disease, 1980–2000. N Engl J Med. 2007;356(23): 2388–98.
2. Boden WE, O'Rourke RA, Teo KK, Hartigan PM, Maron DJ, Kostuk WJ, et al. Optimal medical therapy with or without PCI for stable coronary disease. N Engl J Med. 2007;356(15): 1503–16.
3. Weintraub WS, Spertus JA, Kolm P, Maron DJ, Zhang Z, Jurkovitz C, et al. Effect of PCI on quality of life in patients with stable coronary disease. N Engl J Med. 2008;359(7): 677–87.
4. Wijeysundera HC, Nallamothu BK, Krumholz HM, Tu JV, Ko DT. Meta-analysis: effects of percutaneous coronary intervention versus medical therapy on angina relief. Ann Intern Med. 2010;152(6):370–9.

5. Heidenreich PA, McDonald KM, Hastie T, Fadel B, Hagan V, Lee BK, et al. Meta-analysis of trials comparing beta-blockers, calcium antagonists, and nitrates for stable angina. JAMA. 1999;281(20):1927–36.
6. Pepine CJ, Abrams J, Marks RG, Morris JJ, Scheidt SS, Handberg E. Characteristics of a contemporary population with angina pectoris. TIDES investigators. Am J Cardiol. 1994;74(3):226–31.
7. Mannheimer C, Camici P, Chester MR, Collins A, DeJongste M, Eliasson T, et al. The problem of chronic refractory angina; report from the ESC joint study group on the treatment of refractory angina. Eur Heart J. 2002;23(5):355–70.
8. Palmer RMJ, Ashton DS, Moncada S. Vascular endothelial cells synthesize nitric oxide from L-arginine. Nature. 1988;333(6174):664–6.
9. Casino PR, Kilcoyne CM, Quyyumi AA, Hoeg JM, Panza JA. Investigation of decreased availability of nitric oxide precursor as the mechanism responsible for impaired endothelium-dependent vasodilation in hypercholesterolemic patients. J Am Coll Cardiol. 1994;23(4):844–50.
10. Campisi R, Czernin J, Schoder H, Sayre JW, Schelbert HR. L-arginine normalizes coronary vasomotion in long-term smokers. Circulation. 1999;99(4):491–7.
11. Chauhan MDMA, More MRS, Mullins MDMPA, Taylor G, Petch MDFFMC, Schofield MDFFPM. Aging-associated endothelial dysfunction in humans is reversed by L-Arginine. J Am Coll Cardiol. 1996;28(7):1796–804.
12. Higashi Y, Oshima T, Sasaki S, Nakano Y, Kambe M, Matsuura H, et al. Angiotensin-converting enzyme inhibition, but not calcium antagonism, improves a response of the renal vasculature to L-arginine in patients with essential hypertension. Hypertension. 1998;32(1):16–24.
13. Tousoulis D, Tentolouris C, Crake T, Katsimaglis G, Stefanadis C, Toutouzas P, et al. Effects of l- and d-arginine on the basal tone of human diseased coronary arteries and their responses to substance P. Heart. 1999;81(5):505–11.
14. Tentolouris C, Tousoulis D, Toutouzas P, Davies G. Effects of acute L-arginine administration in coronary atherosclerosis. Circulation. 1999;99(12):1648–9.
15. Tentolouris C, Tousoulis D, Davies GJ, Stefanadis C, Toutouzas P. Serum cholesterol level, cigarette smoking, and vasomotor responses to L-arginine in narrowed epicardial coronary arteries. Am J Cardiol. 2000;85(4):500–3.
16. Tousoulis D, Davies G, Tentolouris C, Crake T, Toutouzas P. Coronary stenosis dilatation induced by L-arginine. Lancet. 1997;349(9068):1812–3.
17. Egashira K, Hirooka Y, Kuga T, Mohri M, Takeshita A. Effects of L-arginine supplementation on endothelium-dependent coronary vasodilation in patients with angina pectoris and normal coronary arteriograms. Circulation. 1996;94(2):130–4.
18. Böger RH, Bode-Böger SM, Thiele W, Creutzig A, Alexander K, Frölich JC. Restoring vascular nitric oxide formation by l-arginine improves the symptoms of intermittent claudication in patients with peripheral arterial occlusive disease. J Am Coll Cardiol. 1998;32(5):1336–44.
19. Hamon M, Vallet B, Bauters C, Wernert N, McFadden E, Lablanche J, et al. Long-term oral administration of L-arginine reduces intimal thickening and enhances neoendothelium-dependent acetylcholine-induced relaxation after arterial injury. Circulation. 1994;90(3):1357–62.
20. Szabó G, Bährle S, Bátkai S, Stumpf N, Dengler TJ, Zimmermann R, et al. l-arginine: effect on reperfusion injury after heart transplantation. World J Surg. 1998;22(8):791–8.
21. Drexler H, Zeiher AM, Meinzer K, Just H. Correction of endothelial dysfunction in coronary microcirculation of hypercholesterolaemic patients by L-arginine. Lancet. 1991;338(8782–8783):1546–50.
22. Walker HA, McGing E, Fisher I, Böger RH, Bode-Böger SM, Jackson G, et al. Endothelium-dependent vasodilation is independent of the plasma L-arginine/ADMA ratio in men with stable angina: lack of effect of oral l-arginine on endothelial function, oxidative stress and exercise performance. J Am Coll Cardiol. 2001;38(2):499–505.
23. Ceremuzynski MDPL, Chamiec MDT, Herbaczynska-Cedro MDPK. Effect of supplemental oral L-arginine on exercise capacity in patients with stable angina pectoris. Am J Cardiol. 1997;80(3):331–3.
24. Blum A, Porat R, Rosenschein U, Keren G, Roth A, Laniado S, et al. Clinical and inflammatory effects of dietary L-arginine in patients with intractable angina pectoris. Am J Cardiol. 1999;83(10):1488–90.
25. Chaitman BR, Pepine CJ, Parker JO, Skopal J, Chumakova G, Kuch J, et al. Effects of ranolazine with atenolol, amlodipine, or diltiazem on exercise tolerance and angina frequency in patients with severe chronic angina: a randomized controlled trial. JAMA. 2004;291(3):309–16.
26. Pauly DF, Pepine CJ. Ischemic heart disease: metabolic approaches to management. Clin Cardiol. 2004;27(8):439–41.
27. Chaitman BR, Skettino SL, Parker JO, Hanley P, Meluzin J, Kuch J, et al. Anti-ischemic effects and long-term survival during ranolazine monotherapy in patients with chronic severe angina. J Am Coll Cardiol. 2004;43(8):1375–82.
28. Chaitman BR. Ranolazine for the treatment of chronic angina and potential use in other cardiovascular conditions. Circulation. 2006;113(20):2462–72.
29. Rousseau MF, Pouleur H, Cocco G, Wolff AA. Comparative efficacy of ranolazine versus atenolol for chronic angina pectoris. Am J Cardiol. 2005;95(3):311–6.
30. Suryapranata H, MacLeod D. Nicorandil and cardiovascular performance in patients with coronary artery disease. J Cardiovasc Pharmacol. 1992;20 Suppl 3:S45–51.
31. Holzmann S. Cyclic GMP as possible mediator of coronary arterial relaxation by nicorandil (SG-75). J Cardiovasc Pharmacol. 1983;5(3):364–70.
32. Thormann J, Schlepper M, Kramer W, Gottwik M, Kindler M. Effectiveness of nicorandil (SG-75), a new long-acting drug with nitroglycerin effects, in patients with coronary artery disease: improved left ventricular function and regional wall motion and abolition of pacing-induced angina. J Cardiovasc Pharmacol. 1983;5(3):371–7.
33. Akai K, Wang Y, Sato K, Sekiguchi N, Sugimura A, Kumagai T, et al. Vasodilatory effect of nicorandil on coronary arterial microvessels: its dependency on vessel size and the involvement of the ATP-sensitive potassium channels. J Cardiovasc Pharmacol. 1995;26(4):541–7.
34. The IONA Study Group. Trial to show the impact of nicorandil in angina (IONA): design, methodology, and management. Heart. 2001;85(6):e9.
35. The IONA Study Group. Effect of nicorandil on coronary events in patients with stable angina: the Impact of

Nicorandil in Angina (IONA) randomised trial. Lancet. 2002;359(9314):1269–75.
36. DiFrancesco D. Cardiac pacemaker I(f) current and its inhibition by heart rate-reducing agents. Curr Med Res Opin. 2005;21(7):1115–22.
37. DiFrancesco D. The cardiac hyperpolarizing-activated current, i_f. Origins and developments. Prog Biophys Mol Biol. 1985;46(3):163–83.
38. DiFrancesco D, Tortora P. Direct activation of cardiac pacemaker channels by intracellular cyclic AMP. Nature. 1991;351(6322):145–7.
39. Ludwig A, Zong X, Jeglitsch M, Hofmann F, Biel M. A family of hyperpolarization-activated mammalian cation channels. Nature. 1998;393(6685):587–91.
40. Thollon C, Bidouard J-P, Cambarrat C, Lesage L, Reure H, Delescluse I, et al. Stereospecific in vitro and in vivo effects of the new sinus node inhibitor (+)-S 16257. Eur J Pharmacol. 1997;339(1):43–51.
41. Bois P, Bescond J, Renaudon B, Lenfant J. Mode of action of bradycardic agent, S 16257, on ionic currents of rabbit sinoatrial node cells. Br J Pharmacol. 1996;118(4):1051–7.
42. Bucchi A, Baruscotti M, DiFrancesco D. Current-dependent block of rabbit sino-atrial node I_f channels by Ivabradine. J Gen Physiol. 2002;120(1):1–13.
43. Borer JS, Fox K, Jaillon P, Lerebours G, for the Ivabradine Investigators Group. Antianginal and antiischemic effects of Ivabradine, an I_f inhibitor, in stable angina: a randomized, double-blind, multicentered, placebo-controlled trial. Circulation. 2003;107(6):817–23.
44. Tardif J-C, Ford I, Tendera M, Bourassa MG, Fox K. Efficacy of ivabradine, a new selective I_f inhibitor, compared with atenolol in patients with chronic stable angina. Eur Heart J. 2005;26(23):2529–36.
45. Tendera M, Borer JS, Tardif J-C. Efficacy of I(f) inhibition with ivabradine in different subpopulations with stable angina pectoris. Cardiology. 2009;114(2):116–25.
46. Marquis-Gravel G, Tardif JC. Ivabradine: the evidence of its therapeutic impact in angina. Core Evid. 2008;3(1):1–12.
47. Manz M, Reuter M, Lauck G, Omran H, Jung W. A single intravenous dose of ivabradine, a novel I(f) inhibitor, lowers heart rate but does not depress left ventricular function in patients with left ventricular dysfunction. Cardiology. 2003;100(3):149–55.
48. DiFrancesco D, Camm JA. Heart rate lowering by specific and selective I(f) current inhibition with ivabradine: a new therapeutic perspective in cardiovascular disease. Drugs. 2004;64(16):1757–65.
49. Pornin M, Harpey C, Allal J, Sellier P, Ourbak P. Lack of effects of trimetazidine on systemic hemodynamics in patients with coronary artery disease: a placebo-controlled study. Clin Trials Metaanal. 1994;29(1):49–56.
50. Kantor PF, Lucien A, Kozak R, Lopaschuk GD. The antianginal drug trimetazidine shifts cardiac energy metabolism from fatty acid oxidation to glucose oxidation by inhibiting mitochondrial long-chain 3-ketoacyl coenzyme A thiolase. Circ Res. 2000;86(5):580–8.
51. MacInnes A, Fairman DA, Binding P, Rhodes Ja, Wyatt MJ, Phelan A, et al. The antianginal agent trimetazidine does not exert its functional benefit via inhibition of mitochondrial long-chain 3-ketoacyl coenzyme A Thiolase. Circ Res. 2003;93(3):e26–32.
52. Lee L, Horowitz J, Frenneaux M. Metabolic manipulation in ischaemic heart disease, a novel approach to treatment. Eur Heart J. 2004;25(8):634–41.
53. Kennedy JA, Horowitz JD. Effect of trimetazidine on carnitine palmitoyltransferase-1 in the rat heart. Cardiovasc Drugs Ther. 1998;12(4):359–63.
54. Szwed H, Sadowski Z, Elikowski W, Koronkiewicz A, Mamcarz A, Orszulak W, et al. Combination treatment in stable effort angina using trimetazidine and metoprolol. Results of a randomized, double-blind, multicentre study (TRIMPOL II). Eur Heart J. 2001;22(24):2267–74.
55. Marzilli M, Klein WW. Efficacy and tolerability of trimetazidine in stable angina: a meta-analysis of randomized, double-blind, controlled trials. Coron Artery Dis. 2003;14(2):171–9.
56. Sellier P, Broustet J-P. Assessment of anti-ischemic and antianginal effect at trough plasma concentration and safety of trimetazidine MR 35 mg in patients with stable angina pectoris: a multicenter, double-blind, placebo-controlled study. Am J Cardiovasc Drugs. 2003;3(5):361–9.
57. Ciapponi A, Pizarro R, Harrison J. Trimetazidine for stable angina. Cochrane Database Syst Rev. 2005;19(4):CD003614.
58. Chazov EI, Lepakchin VK, Zharova EA, Fitilev SB, Levin AM, Rumiantzeva EG, et al. Trimetazidine in Angina Combination Therapy – the TACT study: trimetazidine versus conventional treatment in patients with stable angina pectoris in a randomized, placebo-controlled, multicenter study. Am J Ther. 2005;12(1):35–42.
59. Koylan N, Bilge AK, Adalet K, Mercanoglu F, Buyukozturk K. Comparison of the effects of trimetazidine and diltiazem on exercise performance in patients with coronary heart disease. The Turkish trimetazidine study (TTS). Acta Cardiol. 2004;59(6):644–50.
60. McClellan KJ, Plosker GL. Trimetazidine. A review of its use in stable angina pectoris and other coronary conditions. Drugs. 1999;58(1):143–57.
61. Reaven GM, Chang H, Hoffman BB. Additive hypoglycemic effects of drugs that modify free-fatty acid metabolism by different mechanisms in rats with streptozocin-induced diabetes. Diabetes. 1988;37(1):28–32.
62. Lopaschuk G, Wall S, Olley P, Davies N. Etomoxir, a carnitine palmitoyltransferase I inhibitor, protects hearts from fatty acid-induced ischemic injury independent of changes in long chain acylcarnitine. Circ Res. 1988;63(6):1036–43.
63. Schmidt-Schweda S, Holubarsch C. First clinical trial with etomoxir in patients with chronic congestive heart failure. Clin Sci (Lond). 2000;99(1):27–35.
64. Holubarsch CJ, Rohrbach M, Karrasch M, Boehm E, Polonski L, Ponikowski P, et al. A double-blind randomized multicentre clinical trial to evaluate the efficacy and safety of two doses of etomoxir in comparison with placebo in patients with moderate congestive heart failure: the ERGO (etomoxir for the recovery of glucose oxidation) study. Clin Sci (Lond). 2007;113(4):205–12.
65. Chou TM, Sudhir K, Hutchison SJ, Ko E, Amidon TM, Collins P, et al. Testosterone induces dilation of canine coronary conductance and resistance arteries in vivo. Circulation. 1996;94(10):2614–9.
66. Yue P, Chatterjee K, Beale C, Poole-Wilson PA, Collins P. Testosterone relaxes rabbit coronary arteries and aorta. Circulation. 1995;91(4):1154–60.

67. Jones RD, Pugh PJ, Jones TH, Channer KS. The vasodilatory action of testosterone: a potassium-channel opening or a calcium antagonistic action? Br J Pharmacol. 2003;138(5):733–44.
68. Webb CM, McNeill JG, Hayward CS, de Zeigler D, Collins P. Effects of testosterone on coronary vasomotor regulation in men with coronary heart disease. Circulation. 1999;100(16):1690–6.
69. Jaffe MD. Effect of testosterone cypionate on postexercise ST segment depression. Br Heart J. 1977;39(11): 1217–22.
70. Rosano GMC, Leonardo F, Pagnotta P, Pelliccia F, Panina G, Cerquetani E, et al. Acute anti-ischemic effect of testosterone in men with coronary artery disease. Circulation. 1999;99(13):1666–70.
71. English KM, Steeds RP, Jones TH, Diver MJ, Channer KS. Low-dose transdermal testosterone therapy improves angina threshold in men with chronic stable angina: a randomized, double-blind, placebo-controlled study. Circulation. 2000; 102(16):1906–11.
72. Wu SZ, Weng XZ. Therapeutic effects of an androgenic preparation on myocardial ischemia and cardiac function in 62 elderly male coronary heart disease patients. Chin Med J (Engl). 1993;106(6):415–8.
73. Webb CM, Adamson DL, de Zeigler D, Collins P. Effect of acute testosterone on myocardial ischemia in men with coronary artery disease. Am J Cardiol. 1999;83(3):437–9.
74. Thompson PD, Ahlberg AW, Moyna NM, Duncan B, Ferraro-Borgida M, White CM, et al. Effect of intravenous testosterone on myocardial ischemia in men with coronary artery disease. Am Heart J. 2002;143(2):249–56.
75. Malkin CJ, Pugh PJ, Morris PD, Kerry KE, Jones RD, Jones TH, et al. Testosterone replacement in hypogonadal men with angina improves ischaemic threshold and quality of life. Heart. 2004;90(8):871–6.
76. Magness RR, Rosenfeld CR. Local and systemic estradiol-17 beta: effects on uterine and systemic vasodilation. Am J Physiol Endocrinol Metab. 1989;256(4):E536–42.
77. E. Sanderson J, Sanderson J, Haines CJ, Yeung L, W. K. Yip G, Tang K, et al. Anti-ischemic action of estrogen-progestogen continuous combined hormone replacement therapy in postmenopausal women with established angina pectoris: a randomized, placebo-controlled, double-blind, parallel-group trial. J Cardiovasc Pharmacol. 2001;38(3):372–83.
78. Writing Group for the Women's Health Initiative Investigators. Risks and benefits of estrogen plus progestin in healthy postmenopausal women. JAMA. 2002;288(3):321–33.
79. Hulley S, Grady D, Bush T, Furberg C, Herrington D, Riggs B, et al. Randomized trial of estrogen plus progestin for secondary prevention of coronary heart disease in postmenopausal women. JAMA. 1998;280(7):605–13.
80. Yang E, Barsness G. Evolving treatment strategies for chronic refractory angina. Expert Opin Pharmacother. 2006;7(3):259–66.

EECP

6

Bradley A. Bart

External counterpulsation is a noninvasive, device-based treatment for patients with coronary artery disease and medically refractory angina. This chapter will review the initial development, clinical applications, and possible mechanisms of action of counterpulsation therapy for ischemic heart disease.

Counterpulsation for Ischemic Heart Disease

Counterpulsation therapy was developed to reduce myocardial ischemia by favorably altering myocardial oxygen supply and demand [1–4]. Early cardiac assist devices withdrew a volume of blood from the aorta during systole (ventricular unloading phase) and rapidly returned it during diastole (diastolic augmentation/counterpulsation) [5]. Ventricular unloading reduced myocardial oxygen demand and counterpulsation increased diastolic pressure in the aorta leading to an increase in coronary artery perfusion pressure during diastole. Experience with this approach was promising – counterpulsation therapy increased survival in a canine model of acute myocardial infarction and stimulated the development of collateral coronary vessels [1, 6].

The intra-aortic balloon pump (IABP) was developed as a simplified form of cardiac assist device [7, 8]. Diastolic augmentation was achieved by the rapid inflation of a balloon positioned in the descending aorta rather than an infusion of blood. Left ventricular unloading was achieved by the rapid deflation of the balloon at the onset of systole, creating a vacuum in the aorta in the area previously occupied by the gas-filled balloon. This modification in design allowed for relatively easy instrumentation and did not require volumes of blood to be rapidly removed from and returned to the aorta [1, 7, 9–11].

Today, the IABP is used to relieve intractable angina, to treat acute myocardial infarction complicated by cardiogenic shock, to enhance coronary artery perfusion pressure in the setting of thrombolytic therapy [9, 12–14] and percutaneous coronary intervention (PCI) [15] and to stabilize hemodynamically compromised patients until definitive therapies can be rendered [1, 12]. Use of the IABP is limited to the hospital setting and is associated with numerous complications, many of which can be life threatening [12].

External Counterpulsation

External counterpulsation, the application of a positive pressure pulse to the lower extremities without direct instrumentation of the vasculature, was developed in the 1950s and 1960s [16–19]. Fluid-filled bladders delivered a positive pressure pulse to the lower extremities during diastole, and released pressure (or applied a negative pressure) during systole thereby increasing diastolic blood pressure 40–50% and decreasing systolic blood pressure 30% [20]. These hydraulic devices were cumbersome and had variable effects on diastolic augmentation. Some investigators hypothesized that simultaneous external compression of the entire lower

B.A. Bart
Hennepin County Medical Center,
University of Minnesota, Minneapolis,
MN, USA
e-mail: bartx006@umn.edu

G.W. Barsness and D.R. Holmes Jr. (eds.), *Coronary Artery Disease*,
DOI 10.1007/978-1-84628-712-1_6, © Springer-Verlag London Limited 2012

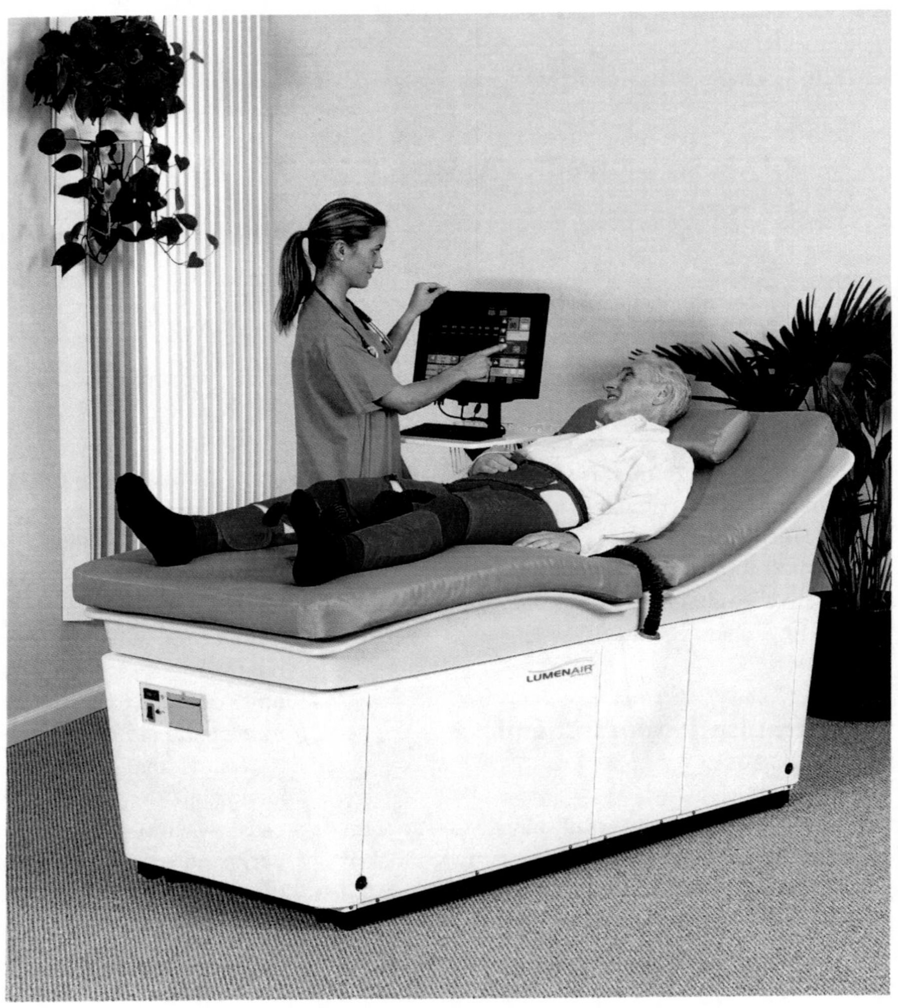

Fig. 6.1 EECP treatment console and table (Graphics courtesy of Vasomedical, Inc., Westbury, NY)

extremity could cause early collapse of proximal vessels such that reversal of aortic blood flow and diastolic augmentation would be adversely affected [20, 21].

In the 1980s, a pneumatic device was developed with a series of air-filled cuffs that applied pressure to the lower extremities sequentially from calves to thighs to buttocks [22, 23]. The cuffs inflated sequentially during diastole causing retrograde aortic flow, diastolic augmentation, and increased venous return. During systole, the cuffs rapidly deflated resulting in unloading of the left ventricle and a decrease in systolic blood pressure (Figs. 6.1 and 6.2). This counterpulsation device markedly enhanced diastolic augmentation due to the sequential inflation of the cuffs and compression of the upper thighs and buttocks (an area not accessible to the older hydraulic systems). To distinguish this form of external counterpulsation from the nonsequential hydraulic systems, it was called sequential external counterpulsation, or SECP [23].

The initial American experience with a sequential pneumatic system was published by the group at State University of New York (SUNY), Stony Brook by Lawson et al. [24]. This group was supported by a company (Vasomedical) that manufactured the counterpulsation device, registering the name "enhanced external counterpulsation" (EECP). EECP results in retrograde aortic blood flow during the diastolic

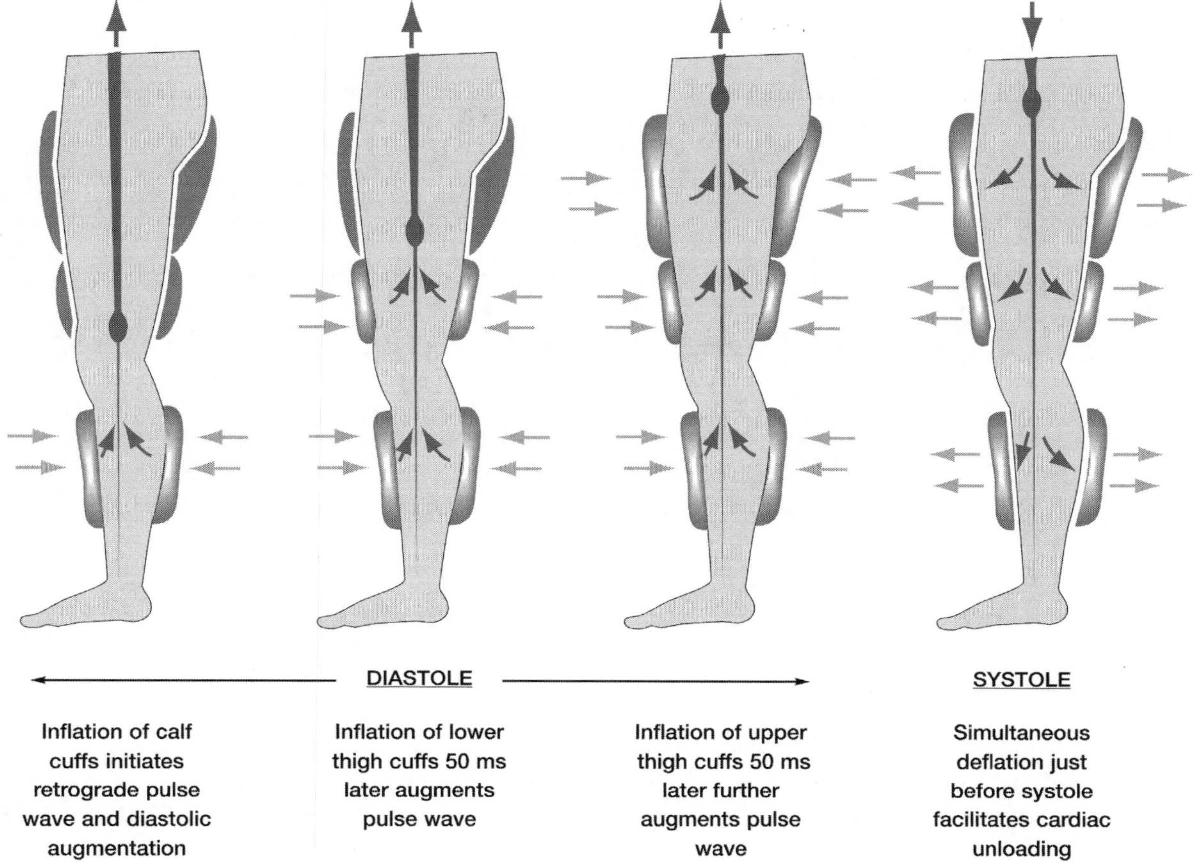

Fig. 6.2 Sequential external counterpulsation. At the onset of diastole, pneumatic cuffs sequentially inflate from calves to lower thighs to upper thighs and buttocks causing retrograde blood flow in the aorta, increased diastolic pressure and increased venous return. During systole, the cuffs rapidly deflate resulting in unloading of the left ventricle and decreased systolic blood pressure (Graphics courtesy of Vasomedical, Inc., Westbury, NY)

compression phase [15, 25] and increases coronary artery mean pressure 16% and peak diastolic pressure 93% (Fig. 6.3) [26]. Coronary artery Doppler studies show an increase in flow velocity of 150% and TIMI frame counts during angiography show that coronary flow increases 28% [26]. Systolic blood pressure and systemic vascular resistance decrease [26, 27] and cardiac output increases during EECP [27, 28].

Compared to the more invasive IABP, EECP produces similar diastolic augmentation and higher cardiac output [29]. The increased cardiac output is felt to be due, in part, to increased venous return and augmentation of atrial preload that occurs with EECP and not IABP [28, 29].

Clinical Applications of External Counterpulsation

Acute Myocardial Infarction and Cardiogenic Shock

Cardiac support devices were developed in an era when optimizing myocardial blood flow and minimizing left ventricular work were the primary therapeutic goals for patients with myocardial infarction. Indeed, the occluded infarct-related artery was not viewed as an attractive therapeutic target: "The primary concern in acute coronary occlusion is not the occlusion but the resultant condition of the myocardium. Once this

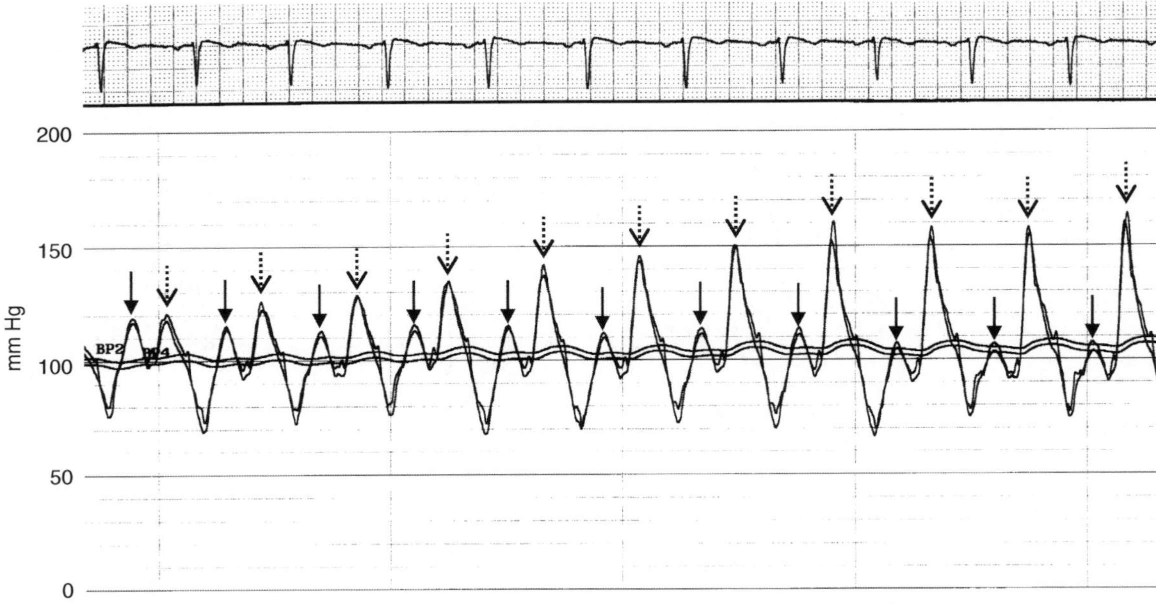

Fig. 6.3 Simultaneous aortic and coronary artery pressures at the onset of EECP. Diastolic pressure increases (*dashed arrows*) and systolic pressure decreases (*solid arrows*) in both aorta and coronary artery as cuff pressure is gradually increased (From Micheals et al. [26], by permission of Circulation)

simple conceptual alteration in emphasis is made, promising new avenues of therapy evolve [5]."

External counterpulsation in the setting of uncomplicated myocardial infarction increases diastolic blood pressure and cardiac index [30], limits infarct size measured by precordial ST-segment mapping and serum levels of creatine phosphokinase-myoglobin [31], and is associated with improved survival [22, 31, 32]. Cardiac output, right atrial pressure, and atrial natriuretic peptide levels increase while brain natriuretic peptide levels are not affected suggesting that the increase in cardiac output is due, in part, to increased venous return and enhanced pre-load [28].

External counterpulsation has also been used in patients with cardiogenic shock [33, 34]. In 1974, Soroff et al. performed external counterpulsation in 20 patients with myocardial infarction complicated by cardiogenic shock for up to 4 h within 24 h of the onset of shock [20]. Treatment was effective in the majority of patients with only one patient failing to achieve at least a 50% increase in diastolic pressure. The overall in-hospital survival rate was 45%, which was significantly greater than the anticipated survival based on historical controls. In another study, 52 patients with acute myocardial infarction were treated with external counterpulsation immediately after arrival to the hospital [22]. Compared to controls, patients treated with external counterpulsation experienced significant improvements in chest pain and ST-T changes. Five patients with acute myocardial infarction and cardiogenic shock were treated with external counterpulsation and had invasive hemodynamic measurements performed. Four of the five patients experienced hemodynamic improvements in cardiac index, systolic blood pressure, and pulmonary capillary wedge pressure. The one patient without hemodynamic improvement failed to achieve significant diastolic augmentation. The authors concluded that diastolic augmentation is critical to achieving good clinical outcomes in the setting of acute myocardial infarction and cardiogenic shock. Indeed, the effectiveness of EECP in this setting is largely predicted by the degree of diastolic augmentation [22].

Angina Pectoris

Advances in the treatment of acute myocardial infarction, such as thrombolytics and PCI, redirected the focus of EECP to the treatment of chronic angina.

Early investigators hypothesized that EECP could lead to sustained increases in myocardial perfusion, improved exercise tolerance, and reduced angina [21].

Results of external counterpulsation for the treatment of angina using the early nonsequential hydraulic systems were mixed [21, 22]. External counterpulsation therapy was effective in relieving symptoms of angina in studies that documented effective diastolic augmentation [35, 36]; however, other studies that failed to achieve significant diastolic augmentation did not have any effect on angina [37, 38].

In 1983, Zheng et al. used sequential external counterpulsation in 200 patients with chronic angina [23]. Patients were treated for 1 h each day over 12 days; 97% experienced reductions in angina (compared to 73% in a control group treated with antianginal medications), and patients experienced less ischemia, fewer episodes of recurrent ischemia, and increased exercise tolerance. Sham treatments were delivered in a subset of patients without clinical improvement. The clinical success in this patient population and in earlier studies was attributed to effective diastolic augmentation during external counterpulsation [21–23].

Lawson et al. were the first Americans to publish their experience with modern EECP using pneumatic cuffs and sequential inflation [24]. Eighteen patients were treated 1 h daily for a total of 36 h. All patients had chronic, incapacitating angina despite optimal medical and surgical therapy, and evidence of ischemia by thallium-201 perfusion imaging. All patients experienced symptomatic improvement immediately following EECP and 16 of 18 had complete relief from angina during activities of daily living. Exercise tolerance and rate-pressure product during maximal treadmill testing increased significantly compared to baseline. Myocardial perfusion studies, performed to the same stress end point to provide comparative information on ischemic burden, showed complete resolution of ischemia in 67% of patients, improvement in 11%, and no change in 22%. These improvements were sustained 3 years after completion of EECP suggesting that the benefit is maintained long term [5, 39, 40].

Other small studies demonstrated significant improvements in exercise tolerance [24, 41–48], time to ST depression during treadmill exercise testing [43, 44, 46], angina [23, 24, 39, 41–43, 45–53], nitroglycerin use [24, 39, 42, 43, 47–49, 52], myocardial perfusion [24, 39, 41, 42, 44, 46, 54], and quality of life [55, 56] (Table 6.1).

Randomized, Controlled Trial of EECP for Angina

The nature of EECP precludes a double-blind, placebo controlled trial design. However, EECP has been compared to "sham" treatments involving low cuff inflation pressures such that diastolic augmentation does not occur [23, 36, 43]. The Multicenter Study of Enhanced External Counterpulsation (MUST-EECP) was a prospective, multicenter, randomized, "sham"-controlled trial to assess the safety and efficacy of EECP in patients with stable angina [43]. Patients were enrolled in the study if they had class I, II, or III angina; evidence of ischemia on an exercise treadmill test; and documented evidence of coronary artery disease. Important exclusion criteria included revascularization in the preceding 3 months, overt congestive heart failure or a left ventricular ejection fraction ≤30%, significant valvular heart disease, uncontrolled hypertension, a permanent pacemaker or implantable cardiac defibrillator, uncontrolled arrhythmias, and significant stenosis of the left main coronary artery without bypass. Patients were randomized to 35 h of active counterpulsation achieving a mean diastolic augmentation ratio (systolic:diastolic blood pressure) of 1.41 or "sham" therapy with cuff pressures inflated to 75 mmHg (enough to preserve the appearance and feel of EECP treatment, but not achieving significant diastolic augmentation). The primary end points of the study were changes in exercise duration and time to ≥1 mm ST segment depression during exercise treadmill testing. Patients in the active treatment arm had a significant increase in time to ≥1 mm ST depression and a decrease in the frequency of angina compared to controls (Fig. 6.4). However, there was no significant difference in exercise duration or in the amount of sublingual nitroglycerin used. Health-related quality of life was assessed at baseline, immediately after EECP and at 1 year. Compared to sham-control patients, patients in the active treatment group had significant improvements in all quality of life scales immediately after EECP and these improvements persisted for 1 year [64].

International Registry and Consortium Experience: EECP in the General Population

The International EECP Patient Registry (IEPR) and the External Counterpulsation Consortium were established to assess the safety, efficacy, and long-term outcomes of patients undergoing EECP [49, 50].

Table 6.1 Authors, year of publication, study size, and outcomes of EECP for angina

Authors	Year	Number of patients	Angine↓≥1 class (%)	Nitroglycerin use	Exercise tolerance	Myocardial perfusion (%)
Zheng et al. [23]	1983	200	↓(97)	NA	NA	NA
Lawson et al. [24]	1992	18	↓ (100)	↓	↑	↑ (78)
Lawson et al. [42]	1996	27	NA	NA	↑	↑ (78)
Lawson et al. [54]	1996	50	↓ (100)	NA	NA	↑ (80)
Lawson et al. [41]	1998	60	↓	NA	↑	↑ (75)
Aurora et al. [43]	1999	139	↓	↓	↑	NA
Lawson et al. [39]	2000	33	↓ (100)	↓	NA	↑ (79)
Lawson et al. [50]	2000	2,289	↓ (73)	NA	NA	NA
Urano et al. [46]	2001	12	NA	NA	↑	↑
Masuda et al. [44]	2001	11	NA	NA	↑	↑
Stys et al. [51]	2001	395	↓ (88)	NA	NA	NA
Springer et al. [56]	2001	27	↓	↓	NA	↑ (63)
Stys et al. [45]	2002	175	↓ (85)	NA	↑	↑ (83)
Lawson et al. [57]	2003	4,592	↓ (73)	↓	NA	NA
Bagger et al. [58]	2004	23	↓	↓	↑	↑[a]
Masuda et al. [59]	2004	18	NA	↓	↑	↑
Dockery et al. [60]	2004	23	NA	NA	↑	NA
Shechter et al. [61]	2003	20	↓	↓	NA	NA
Tartaglia et al. [62]	2003	25	↓ (93)	NA	↑	↑
Bonetti et al. [63]	2003	23	↓ (74)	NA	NA	NA
Loh et al. [47]	2006	61	↓(86)	↓	↑	NA
Novo et al. [48]	2006	25	↓(84)	↓	↑	↑[a]
Pettersson et al. [52]	2006	55	↓(79)	↓	NA	NA

[a]Wall motion score by dobutamine echocardiography. The percent of patients experiencing improvement in angina class and myocardial perfusion are indicated in parentheses when known

NA not assessed, ↓ = decrease, ↑ = increase

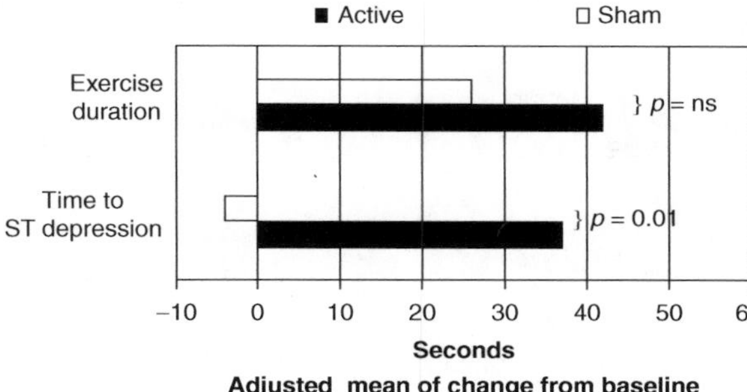

Fig. 6.4 Time to ischemic ST-depression and total exercise duration in chronic angina patients treated with active or "sham" EECP [43] (Graphics courtesy of Vasomedical, Inc., Westbury, NY)

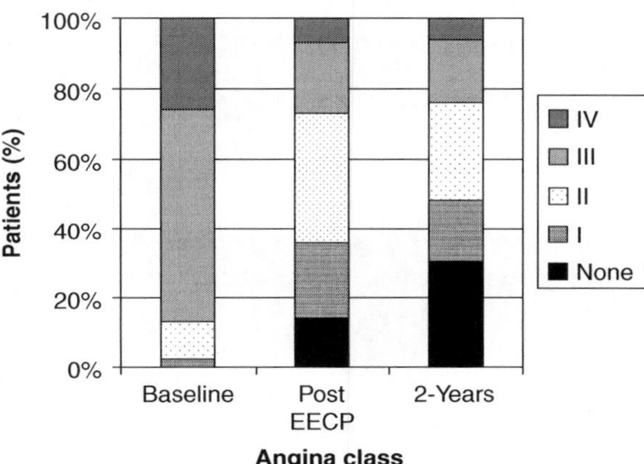

Fig. 6.5 CCS angina classification in 1,097 patients before, immediately, and 2 years after EECP (From Micheals et al. [66], by permission of American Journal of Cardiology)

These programs represent a broad spectrum of patients reflecting the diversity encountered in the community setting. Based on clinical responses assessed in over 7,000 patients, 73% experienced improved angina ≥1 Canadian Cardiovascular Society (CCS) class following EECP and this improvement was sustained over a 2-year period [49, 50, 65] (Fig. 6.5). Adverse cardiac events occurring during EECP are uncommon and include death 0.3%, myocardial infarction 0.3–0.9%, unstable angina 3.4%, and worsening heart failure 2.4% [49, 50]. In the IEPR, 18% of patients returned for a repeat course of therapy during the 2-year follow-up period. Of these, the majority (70%) responded to the additional course of EECP with improved angina symptoms and decreased nitroglycerin use [65].

Comparisons to Traditional Revascularization: Safety and Efficacy

Comparisons between EECP and PCI for the treatment of chronic angina are difficult because referral patterns for these two interventions define patient populations that differ considerably from one another. Medicare reimbursement requires that patients undergoing EECP must have advanced angina (class III–IV) and not be optimal candidates for revascularization. For this reason, patients referred for EECP have a high prevalence of comorbid conditions including: multivessel coronary artery disease (75.2%), previous revascularization (85.7%), prior myocardial infarction (67.3%), congestive heart failure (31.6%), diabetes (41.4%), and peripheral arterial disease (3.3%) [57].

Holubkov et al. [67] compared baseline characteristics and 1 year outcomes among 323 patients treated with EECP in the IEPR to 448 patients treated with elective PCI in the NHLBI Dynamic Registry. All patients had stable angina and were felt to be acceptable candidates for PCI. Compared to patients treated with PCI, patients undergoing EECP had a higher prevalence of prior coronary revascularization, myocardial infarction, congestive heart failure, left ventricular dysfunction, and diabetes mellitus. Despite these comorbidities, there was no significant difference in survival between the two groups during 1-year follow-up. Patients undergoing PCI had more symptom relief (73.4% of Dynamic Registry patients reported no angina symptoms at 1 year compared to 47.3% of EECP patients) and patients undergoing EECP were more likely to be taking antianginal medications. However, patients treated with PCI were more likely to undergo repeat revascularization procedures during 1-year follow-up than patients initially treated with EECP (17.2% vs 6.3%). Given the higher risk profile among the EECP patients and the low complication rate, the authors conclude that EECP may be a safe alternative to PCI in patients with stable angina.

In another study, the IEPR was used to examine EECP as a primary treatment strategy for angina [68]. Baseline characteristics and clinical outcomes were assessed in two patient groups. The first group (primary intervention group) included 215 patients without prior revascularization who were considered suitable candidates for PCI or bypass graft surgery but had chosen EECP as a primary treatment strategy. The second group included 4,239 patients who had undergone traditional revascularization prior to EECP.

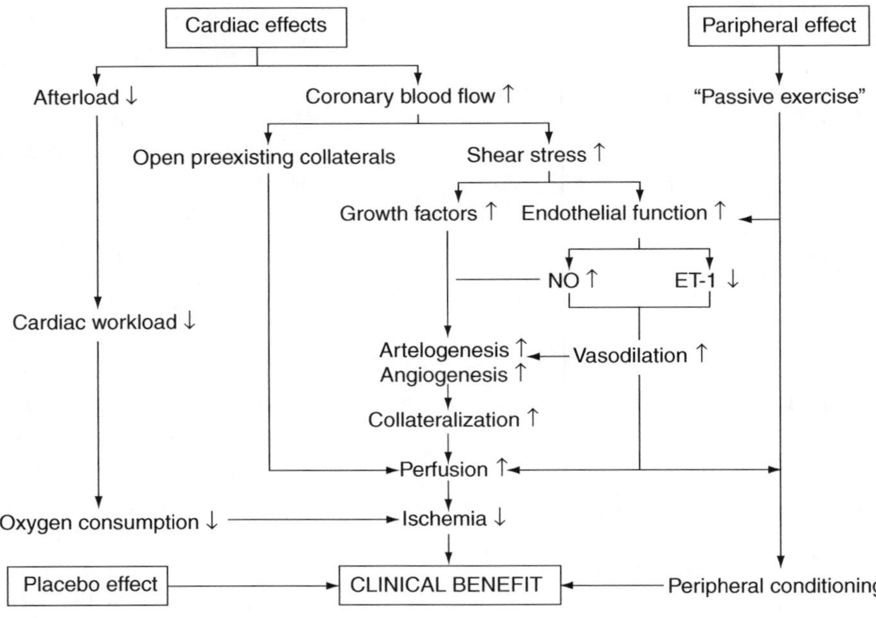

Fig. 6.6 Possible mechanisms of clinical benefit of EECP. *NO* nitric oxide, *ET-1* endothelin-1 (From Bonetti et al. [69], by permission of the Journal of the American College of Cardiology)

Immediately following EECP, patients in both groups experienced similar improvements in CCS angina class. However, patients in the primary intervention group experienced significantly greater improvements in angina frequency and nitroglycerin usage. Six months following completion of EECP, patients in the primary intervention group continued to have improved symptomatic relief compared to the control group of patients who had undergone traditional revascularization prior to initiating EECP.

Possible Mechanisms Explaining Antianginal Effect

Clinical benefit following EECP may be the result of improved cardiac hemodynamics, enhance coronary blood flow, peripheral conditioning, and placebo effect [69] (Fig. 6.6). However, the precise mechanisms involved in symptom relief following EECP have not been clearly defined [69–72].

Improved Cardiac Hemodynamics

Acutely, EECP improves cardiac output, decreases afterload and cardiac work, and improves coronary artery perfusion. Some of the clinical benefit of EECP may be the result of these hemodynamic changes that favorably affect the balance between myocardial oxygen supply and demand.

Improved Coronary Blood Flow

EECP may improve myocardial perfusion directly as a result of hemodynamic effects, or indirectly through the formation of vasoactive and angiogenic substances. Preformed collateral vessels could be directly recruited and enhanced during EECP as a result of diastolic augmentation and increased coronary artery perfusion pressure. EECP increases collateral blood vessel formation in a canine model after 1 h of treatment [73] and there is indirect evidence in humans that the hemodynamic changes produced by EECP could influence the formation of collateral vessels. In one study, patients with severe 3-vessel disease and no patent bypass conduits were less likely to benefit from EECP than patients with less severe coronary artery disease [54]. In this clinical setting, increased diastolic pressures experienced during EECP would be less likely to recruit extant collateral vessels because increases in intraluminal pressures would not reach the majority of the coronary arterial tree.

Indirect mechanisms by which EECP may improve myocardial perfusion include enhanced production of angiogenic growth factors, vasoactive substances, and improved endothelial function. Intravascular shear stress, which is increased during EECP, is recognized as a potent stimulus for the formation of vasodilators such as nitric oxide [74–77] and may modulate the production of endothelin-1, a potent vasoconstrictor [76]. In addition to being a potent vasodilator, nitric oxide is an important cofactor in angiogenesis [69]. Increased levels of nitric oxide have been reported following EECP as have increased levels of angiogenic growth factors including vascular endothelial growth factor, basic fibroblast growth factor, and hepatocyte growth factor [72, 78–81]. These vasoactive and angiogenic substances could stimulate the formation of collateral vessels and promote coronary artery vasodilation resulting in improved myocardial perfusion [69, 72]. In one study, 12 dogs were randomly assigned to EECP or control after occlusion of the mid-left anterior descending coronary artery [80]. EECP was performed 1 h each day in the intervention animals for a total of 6 weeks. Compared to dogs in the control group, EECP resulted in increased microvessel formation in the infarct zone on immunohistochemical analysis of alpha-actin and von Willebrand factor; increased VEGF levels and VEGF expression by ELISA, immunohistochemical staining, and reverse transcriptase PCR analysis; improved perfusion by Tc99-single photon emission computer tomography (SPECT); and increased ejection fraction [80].

In humans, radionuclide myocardial perfusion studies provide indirect evidence of collateral formation following EECP. A cooperative study group performed blinded interpretations of radionuclide myocardial perfusion studies at baseline and 6 months following EECP on 175 consecutive patients with chronic angina [45]. Eighty-three percent of patients undergoing the same level of exercise pre- and post-EECP experienced significant improvement in myocardial perfusion. Patients undergoing maximal stress testing at baseline and at the 6-month visit experienced an increase in exercise duration without a change in rate-pressure product and 54% showed improved myocardial perfusion. Other studies have documented substantial improvement in myocardial perfusion following EECP using radionuclide myocardial perfusion imaging [24, 46, 54] and positron emission tomography [44, 59].

Peripheral Effects

In addition to favorably altering cardiac hemodynamics and myocardial perfusion, EECP may result in beneficial peripheral adaptations. Systemic changes in vascular and endothelial function could result from the shear forces produced during EECP [82]. This "peripheral conditioning" may be similar to the effect exercise has on vascular function. For example, bicycle exercise in heart failure patients with impaired endothelial function leads to improved endothelial function in the upper extremities, indicating a systemic effect of exercise training [83]. In a similar fashion, EECP increases nitric oxide levels [44, 72, 81], improves systemic and coronary endothelial function [61, 69, 84, 85], and reduces arterial stiffness and improves wave reflection characteristics [86]. Clinically, EECP improves exercise capacity and myocardial perfusion without significant changes in the rate-pressure product suggesting a decrease in peripheral resistance and heart rate response to exercise consistent with a "training effect" [42, 45].

The degree of diastolic augmentation and the ratio of systolic to diastolic pressure (diastolic augmentation ratio) produced by EECP is another indirect means by which improvements in endothelial function may be observed. Indeed, older patients with more advanced disease and comorbid conditions have lower diastolic augmentation ratios at baseline compared to younger, healthier patients and are less likely to derive clinical benefits [87]. However, patients with the greatest improvement in diastolic augmentation ratio during EECP are most likely to experience symptom relief [87].

Placebo Effect

There may be nonspecific contributors to the clinical benefits of EECP. Patients experience an intensive treatment program over a 4–6 week period that involves daily contact with health care personnel. The meaning of this form of treatment in the context of a patient's clinical condition could elicit a "meaning response" or placebo effect [88, 89]. Indeed, patients receiving sham bypass graft surgery did as well as those receiving the actual procedure in two randomized trials [90, 91]. More recently, patients treated with placebo experienced similar improvements in exercise time and angina compared to patients receiving angiogenesis growth factors or the gene that encodes for vascular endothelial growth factor in randomized, double-blind controlled studies [92–94]. Concerns have also been raised about the influence of a placebo effect following transmyocardial laser revascularization [95]. The results of MUST-EECP suggest that not all the clinical effectiveness of EECP can be attributed to a placebo effect. Patients receiving active treatment experienced a significant decrease in the time to ischemic ST depression compared to patients in the "sham" treated group. In addition, patients in the active treatment group experienced significant improvements in health-related quality of life that persisted during a 1-year follow-up interval while patients in the control group did not [43, 64].

Indications for and Prescription of EECP

EECP is approved by the FDA for the treatment of acute myocardial infarction, cardiogenic shock, congestive heart failure, and stable angina. Approval for the former two indications dates to an era that preceded the advent of thrombolytic therapy and PCI. For this reason, EECP is most commonly applied in the setting of stable angina. However, it is also indicated for patients with class II-III heart failure.

The usual EECP treatment regimen is 35 h administered 1–2 h/day [96]. Contraindications to EECP include the following: arrhythmias that interfere with the triggering of the EECP system, bleeding diathesis or warfarin therapy with INR ≥3.0, current or recent (within 2 months) lower extremity thrombophlebitis, severe lower extremity vaso-occlusive disease, severe pulmonary hypertension (pulmonary artery mean pressure >50 mmHg), and presence of a documented aortic aneurysm requiring surgical repair and pregnancy [96]. Patients with uncontrolled hypertension should receive effective treatment for their hypertension prior to initiating therapy. Patients with congestive heart failure or at risk of complications from increased venous return during EECP should be medically optimized before initiating treatment. Patients with significant valvular heart disease such as aortic insufficiency or severe mitral or aortic stenosis should be carefully chosen and monitored [71, 96]. Medicare reimbursement is available for EECP in patients with functional class III or IV angina who are not readily amenable to revascularization. Coronary angiography and stress testing is not required but may be helpful in determining whether or not patients qualify for reimbursement under Medicare guidelines.

Future Directions: EECP for Heart Failure

The hemodynamic, neurohormonal, and vascular effects of EECP suggest that it may be useful for patients with heart failure [97]. In a retrospective IEPR study, 548 patients with a history of congestive heart failure tolerated EECP without any increase in the overall rate of adverse experiences and 68% reported a significant reduction in angina [98]; decreased angina and improved quality of life were maintained at 2 years [99]. Other studies show that EECP in patients with heart failure improves left ventricular ejection fraction, decreases pro-BNP levels, and improves NYHA functional class [100, 101]. EECP is associated with a reduction in the number of hospitalizations and emergency department visits [100, 102]. EECP is an effective treatment for angina in patients with systolic and diastolic dysfunction and the clinical benefits persist for up to 1 year [103].

A small, prospective feasibility study of EECP for patients with heart failure and ejection fractions ≤35% showed that EECP was well tolerated and was associated with significant improvements in peak VO_2, exercise duration, and quality of life [104].

The Prospective Evaluation of EECP in Heart failure trial (PEECH) was a prospective, multicenter, randomized, controlled, single-blind study enrolling 187 patients with mild to moderate congestive heart failure and left ventricular dysfunction with ejection fractions ≤35% [105, 106]. Stable patients treated with optimal heart failure medications including ACE inhibitors and beta-blockers were randomly assigned to undergo standard EECP treatment for 35 h or continued medical therapy. Research personnel evaluating study subjects at baseline and during the follow-up visits were blinded to treatment allocation. The co-primary end points were the percent of subjects with at least 1.25 mL/kg/min increase in peak VO_2 and the percent of patients with at least a 60 s increase in exercise duration from baseline at the 6-month follow-up visit. Patients tolerated EECP well and there were no significant differences in the frequency of adverse events between the EECP and control groups. EECP treated patients were more likely to experience an increase in exercise duration ≥ 60 s at the 6-month visit compared to the control group (35.4% vs 25.3%, $p=0.016$). There was no significant difference in the percentage of patients experiencing ≥1.25 mL/kg/min in peak VO_2. Patients in the EECP group experienced significant improvements in exercise duration, NYHA symptoms, and quality of life [105].

Summary

EECP results in diastolic augmentation, increased coronary artery perfusion pressure, and decreased left ventricular work. It is associated with improved myocardial perfusion during stress testing, increased levels of nitric oxide and angiogenic growth factors, and improved endothelial function. Clinically, EECP reduces angina by ≥1 CCS class in over 70% of patients and is an attractive, noninvasive, and safe therapeutic intervention for patients with angina who are not optimal candidates for revascularization. The effectiveness of EECP for the treatment of heart failure symptoms is still under investigation.

References

1. Harken DE, Soroff HS, Birtwell WC. Assisted circulation: counterpulsation and coronary artery disease. Surg Annu. 1972;4:165–89.
2. Clauss RH, Birtwell WC, Albertal G, et al. Assisted circulation. I. The arterial counterpulsator. J Thorac Cardiovasc Surg. 1961;41:447–58.
3. Nachlas MM, Siedband MP. The influence of diastolic augmentation on infarct size following coronary artery ligation. J Thorac Cardiovasc Surg. 1967;53(5):698–706.
4. Soroff HS, Ruiz U, Birtwell WC, Many M, Giron F, Deterling Jr RA. Assisted circulation by external pressure variation. Isr J Med Sci. 1969;5(4):506–14.
5. Jacobey JA, Taylor WJ, Smith GT, Gorlin R, Harken DE. A new therapeutic approach to acute coronary occlusion. II. Opening dormant coronary collateral channels by counterpulsation. Am J Cardiol. 1963;11:218–27.
6. Jacobey JA, Taylor W, Smith G, Gorlin R, Harken DE. A new therapeutic approach to acute coronary occlusion. I. Production of standardized coronary occlusion with microspheres. Am J Cardiol. 1962;9:60–73.
7. Kantrowitz A, Tjonneland S, Freed PS, Phillips SJ, Butner AN, Sherman Jr JL. Intraaortic balloon pumping. JAMA. 1968;203(11):988.
8. Moulopoulos SD, Topaz S, Kolff W. Diastolic balloon pumping (with carbon dioxide) in the aorta – a mechanical assistance to the failing circulation. Am Heart J. 1962;63:669–75.
9. Scheidt S, Wilner G, Mueller H, et al. Intra-aortic balloon counterpulsation in cardiogenic shock. Report of a co-operative clinical trial. N Engl J Med. 1973;288(19):979–84.
10. Kern MJ, Aguirre FV, Tatineni S, et al. Enhanced coronary blood flow velocity during intraaortic balloon counterpulsation in critically ill patients. J Am Coll Cardiol. 1993;21(2):359–68.
11. Kern MJ, Aguirre F, Bach R, Donohue T, Siegel R, Segal J. Augmentation of coronary blood flow by intra-aortic balloon pumping in patients after coronary angioplasty. Circulation. 1993;87(2):500–11.
12. Ferguson III JJ, Cohen M, Freedman Jr RJ, et al. The current practice of intra-aortic balloon counterpulsation: results from the Benchmark Registry. J Am Coll Cardiol. 2001;38(5):1456–62.
13. Ohman EM, Califf RM, George BS, et al. The use of intraaortic balloon pumping as an adjunct to reperfusion therapy in acute myocardial infarction. The Thrombolysis and Angioplasty in Myocardial Infarction (TAMI) study group. Am Heart J. 1991;121(3 Pt 1):895–901.
14. Ohman EM, George BS, White CJ, et al. Use of aortic counterpulsation to improve sustained coronary artery patency during acute myocardial infarction. Results of a randomized trial. The randomized IABP study group. Circulation. 1994;90(2):792–9.
15. Lincoff AM, Popma JJ, Ellis SG, Vogel RA, Topol EJ. Percutaneous support devices for high risk or complicated coronary angioplasty. J Am Coll Cardiol. 1991;17(3):770–80.
16. Birtell W, Giron F, Soroff H, Ruiz U, Collins J, Deterling R. Support of the systemic circulation and left ventricular assist by synchronous pulsation of extramural pressure. Trans Am Soc Artif Intern Organs. 1965;11:43–51.
17. Dennis C, Moreno J, Hall D, et al. Studies external counterpulsation as a potential measure for acute left heart failure. Trans Am Soc Artif Intern Organs. 1963;9:186–91.
18. Soroff HS, Birtwell WC, Giron F, Collins JA, Deterling Jr RA. Support of the systemic circulation and left ventricular assist by synchronous pulsation of extramural pressure. Surg Forum. 1965;16:148–50.
19. Osborn JJ, Main FB, Gerobe FL. Circulatory support by leg or airway pulses in experimental mitral insufficiency. Circulation. 1963;28:781.
20. Soroff HS, Cloutier CT, Birtwell WC, Begley LA, Messer JV. External counterpulsation. Management of cardiogenic shock after myocardial infarction. JAMA. 1974;229(11):1441–50.
21. Soroff HS, Hui J, Giron F. Current status of external counterpulsation. Crit Care Clin. 1986;2(2):277–95.
22. Zheng ZS, Yu LQ, Cai SR, et al. New sequential external counterpulsation for the treatment of acute myocardial infarction. Artif Organs. 1984;8(4):470–7.
23. Zheng ZS, Li TM, Kambic H, et al. Sequential external counterpulsation (SECP) in China. Trans Am Soc Artif Intern Organs. 1983;29:599–603.
24. Lawson WE, Hui JC, Soroff HS, et al. Efficacy of enhanced external counterpulsation in the treatment of angina pectoris. Am J Cardiol. 1992;70(9):859–62.
25. Lawson WE, Hui JCK. Enhanced external counterpulsation for chronic myocardial ischemia. J Crit Illn. 2000;15(11):629–36.

26. Michaels AD, Accad M, Ports TA, Grossman W. Left ventricular systolic unloading and augmentation of intracoronary pressure and Doppler flow during enhanced external counterpulsation. Circulation. 2002;106(10):1237–42.
27. Strobeck JE. Enhanced external counterpulsation in congestive heart failure: possibly the most potent inodilator to date. Congest Heart Fail. 2002;8(4):201–3.
28. Taguchi I, Ogawa K, Kanaya T, Matsuda R, Kuga H, Nakatsugawa M. Effects of enhanced external counterpulsation on hemodynamics and its mechanism. Circ J. 2004;68(11):1030–4.
29. Taguchi I, Ogawa K, Oida A, Abe S, Kaneko N, Sakio H. Comparison of hemodynamic effects of enhanced external counterpulsation and intra-aortic balloon pumping in patients with acute myocardial infarction. Am J Cardiol. 2000;86(10):1139–41, A9.
30. Parmley WW, Chatterjee K, Charuzi Y, Swan HJ. Hemodynamic effects of noninvasive systolic unloading (nitroprusside) and diastolic augmentation (external counterpulsation) in patients with acute myocardial infarction. Am J Cardiol. 1974;33(7):819–25.
31. Triulzi E, Devizzi S, Rovelli G, Grieco A. Efficacy of enhanced aortic diastolic pressure with an external counterpulsation method in the acute myocardial infarction (author's transl). G Ital Cardiol. 1980;10(6):690–702.
32. Amsterdam EA, Banas J, Criley JM, et al. Clinical assessment of external pressure circulatory assistance in acute myocardial infarction. Report of a cooperative clinical trial. Am J Cardiol. 1980;45(2):349–56.
33. Beckman CB, Romero L, Shatney C, Nicoloff D, Lillehei R, Dietzman R. Clinical comparison of the intra-aortic balloon pump and external counterpulstion for cardiogenic shock. Trans Am Soc Artif Intern Organs. 1973;19:414–8.
34. Soroff HS, Giron F, Ruiz U, Birtwell WC, Hirsch LJ, Deterling Jr RA. Physiologic support of heart action. N Engl J Med. 1969;280(13):693–704.
35. Banas J, Brilla A, Soroff H, Levine H. Evaluation of external counterpulsation for the treatment of severe angina pectoris. Circulation. 1972;46(Suppl II):II-74. Ref Type: Abstract.
36. Clapp J, Banas J, Stickley L, Salem D, Pollak R, Levine H. Evaluation of sham and true external counterpulsation in patients with angina pectoris. Circulation. 1974;50(Suppl III):III-108. Ref Type: Abstract.
37. Loeb HS, Khan M, Towne W, Gunnar R. Effects of external counter-pulsation; management of cardiogenic shock after myocardial infarction. Circulation. 1974;49–50(Suppl II):II-255. Ref Type: Abstract.
38. Solignac A, Ferguson R, Bourassa M. External counterpulsation: coronary hemodynamics and use in treatment of patients with stable angina pectoris. Cathet Cardiovasc Diagn. 1977;3:37. Ref Type: Abstract.
39. Lawson WE, Hui JC, Cohn PF. Long-term prognosis of patients with angina treated with enhanced external counterpulsation: five-year follow-up study. Clin Cardiol. 2000;23(4):254–8.
40. Lawson WE, Hui JC, Zheng ZS, et al. Three-year sustained benefit from enhanced external counterpulsation in chronic angina pectoris. Am J Cardiol. 1995;75(12):840–1.
41. Lawson WE, Hui JC, Guo T, Burger L, Cohn PF. Prior revascularization increases the effectiveness of enhanced external counterpulsation. Clin Cardiol. 1998;21(11): 841–4.
42. Lawson WE, Hui JC, Zheng ZS, et al. Improved exercise tolerance following enhanced external counterpulsation: cardiac or peripheral effect? Cardiology. 1996;87(4):271–5.
43. Arora RR, Chou TM, Jain D, et al. The multicenter study of enhanced external counterpulsation (MUST-EECP): effect of EECP on exercise-induced myocardial ischemia and anginal episodes. J Am Coll Cardiol. 1999;33(7):1833–40.
44. Masuda D, Nohara R, Hirai T, et al. Enhanced external counterpulsation improved myocardial perfusion and coronary flow reserve in patients with chronic stable angina; evaluation by(13)N-ammonia positron emission tomography. Eur Heart J. 2001;22(16):1451–8.
45. Stys TP, Lawson WE, Hui JC, et al. Effects of enhanced external counterpulsation on stress radionuclide coronary perfusion and exercise capacity in chronic stable angina pectoris. Am J Cardiol. 2002;89(7):822–4.
46. Urano H, Ikeda H, Ueno T, Matsumoto T, Murohara T, Imaizumi T. Enhanced external counterpulsation improves exercise tolerance, reduces exercise-induced myocardial ischemia and improves left ventricular diastolic filling in patients with coronary artery disease. J Am Coll Cardiol. 2001;37(1):93–9.
47. Loh PH, Louis AA, Windram J, et al. The immediate and long-term outcome of enhanced external counterpulsation in treatment of chronic stable refractory angina. J Intern Med. 2006;259(3):276–84.
48. Novo G, Bagger JP, Carta R, Koutroulis G, Hall R, Nihoyannopoulos P. Enhanced external counterpulsation for treatment of refractory angina. J Cardiovasc Med. 2006; 7(5):335–9.
49. Barsness G, Feldman AM, Holmes Jr DR, Holubkov R, Kelsey SF, Kennard ED. The International EECP Patient Registry (IEPR): design, methods, baseline characteristics, and acute results. Clin Cardiol. 2001;24(6):435–42.
50. Lawson WE, Hui JC, Lang G. Treatment benefit in the enhanced external counterpulsation consortium. Cardiology. 2000;94(1):31–5.
51. Stys T, Lawson WE, Hui JC, Lang G, Liuzzo J, Cohn PF. Acute hemodynamic effects and angina improvement with enhanced external counterpulsation. Angiology. 2001; 52(10):653–8.
52. Pettersson T, Bondesson S, Cojocaru D, Ohlsson O, Wackenfors A, Edvinsson L. One year follow-up of patients with refractory angina pectoris treated with enhanced external counterpulsation. BMC Cardiovasc Disord. 2006;6(28). doi:10.1186/1471-2261-6-28.
53. Cohn PF. External counterpulsation for the treatment of myocardial ischemia. Heart Dis. 1999;1(4):221–5.
54. Lawson WE, Hui JC, Zheng ZS, et al. Can angiographic findings predict which coronary patients will benefit from enhanced external counterpulsation? Am J Cardiol. 1996;77(12):1107–9.
55. Fricchione GL, Jaghab K, Lawson W, et al. Psychosocial effects of enhanced external counterpulsation in the angina patient. Psychosomatics. 1995;36(5):494–7.
56. Springer S, Fife A, Lawson W, et al. Psychosocial effects of enhanced external counterpulsation in the angina patient: a second study. Psychosomatics. 2001;42(2):124–32.
57. Lawson WE, Kennard ED, Hui JC, Holubkov R, Kelsey SF. Analysis of baseline factors associated with reduction in chest pain in patients with angina pectoris treated by

enhanced external counterpulsation. Am J Cardiol. 2003;92(4):439–43.

58. Bagger JP, Hall RJ, Koutroulis G, Nihoyannopoulos P. Effect of enhanced external counterpulsation on dobutamine-induced left ventricular wall motion abnormalities in severe chronic angina pectoris. Am J Cardiol. 2004;93(4):465–7.
59. Masuda D, Fujita M, Nohara R, Matsumori A, Sasayama S. Improvement of oxygen metabolism in ischemic myocardium as a result of enhanced external counterpulsation with heparin pretreatment for patients with stable angina. Heart Vessels. 2004;19(2):59–62.
60. Dockery F, Rajkumar C, Bulpitt CJ, Hall RJ, Bagger JP. Enhanced external counterpulsation does not alter arterial stiffness in patients with angina. Clin Cardiol. 2004;27(12): 689–92.
61. Shechter M, Matetzky S, Feinberg MS, Chouraqui P, Rotstein Z, Hod H. External counterpulsation therapy improves endothelial function in patients with refractory angina pectoris. J Am Coll Cardiol. 2003;42(12):2090–5.
62. Tartaglia J, Stenerson Jr J, Charney R, et al. Exercise capability and myocardial perfusion in chronic angina patients treated with enhanced external counterpulsation. Clin Cardiol. 2003;26(6):287–90.
63. Bonetti PO, Barsness GW, Keelan PC, et al. Enhanced external counterpulsation improves endothelial function in patients with symptomatic coronary artery disease. J Am Coll Cardiol. 2003;41(10):1761–8.
64. Arora RR, Chou TM, Jain D, et al. Effects of enhanced external counterpulsation on health-related quality of life continue 12 months after treatment: a substudy of the Multicenter Study of Enhanced External Counterpulsation. J Investig Med. 2002;50(1):25–32.
65. Michaels AD, Barsness GW, Soran O, et al. Frequency and efficacy of repeat enhanced external counterpulsation for stable angina pectoris (from the International EECP Patient Registry). Am J Cardiol. 2005;95(3):394–7.
66. Michaels AD, Linnemeier G, Soran O, Kelsey SF, Kennard ED. Two-year outcomes after enhanced external counterpulsation for stable angina pectoris (from the International EECP Patient Registry [IEPR]). Am J Cardiol. 2004;93(4):461–4.
67. Holubkov R, Kennard ED, Foris JM, et al. Comparison of patients undergoing enhanced external counterpulsation and percutaneous coronary intervention for stable angina pectoris. Am J Cardiol. 2002;89(10):1182–6.
68. Fitzgerald CP, Lawson WE, Hui JC, Kennard ED. Enhanced external counterpulsation as initial revascularization treatment for angina refractory to medical therapy. Cardiology. 2003;100(3):129–35.
69. Bonetti PO, Holmes Jr DR, Lerman A, Barsness GW. Enhanced external counterpulsation for ischemic heart disease: what's behind the curtain? J Am Coll Cardiol. 2003;41(11):1918–25.
70. Shea ML, Conti CR, Arora RR. An update on enhanced external counterpulsation. Clin Cardiol. 2005;28(3):115–8.
71. Sinvhal RM, Gowda RM, Khan IA. Enhanced external counterpulsation for refractory angina pectoris. Heart. 2003;89(8):830–3.
72. Barsness GW. Enhanced external counterpulsation in unrevascularizable patients. Curr Interv Cardiol Rep. 2001; 3(1):37–43.
73. Cai D, Wu R, Shao Y. Experimental study of the effect of external counterpulsation on blood circulation in the lower extremities. Clin Invest Med. 2000;23(4):239–47.
74. Corson MA, James NL, Latta SE, Nerem RM, Berk BC, Harrison DG. Phosphorylation of endothelial nitric oxide synthase in response to fluid shear stress. Circ Res. 1996;79(5):984–91.
75. Dimmeler S, Fleming I, Fisslthaler B, Hermann C, Busse R, Zeiher AM. Activation of nitric oxide synthase in endothelial cells by Akt-dependent phosphorylation. Nature. 1999;399(6736):601–5.
76. Kuchan MJ, Frangos JA. Shear stress regulates endothelin-1 release via protein kinase C and cGMP in cultured endothelial cells. Am J Physiol. 1993;264(1 Pt 2):H150–6.
77. Tseng H, Peterson TE, Berk BC. Fluid shear stress stimulates mitogen-activated protein kinase in endothelial cells. Circ Res. 1995;77(5):869–78.
78. Masuda D, Nohara R, Kataoka K, et al. Enhanced external counterpulsation promotes angiogenesis factors in patients with chronic stable angina. Circulation. 2001;104(Suppl II): II-445. Ref Type: Abstract.
79. Werner D, Friedel C, Kropp J, et al. Pneumatic external counterpulsation – a new treatment for selected patients with symptomatic coronary artery disease. Circulation. 1998; 98(17):I-350. Ref Type: Abstract.
80. Wu G, Du Z, Hu C, et al. Angiogenic effects of long-term enhanced external counterpulsation in a dog model of myocardial infarction. Am J Physiol Heart Circ Physiol. 2006;290(1):H248–54.
81. Akhtar M, Wu GF, Du ZM, Zheng ZS, Michaels AD. Effect of external counterpulsation on plasma nitric oxide and endothelin-1 levels. Am J Cardiol. 2006;98(1):28–30.
82. O'Rourke MF, Hashimoto J. Enhanced external counterpulsation why the benefit? J Am Coll Cardiol. 2006; 48(6):1215–6.
83. Linke A, Schoene N, Gielen S, et al. Endothelial dysfunction in patients with chronic heart failure: systemic effects of lower-limb exercise training. J Am Coll Cardiol. 2001; 37(2):392–7.
84. Bonetti PO, Gadasalli SN, Lerman A, Barsness GW. Successful treatment of symptomatic coronary endothelial dysfunction with enhanced external counterpulsation. Mayo Clin Proc. 2004;79(5):690–2.
85. Tao J, Tu C, Yang Z, et al. Enhanced external counterpulsation improves endothelium-dependent vasorelaxation in the carotid arteries of hypercholesterolemic pigs. Int J Cardiol. 2006;112(3):269–74.
86. Nichols WW, Estrada JC, Braith RW, Owens K, Conti CR. Enhanced external counterpulsation treatment improves arterial wall properties and wave reflection characteristics in patients with refractory angina. J Am Coll Cardiol. 2006;48(6):1208–14.
87. Lakshmi MV, Kennard ED, Kelsey SF, Holubkov R, Michaels AD. Relation of the pattern of diastolic augmentation during a course of enhanced external counterpulsation (EECP) to clinical benefit (from the International EECP Patient Registry [IEPR]). Am J Cardiol. 2002;89(11): 1303–5.
88. Moerman DE, Jonas WB. Deconstructing the placebo effect and finding the meaning response. Ann Intern Med. 2002;136(6):471–6.

89. Gottlieb SS, Pina IL. Enhanced external counterpulsation: what can we learn from the treatment of neurasthenia? J Am Coll Cardiol. 2006;48(6):1206–7.
90. Thomas GI, Cobb LA, Dillard DH, Bruce RA, Merendino KA. An evaluation of internal-mammary-artery ligation by a double-blind technic. N Engl J Med. 1959;260(22):1115–8.
91. Dimond EG, Kittle CF, Crockett JE. Comparison of internal mammary artery ligation and sham operation for angina pectoris. Am J Cardiol. 1960;5:483–6.
92. Henry TD, Annex BH, McKendall GR, et al. The VIVA trial: vascular endothelial growth factor in ischemia for vascular angiogenesis. Circulation. 2003;107(10):1359–65.
93. Kastrup J, Jorgensen E, Ruck A, et al. Direct intramyocardial plasmid vascular endothelial growth factor-A165 gene therapy in patients with stable severe angina pectoris: a randomized double-blind placebo-controlled study: the euroinject one trial. J Am Coll Cardiol. 2005;45(7):982–8.
94. Simons M, Annex BH, Laham RJ, et al. Pharmacological treatment of coronary artery disease with recombinant fibroblast growth factor-2: double-blind, randomized, controlled clinical trial. Circulation. 2002;105(7):788–93.
95. Lange RA, Hillis LD. Transmyocardial laser revascularization. N Engl J Med. 1999;341(14):1075–6.
96. Michaels AD, McCullough PA, Soran OZ, et al. Primer: practical approach to the selection of patients for and application of EECP. Nat Clin Pract Cardiovasc Med. 2006;3(11):623–32.
97. Silver MA. Mechanisms and evidence for the role of enhanced external counterpulsation in heart failure management. Curr Heart Fail Rep. 2006;3(1):25–32.
98. Lawson WE, Kennard ED, Holubkov R, et al. Benefit and safety of enhanced external counterpulsation in treating coronary artery disease patients with a history of congestive heart failure. Cardiology. 2001;96(2):78–84.
99. Soran O, Kennard ED, Kfoury AG, et al. Two-year clinical outcomes after enhanced external counterpulsation (EECP) therapy in patients with refractory angina pectoris and left ventricular dysfunction (report from The International EECP Patient Registry). Am J Cardiol. 2006;97(1):17–20.
100. Vijayaraghavan K, Santora L, Kahn J, Abbott N, Torelli J, Vardi G. New graduated pressure regimen for external counterpulsation reduces mortality and improves outcomes in congestive heart failure: a report from the cardiomedics external counterpulsation patient registry. Congest Heart Fail. 2005;11(3):147–52.
101. Kaluski E, Gabara Z, Uriel N, et al. The benefits and safety of external counterpulsation in symptomatic heart failure. IMAJ. 2006;8(10):687–90.
102. Soran O, Kennard ED, Bart BA, Kelsey SF. Impact of external counterpulsation treatment on emergency department visits and hospitalizations in refractory angina patients with left ventricular dysfunction. Congest Heart Fail. 2007;13(1):36–40.
103. Lawson WE, Silver MA, Hui JC, Kennard ED, Kelsey SF. Angina patients with diastolic versus systolic heart failure demonstrate comparable immediate and one-year benefit from enhanced external counterpulsation. J Card Fail. 2005;11(1):61–6.
104. Soran O, Kennard ED, Kelsey SF, Holubkov R, Strobeck J, Feldman AM. Enhanced external counterpulsation as treatment for chronic angina in patients with left ventricular dysfunction: a report from the International EECP Patient Registry (IEPR). Congest Heart Fail. 2002;8(6):297–302.
105. Bashore TM, Faxon DP, Fonarow GC, et al. Best of the ACC scientific session 2005. Rev Cardiovasc Med. 2005;6(2):98–117.
106. Feldman AM, Silver MA, Francis GS, De Lame PA, Parmley WW. Treating heart failure with enhanced external counterpulsation (EECP): design of the Prospective Evaluation of EECP in Heart Failure (PEECH) trial. J Card Fail. 2005;11(3):240–5.

7 Therapeutic Angiogenesis

Timothy D. Henry and Daniel Satran

Introduction

Therapeutic angiogenesis is the use of angiogenic growth factors, genes that encode for growth factors, or cell-based therapies to enhance the natural process of collateral vessel development in ischemic tissue [1]. The goal of therapeutic angiogenesis is to increase proangiogenic signals to alter the balance in favor of new blood vessel growth and vascular remodeling. This chapter reviews therapeutic agents used in myocardial angiogenesis, randomized placebo-controlled clinical trials in the field, and expectations for future research and therapy.

In recent years, improvements in both pharmacologic and revascularization therapies have greatly increased the life expectancy for patients with coronary artery disease (CAD). As patients live longer with more extensive CAD, an increasing number develop myocardial ischemia not amenable to conventional revascularization techniques. In a series of 500 patients from the Cleveland Clinic who underwent coronary angiography, 12% had evidence for ischemia and were not candidates for conventional revascularization [2]. The European Society of Cardiology estimates as many as 15% of patients with angina have a diagnosis of refractory angina [3]. There is limited data regarding the natural history of refractory angina. We recently reported an overall mortality of 11.7% (6.2% cardiovascular) at a mean follow-up of 5.4 years in 1,098 patients with refractory ischemia followed at the Minneapolis Heart Institute [4]. This overall low mortality is consistent with randomized clinical trials. Therefore the major challenge for these patients is not high mortality but persistent angina and poor quality of life. For these "no option" patients, the investigation of novel angiogenic therapies offers hope for an improved quality of life by relieving angina symptoms.

Protein and Gene Therapy

The natural process of angiogenesis is complex with a large number of angiogenic growth factors, as well as inhibitors of angiogenesis, having been identified [5, 6]. Clinical experience with protein growth factors and genes encoding for these growth factors to enhance myocardial angiogenesis primarily involves vascular endothelial growth factor (VEGF) and fibroblast growth factor (FGF). Protein alone, plasmid, and adenoviral vectors using a variety of delivery methods (intravenous, intracoronary, and intramyocardial) have been used in clinical trials of angiogenesis.

VEGFs are naturally occurring angiogenic glycoproteins that vary in vascular permeability depending on the isoform [7, 8]. Seven isoforms have been identified (121, 145, 148, 165, 183, 189, and 206 amino acids, respectively) but VEGF165 is the most common in humans. Endothelium responds to VEGF with

T.D. Henry (✉)
Minneapolis Heart Institute Foundation
at Abbott Northwestern Hospital,
University of Minnesota, Minneapolis,
MN, USA
e-mail: henry003@umn.edu

D. Satran
Department of Internal Medicine,
University of Minnesota, Minneapolis, MN, USA
e-mail: danielsatran@yahoo.com

G.W. Barsness and D.R. Holmes Jr. (eds.), *Coronary Artery Disease*,
DOI 10.1007/978-1-84628-712-1_7,

proliferation, migration, vascular tube formation, and production of proteases such as plasminogen activator and interstitial collagenase, all important steps in capillary sprout formation.

FGF is a family of more than 20 potent angiogenic cytokines. Unlike VEGF, FGF is not associated with permeability and lacks specificity for endothelial cells, binding to cells as diverse as fibroblasts and vascular smooth muscle cells [9]. FGF is similar to VEGF in that it produces nitric-oxide-mediated vasodilation and stimulates endothelial production of proteases. FGF-1 (acidic FGF), FGF-2 (basic FGF), and FGF-4 have been used in human clinical trials.

Clinical Trials

Successful preclinical models [7, 10] exploring the effect of a variety of agents led to Phase 1 clinical trials [11–13] which were positive and stimulated considerable excitement (please see Chap. 2). These initial trials laid the groundwork for a number of Phase 2 randomized placebo-controlled trials with disappointing results (Table 7.1). The lessons learned in these trials, however, have helped to provide the framework for future investigations and ongoing therapeutic development.

Protein Therapy

There have been two large randomized placebo-controlled trials using intracoronary protein delivery for angiogenesis: the Vascular Endothelial Growth Factor in Ischemia for Vascular Angiogenesis (VIVA) trial [14] and the FGF Initiating RevaScularization Trial (FIRST) [15].

The VIVA trial was the first large phase 2, double-blind, placebo-controlled trial using recombinant human VEGF165 (rhVEGF165) [14]. A total of 178 patients with Canadian Cardiovascular Society (CCS) class 2–4 angina were randomized to intracoronary infusions of placebo, low-dose (17 ng/kg/min), or high-dose (50 ng/kg/min) rhVEGF165 protein for 20 min followed by 4-h intravenous infusions of the same dose on days 3, 6, and 9. The primary endpoint of this trial was change in exercise duration from baseline to 60 days and did not differ between placebo and either infusion group (placebo, +48 s; low dose, +30 s; high dose, +30 s). However, while VEGF offered no benefit beyond placebo at day 60, improvement in the placebo group had diminished by day 120 while the high-dose VEGF group (50 ng/kg/min) showed ongoing improvement. This resulted in a significant reduction in angina ($p=0.05$) and trends for improvement in exercise time (placebo +24 s, high dose +48 s, $p=0.15$) and quality of life at day 120. At 1-year follow-up in 106 patients at 13 sites there was no significant difference in death or myocardial infarction in the three groups [10]. Overall, however, 31.6% of patients in the placebo group, 16.1% of patients in the low-dose, and 11.8% ($p<0.04$ compared with placebo) of patients in the high-dose group sustained clinical events (primarily revascularization) at 1 year. With regard to CCS class, the placebo effect – so prominent at 60 days – was negligible at 1 year (mean CCS class 2.4 ± 1.6 compared to a baseline of 2.8 ± 0.6, $p=\text{NS}$). Mean CCS class in the low-dose group at 1 year was 2.3 ± 1.4 ($p<0.05$ compared to a baseline of 2.9 ± 0.6), and patients treated with high-dose VEGF had a sustained response to therapy with significantly reduced CCS class of 1.9 ± 1.3 ($p<0.001$ compared to a baseline of 2.7 ± 0.8).

The FIRST Trial was a multicenter, double-blind, placebo-controlled angiogenesis trial of 337 patients with CCS class 2–4 angina randomized to a single intracoronary infusion of 0, 0.3, 3, or 30 ug/kg of recombinant FGF2 (rFGF2) [15]. Efficacy was evaluated at 90 and 180 days by exercise tolerance test (ETT), myocardial nuclear perfusion imaging, and quality-of-life questionnaires. At 90 days, exercise duration was increased in all groups with no significant differences between groups. Nuclear perfusion evaluation also demonstrated no significant difference between groups. Patients treated with rFGF2 had reduced angina, as assessed by the Seattle Angina Questionnaire score and Short-Form 36 scale; these differences were more prominent in patients with CCS class 3–4 angina at baseline. However, none of the differences were significant at 180 days due to continued improvement in the placebo group.

Two other small randomized trials have utilized FGF protein in conjunction with coronary artery bypass grafting (CABG) and angiogenic growth factors. A randomized, placebo-controlled study in 20 patients evaluated the safety of injecting FGF-1 (0.01 mg/kg) close to a severely diseased LAD grafted by an internal mammary artery [16]. Angiography of the internal mammary artery 12 weeks after surgery

Table 7.1 Therapeutic myocardial angiogenesis: summary of randomized placebo-controlled clinical trials

	N	CCS class	Mean age (years)	Angiogenic agent	Delivery method	Primary endpoint	Results
Protein trial							
VIVA [14]	178	2–4	61(placebo) 61 (low) 58 (high)	rhVEGF165	Intracoronary, Intravenous	Change in ETT duration at 60 days	No improvement in treatment group at day 60. By day 120, high-dose group showed improvement in angina and a trend toward improved ETT.
FIRST [15]	337	2–4	63	rFGF2	Intracoronary	Change in ETT duration at 90 days	ETT improved and angina decreased at 90 days (effect more pronounced in high-risk groups). No improvement (ETT or SPECT) at 180 days due to continued improvement in placebo group.
Schumacher et al. [16]	40	n/a	n/a	FGF-1	Intramyocardial (at CABG)	Angiographic capillary formation at 12 weeks	Enhanced capillary formation in the treatment group
Laham et al. [17]	24	n/a	55	FGF-2	Intramyocardial (at CABG)	Safety	No adverse events with therapy; improved SPECT scores in high-dose treatment group at 3 months
Gene trial							
AGENT-1 [18]	79	2–3	62 (placebo) 59 (active)	Ad5-FGF4	Intracoronary	Safety, change in ETT duration at 4 and 12 weeks	No adverse events with therapy; treatment group with trend toward improvement in ETT (1.3 versus 0.7 min, p=NS) at 4 weeks
AGENT-2 [19]	52	2–3	57 (placebo) 59 (active)	Ad5-FGF4	Intracoronary	Change in magnitude of ischemia with SPECT at 8 weeks	Significant improvement in treatment group, but difference between placebo and treatment group was NS ($p=0.14$) (see text)
AGENT-3 [20]	416	2–4	n/a	Ad5-FGF4	Intracoronary	Change in ETT duration at 3 months, percentage of pts with >30% ETT increase at 3 months	Interim analysis indicated trial would not reach statistical significance→enrollment discontinued. Overall, significant improvement in angina. ETT improved in high-risk subgroups
AGENT-4 [20]	116	2–4	n/a	Ad5-FGF4	Intracoronary	Change in ETT duration at 3 months, percentage of pts with >30% ETT increase at 3 months	Interim analysis indicated trial would not reach statistical significance→enrollment discontinued. See AGENT 3/4 meta-analysis.
VEGF-2 [21]	19	3–4	61	phVEGF2	Intramyocardial	CCS angina class at 12 weeks	Statistically significant improvement for treatment group versus placebo (–1.3 versus 0.1, $p=0.04$)

(continued)

Table 7.1 (continued)

	N	CCS class	Mean age (years)	Angiogenic agent	Delivery method	Primary endpoint	Results
Euroinject-One [22]	80	3–4	61	phVEGF2	Intramyocardial	Change in magnitude of ischemia by SPECT at 3 months	No significant improvement for treatment group versus placebo in SPECT score; improvement in angina in both treatment and placebo groups; improvement in wall motion in treatment group
GENASIS [23]	295	3–4	n/a	phVEGF2	Intramyocardial	Change in ETT duration at 3 months	Interim analysis indicated trial would not reach statistical significance → enrollment discontinued
Northern [24]	120	3–4	n/a	adVEGF165	Intramyocardial	Change in myocardial perfusion (stress/rest and summed stress scores) at 12 weeks	Results pending
NOVA [25]	129	2–4	n/a	adVEGF121	Intramyocardial	Change in ETT duration at 26 weeks	Results pending
Cell trial							
Losordo et al. [26]	24	3–4	62	G-CSF-mobilized CD34+ cells	Intramyocardial	Safety	No increase in adverse events in treatment group; trend toward reduction in angina frequency and CCS class in treatment group

demonstrated enhanced capillary formation and this was also demonstrated at 3-year follow-up [27]. A phase 1, double-blind, randomized placebo-controlled trial of 24 patients evaluated periepicardial coronary placement of heparin-alginate pellets containing 10 ug of FGF-2 ($n=8$), 100 ug of FGF-2 ($n=8$), or placebo ($n=8$) at the time of CABG in ischemic but viable coronary artery territories [17]. At a mean follow-up of 16 months, there was no increase in clinical events in the FGF-treated patients and all patients in the high-dose FGF-2 group were angina free. Stress nuclear perfusion imaging at baseline and 3 months post-CABG showed worsening of the defect size in the placebo group and significant improvement in the high-dose FGF-2 group. At a mean follow-up of 32 months, nuclear perfusion scans showed a persistent reversible or a new, fixed perfusion defect in the ungraftable territory of 4 of 5 patients given placebo versus 1 of 9 patients treated with FGF-2 ($p=0.02$) and sum-stress scores were lower in FGF-2-treated patients than controls (1.3 ± 1.4 versus 3.9 ± 2.1, respectively; $p=0.04$) suggesting persistent treatment effect [28].

Gene Therapy

Several randomized placebo-controlled trials have investigated gene delivery for angiogenesis including the Angiogenic GENe Therapy (AGENT) [18–20], VEGF-2 [21], and Euroinject-One trials [23].

AGENT-1 evaluated the safety and anti-ischemic effects of five ascending doses of Ad5FGF-4 in 79 patients with chronic stable angina (CCS class 2–3) [18]. Patients were randomized to placebo ($n=19$) or Ad5FGF-4 ($n=60$). The treatment was safe and well tolerated. Patients who received Ad5FGF-4 had nonsignificant improvements in exercise time at 4 weeks compared with patients in the placebo group (1.3 versus 0.7 min). However, the subgroup with a baseline exercise treadmill time of less than 10 min showed significant benefit at 4 weeks compared with placebo (1.6 versus 0.6 min, $p=0.01$, $n=50$) that persisted at 12 weeks.

AGENT-2 randomized 52 patients with CCS class 2–3 angina to placebo ($n=17$) or an injection of 10^{10} Ad5FGF-4 viral particles ($n=35$). This trial was designed to assess whether Ad5FGF-4 would improve myocardial perfusion during stress [19]. Patients who received Ad5FGF-4 showed an improvement in adenosine single-photon emission computed tomography (SPECT) ischemic defect size at 8 weeks (4.2% absolute reduction, $p<0.001$) while there was no change in placebo-treated patients ($p=0.32$). Despite this, the change in reversible perfusion defect size between treatment and placebo arms (4.2% versus 1.6%, $p=0.14$) was not significant. Notably, the outcome was affected by a single outlier in the placebo group who had a 50% decrease in perfusion defect size (felt secondary to noncompliance with antianginal medication). Excluding this patient resulted in a significant change in reversible perfusion defect size between treatment and placebo arms (4.2% versus 0.8%, $p<0.05$).

AGENT-3 and AGENT-4 were phase 2b/3 trials of Ad5FGF4. AGENT-3 was a US-based efficacy study designed to randomize 450 patients with CCS class 2–4 angina not requiring immediate revascularization. The prespecified primary endpoint was change from baseline in ETT at 12 weeks. With 416 patients randomized to intracoronary injection of placebo ($n=139$), 10^9 Ad5FGF-4 viral particles ($n=137$), or 10^{10} viral particles ($n=140$), an interim analysis indicated that as designed, the study was not expected to reach statistical significance for the primary endpoint and enrollment was discontinued. AGENT-4 was an international efficacy study designed to parallel AGENT-3 with the same primary endpoint. AGENT-4 was stopped for the same reason as AGENT-3 with 116 patients enrolled ($n=38$ placebo, $n=43$ in the10^9 viral particle group, and $n=35$ 10^{10} viral particle group). However, there was a significant reduction in CCS class (a prespecified secondary endpoint) in the Ad5FGF-4-treated patients at both 6 and 12 months in AGENT-3. In addition, post-hoc analysis indicated high-risk patients (age greater than 55, CCS class 3–4, baseline exercise time less than 300 s) showed improvement in the primary ETT endpoint. Finally, a meta-analysis of AGENT-3 and AGENT-4 showed a statistically significant increase in ETT duration at 12 weeks in women treated with Ad5FGF-4 (placebo ($n=31$): 2 s; 10^9 viral particles ($n=22$): 60 s ($p=0.04$); 10^{10} viral particles ($n=20$): 69 s ($p<0.05$)) as well as a statistically significant change in CCS class from baseline to 12 months (10^9 viral particles=−0.9 ($p<0.05$), 10^{10} viral particles=−1.3 ($p<0.01$)) when compared to placebo (−0.6, p=NS). These results suggest Ad5FGF-4 may have a clinically meaningful and measurable effect on ETT and other measures of angina in women and potentially both men and women older than age 55 with limited exercise capacity [20]. Definitive identification of a beneficial effect in this or other populations awaits further prospective evaluation.

A phase 1/2, double-blind, randomized placebo-controlled trial to study the safety of percutaneous catheter-based gene transfer of naked plasma DNA encoding for phVEGF-2 [21] randomized 19 patients with CCS angina class 3–4 and chronic myocardial ischemia by SPECT imaging who were not suitable candidates for standard revascularization to receive 6 injections of placebo or phVEGF-2 in doses of 200 ug ($n=9$), 800 ug ($n=9$), or 2000 ug ($n=1$) to LV myocardium guided by LV electromechanical mapping (NOGA). The primary efficacy endpoint, CCS class at 12-week follow-up, showed a statistically significant mean change for phVEGF-2-treated patients versus placebo-treated patients (−1.3 versus 0.1, $p=0.04$). This trial led to the GENASIS trial, a phase 2 randomized placebo-controlled trial to examine the efficacy of percutaneous, intramyocardial injection of phVEGF-2 on ETT at 3 months [23]. The trial originally planned to enroll 404 patients but was stopped prematurely (295 patients) when interim analysis indicated the study as designed was not expected to reach statistical significance for the primary ETT endpoint.

Euroinject-One was a phase 2, double-blind, randomized placebo-controlled trial of percutaneous intramyocardial plasmid gene transfer of phVEGF-165 in 80 patients with CCS angina class 3–4 and evidence of reversible myocardial ischemia by SPECT who were not candidates for revascularization [22]. Patients received 0.5 mg of phVEGF-165 or placebo plasmid by direct injection following NOGA mapping in the myocardial region showing stress-induced myocardial perfusion defects. The primary endpoint, quantitative assessment of myocardial perfusion at 3 months, showed no significant difference between VEGF- and placebo-treated patients (38±3% and 44±2%, respectively). CCS angina class change did not differ significantly between VEGF and placebo-treated patients. Regional wall motion did improve in the VEGF-injected regions as assessed by NOGA and ventriculography [22, 29]. There were five procedure-related complications related to the direct intramyocardial delivery. Subsequently, the same investigators prospectively treated 16 patients (CCS angina class 3–4) with intramyocardial injection of phVEGF-165 followed 1 week later by G-CSF (10 ug/kg/day for 6 days). Two groups from the Euroinject-One cohort

($n=16$ receiving phVEGF-165 alone and $n=16$ receiving placebo) were used as historical controls. The treatment appeared safe, but the primary endpoint – SPECT myocardial perfusion at 3 months – was not significant and unfortunately, data were not available for the entire treatment group [30].

The NOGA Angiogenesis Revascularization Therapy: Evaluation by RadioNuclide Imaging (NORTHERN) Trial is an ongoing trial planning to randomize 120 patients with CCS angina class 3–4 to percutaneous, intramyocardial AdVEGF165 versus placebo [24]. The primary endpoint will be changes in myocardial perfusion rest/stress and summed stress scores from baseline to 12 weeks, repeated at 6 months. Enrollment is expected to be complete in July, 2007. A multicenter, randomized, double-blind, placebo-controlled study evaluating the efficacy of AdVEGF121 delivered by NOGA catheter in 129 patients with CCS 2–4 angina with a primary endpoint of change in ETT at 26 weeks was recently stopped; results are unavailable [25].

Cell-Based Therapy

Cell-based therapy for therapeutic angiogenesis holds great promise for "no option" patients with chronic refractory angina [31, 32]. Although the exact mechanisms underlying how and which stem cells contribute to angiogenesis remain controversial, clinical investigation has begun with unfractionated bone marrow cells (BMCs), which contain both hematopoetic and mesenchymal stem cells, and circulating endothelial progenitor cells (EPCs). EPCs are identified by the cell surface markers CD34, vascular endothelial growth factor receptor 2 (VEGFR2) [33], stem cell marker CD133 (less than 1% of nucleated BMCs), and the ability to differentiate into endothelial cells [34]. EPCs have been shown to contribute directly to blood-vessel formation [33–35]. It is unclear if stem cells participate directly in angiogenesis or via a paracrine effect or both [36, 37].

Five small phase 1 trials have demonstrated excellent initial safety with encouraging preliminary results using unselected BMCs [38–43], but none of these trials were designed to assess efficacy. The only completed randomized trial is a phase 1 double-blind, placebo-controlled trial of intramyocardial injections of granulocyte colony-stimulating factor (G-CSF)-mobilized CD34+ cells in 24 patients [26]. The preliminary results demonstrated a reduction of angina episodes and use of nitroglycerin providing the basis for the first large placebo-controlled stem cell trial in refractory angina. ACT34-CMI is a multicenter, phase 2 double-blind, prospective, randomized, placebo-controlled study to determine the tolerability, efficacy, safety, and dose range of intramyocardial injection of G-CSF-mobilized autologous CD34+ cells for reduction of angina episodes in patients with refractory chronic myocardial ischemia. Similar to the phase 1 trial, patients will receive subcutaneous G-CSF 5 ug/kg/day for 5 days followed by leukoapheresis of CD34+ cells followed by intramyocardial injection of the CD34+ cells using NOGA guidance. Planned enrollment is 150 patients with frequency of angina episodes as the primary endpoint [44]. Two Phase 1 trials using higher dose G-CSF or GM-CSF as a single agent reported an increase in acute coronary syndromes [45]. Therefore, currently the preferred approach appears to be mobilization of cells followed by direct injection of those cells.

Placebo Effect

A major challenge for refractory angina trials is the presence of a prominent placebo effect in these patients [46, 47]. This is an important issue in trial design, affecting choice of endpoints (both primary and secondary, as well as use of surrogate endpoints), selection of higher-risk patient subgroups, and sample size calculation to achieve appropriate power to account for expected improvement in placebo patients. In a meta-analysis of eight randomized placebo-controlled trials for the treatment of refractory angina, the pooled mean change in exercise time and 95% confidence intervals for placebo subjects at 1, 2–3, and 4–6 month intervals was 38 s (21–56), 46 s (29–63), and 54 s (19–88), respectively. None of the trials demonstrated a significant improvement over placebo in the treatment group [47]. In contrast, 5 of 6 myocardial angiogenesis trials demonstrated significant improvement in measures of angina in the treatment group over placebo [47].

Future Directions

Therapeutic angiogenesis has tremendous potential for treating patients with refractory angina not amenable to conventional pharmacologic and interventional therapy. Although current data demonstrate excellent safety with protein, gene, and cell-based therapies for angiogenesis, the evidence for efficacy in placebo-controlled trials is modest at best. There continue to be a large number of unanswered questions. The optimal therapy or combination (protein and/or gene and/or cell), methods of delivery, dose duration, and frequency all remain to be defined and may be different for different treatments. Future trials need to focus on angina and quality-of-life data in this unique and challenging population. A major limitation in the field is the lack of a "gold standard" for myocardial perfusion determination in patients with collateral-dependent ischemia. Advances in cardiac magnetic resonance imaging and positron emission tomography scanning to adequately assess collateral blood flow may allow smaller trials to determine the "optimal" angiogenic agent. Efficacy has not been definitively proven or disproven, and likely will vary depending on the individual growth factor or cell type used and may even need individualization among different patient populations. Safety issues will also need to be readdressed with newer agents or combination therapy. Future trials will need to "embrace diversity" [48] as we deepen our understanding of the underlying mechanisms of angiogenesis and begin to combine biologic modalities. As we learn more about individual variations in collateral development, we may reach the point where a targeted treatment strategy can be achieved for an individual patient.

References

1. Henry TD. Therapeutic angiogenesis. Br Med J. 1999;318:1536–9.
2. Mukherjee D, Bhatt DL, Roe MT, et al. Direct myocardial revascularization and angiogenesis – how many patients might be eligible? Am J Cardiol. 1999;84:598–600.
3. Mannheimer C, Camici P, Chester MR, et al. The problem of chronic refractory angina: report from the ESC Joint Study Group on the Treatment of Refractory Angina. Eur Heart J. 2002;23:355–70.
4. Henry TD, Satran D, Johnson RJ, et al. Natural history of patients with refractory angina. J Am Coll Cardiol. 2006; 47:231A.
5. Carmeliet P. Mechanisms of angiogenesis and arteriogenesis. Nat Med. 2000;6:389–95.
6. Simons M. Angiogenesis: where do we stand now? Circulation. 2005;111:1556–66.
7. Henry TD, Abraham JA. Review of preclinical and clinical results with vascular endothelial growth factors for therapeutic angiogenesis. Curr Interv Cardiol Rep. 2000;2:228–41.
8. Ferrara N, Gerber HP, LeCouter J. The biology of VEGF and its receptors. Nat Med. 2003;9:669–76.
9. Ware JA, Simons M. Angiogenesis in ischemic heart disease. Nat Med. 1997;3:158–64.
10. Cha KS, Schwartz RS, Henry TD. Myocardial angiogenesis: protein growth factors. In: Laham RJ, Baim DS, editors. Angiogenesis and direct myocardial revascularization. Totowa: Humana Press; 2005. p. 190–4.
11. Udelson JE, Dilsizian V, Laham RJ, et al. Therapeutic angiogenesis with recombinant fibroblast growth factor-2 improves stress and rest myocardial perfusion abnormalities in patients with severe symptomatic chronic coronary artery disease. Circulation. 2000;102:1605–10.
12. Hendel RC, Henry TD, Rocha-Singh K, et al. Effect of intracoronary recombinant human vascular endothelial growth factor on myocardial perfusion: evidence for a dose-dependent effect. Circulation. 2000;101:118–21.
13. Henry TD, Rocha-Singh K, Isner JM, et al. Intracoronary administration of recombinant human vascular endothelial growth factor to patients with coronary artery disease. Am Heart J. 2001;142:872–80.
14. Henry TD, Annex BH, McKendall GR, et al. The VIVA Trial: Vascular endothelial growth factor in ischemia for vascular angiogenesis. Circulation. 2003;107(10): 1359–65.
15. Simons M, Annex BH, Laham RJ, et al. Pharmacological treatment of coronary artery disease with recombinant fibroblast growth factor-2: double-blind, randomized, controlled clinical trial. Circulation. 2002;105:788–93.
16. Schumacher B, Pecher P, von Specht BU, et al. Induction of neoangiogenesis in ischemic myocardium by human growth factors: first clinical results of a new treatment of coronary heart disease. Circulation. 1998;97:645–50.
17. Laham RJ, Sellke FW, Edelman ER, et al. Local perivascular delivery of basic fibroblast growth factor in patients undergoing coronary bypass surgery. Circulation. 1999; 100:1865–71.
18. Grines CL, Watkins MW, Helmer G, et al. Angiogenic Gene Therapy (AGENT) trial in patients with stable angina pectoris. Circulation. 2002;105:1291–7.
19. Grines CL, Watkins MW, Mahmarian JJ, et al. A randomized, double-blind, placebo-controlled trial of Ad5FGF-4 gene therapy and its effect on myocardial perfusion in patients with stable angina. J Am Coll Cardiol. 2003;42: 1339–47.
20. Henry TD, Grines CL, Watkins MW, et al. Angiogenic gene therapy: a meta-analysis of intracoronary Ad5FGF-4 from the AGENT-3 and AGENT-4 trials. J Am Coll Cardiol. 2007;50(11):1038–46.
21. Losordo DW, Vale PR, Hendel RC, et al. Phase 1/2 placebo-controlled, double-blind, dose-escalating trial of myocardial vascular endothelial growth factor 2 gene transfer by catheter delivery in patients with chronic myocardial ischemia. Circulation. 2002;105:2012–8.
22. Kastrup J, Jorgenson E, Ruck A, et al. Direct intramyocardial plasmid vascular endothelial growth factor-A165 gene therapy in patients with stable severe angina pectoris: a randomized double-blind placebo-controlled study: the Euroinject One trial. J Am Coll Cardiol. 2005;45:982–8.
23. GENASIS (Genetic Angiogenic Stimulation Investigational Study). www.clinicaltrials.gov (id:NCT00090714).

24. NOGA Angiogenesis revascularization therapy: evaluation by RadioNuclide imaging – The Northern Trial. 2006. www.clinicaltrials.gov (id:NCT001143585).
25. A study to treat patients whose chronic angina symptoms are not relieved by medication and have an area of the heart that cannot be treated by standard therapies. 2006. www.clinicaltrials.gov (id:NCT00215696).
26. Losordo DW, Schatz RA, White CJ, et al. Intramyocardial transplantation of autologous CD34+ stem cells for intractable angina: a phase I/IIa double-blind randomized controlled trial. Circulation. 2007;115(25):3165–72.
27. Pecher P, Schumacher BA. Angiogenesis in ischemic human myocardium: clinical results after 3 years. Ann Thorac Surg. 2000;69:1414–9.
28. Ruel M, Laham RJ, Parker JA, et al. Long-term effects of surgical angiogenic therapy with fibroblast growth factor 2 protein. J Thorac Cardiovasc Surg. 2002;124:28–34.
29. Gyongyosi M, Khorsand A, Zamini S, et al. NOGA-guided analysis of regional myocardial perfusion abnormalities treated with intramyocardial injections of plasmid encoding vascular endothelial growth factor a-165 in patients with chronic myocardial ischemia: subanalysis of the Euroinject-One multicenter double-blind randomized study. Circulation. 2005;112:157–65.
30. Ripa RS, Wang Y, Jorgensen E, et al. Intramyocardial injection of vascular endothelial growth factor-A165 plasmid followed by granulocyte-colony stimulating factor to induce angiogenesis in patients with severe chronic ischaemic heart disease. Eur Heart J. 2006;27:1785–92.
31. Losordo DW, Dimmeler S. Therapeutic angiogenesis and vasculogenesis for ischemic disease: part II: cell-based therapies. Circulation. 2004;109:2692–7.
32. Boyle AJ, Schulman SP, Hare JM. Stem cell therapy for cardiac repair: ready for the next step. Circulation. 2006;114:339–52.
33. Asahara T, Murohara T, Sullivan A, et al. Isolation of putative progenitor endothelial cells for angiogenesis. Science. 1997;275:964–7.
34. Asahara T, Kawamoto A. Endothelial progenitor cells for postnatal vasculogenesis. Am J Physiol Cell Physiol. 2004;287:C572–9.
35. Gunsilius E, Duba HC, Petzer AL, et al. Contribution of endothelial cells of hematopoietic origin to blood vessel formation. Circ Res. 2001;88:E1.
36. Rehman J, Li J, Orschell CM, March KL. Peripheral blood "endothelial progenitor cells" are derived from monocyte/macrophages and secrete angiogenic growth factors. Circulation. 2003;107:1164–9.
37. Kinnaird T, Stabile E, Burnett MS, et al. Marrow-derived stromal cells express genes encoding a broad spectrum of arteriogenic cytokines and promote in vitro and in vivo arteriogenesis through paracrine mechanisms. Circ Res. 2004;94:678–85.
38. Fuchs S, Satler LF, Kornowski R, et al. Catheter-based autologous bone marrow myocardial injection in no-option patients with advanced coronary artery disease: a feasibility study. J Am Coll Cardiol. 2003;41:1721–4.
39. Hamano K, Nishida M, Hirata K, et al. Local implantation of autologous bone marrow cells for therapeutic angiogenesis in patients with ischemic heart disease: clinical trial and preliminary results. Jpn Circ J. 2001;65:845–7.
40. Tse HF, Kwong YL, Chan JK, et al. Angiogenesis in ischaemic myocardium by intramyocardial autologous bone marrow mononuclear cell implantation. Lancet. 2003;361:47–9.
41. Perin EC, Dohmann HF, Borojevic R, et al. Transendocardial, autologous bone marrow cell transplantation for severe, chronic ischemic heart failure. Circulation. 2003;107:2294–302.
42. Perin EC, Dohmann HF, Borojevic R, et al. Improved exercise capacity and ischemia 6 and 12 months after transendocardial injection of autologous bone marrow mononuclear cells for ischemic cardiomyopathy. Circulation. 2004;110:213–8.
43. Briguori C, Reimers B, Sarais C, et al. Direct intramyocardial percutaneous delivery of autologous bone marrow in patients with refractory myocardial angina. Am Heart J. 2006;151:674–80.
44. A double-blind, prospective, randomized, placebo-controlled study to determine the tolerability, efficacy, safety and dose range of intramyocardial injections of G-CSF mobilized auto-CD34+ cells for reduction of angina episodes in patients with refractory chronic myocardial ischemia (ACT34-CMI). www.clinicaltrials.gov (id:NCT00300053).
45. Wilson RF, Henry TD. Granulocyte colony-stimulating factor and granulocyte-macrophage colony-stimulating factor: double-edged swords. J Am Coll Cardiol. 2005;46:1649–50.
46. Rana JS, Mannam A, Donnell-Fink L, et al. Longevity of the placebo effect in the therapeutic angiogenesis and laser myocardial revascularization trials in patients with coronary heart disease. Am J Cardiol. 2005;95:1456–9.
47. Strauss CE, Duval S, Walton DM, et al. A meta-analysis of the placebo effect in the treatment of refractory angina. Am J Cardiol. 2005;96:13H.
48. Gulati R, Simari RD. Cell therapy for angiogenesis: embracing diversity. Circulation. 2005;112:1522–4.

Transmyocardial Laser Revascularization

8

Jignesh S. Shah, Joanna J. Wykrzykowska, and Roger J. Laham

Introduction

Ischemic heart disease remains the leading cause of death in the Western Hemisphere. Despite recent advances in medical therapy and surgical and percutaneous revascularization, the number of so-called no option patients is increasing. These patients are no longer candidates for percutaneous or surgical revascularization but are symptomatic despite maximal medical therapy. A number of investigational therapeutic strategies have been developed to improve the quality of life of "no-option" patients. These, in addition to laser myocardial revascularization discussed here, include angiogenesis and myogenesis approaches, external counterpulsation, as well as spinal cord stimulation. Transmyocardial laser revascularization utilizes a laser to create channels within the myocardium either via the surgical epicardial approach or percutaneous endocardial approach. It was originally proposed that myocardial perfusion could be achieved by the creation of transmyocardial channels, which communicate with the left ventricular cavity, thus mimicking the physiology of blood flow in reptile hearts [1]. Early success of the procedure was followed by closure of the pathways by fibrosis and scarring. Thus, these channels do not remain open for any significant duration and blood does not flow through these channels. However, numerous studies conducted over more than a decade suggested a role of this procedure in unrevascularizable patients who continue to remain symptomatic from their ischemia. Hence, TMR has been performed on over 10,000 patients worldwide [2]. Herein, we review the techniques, proposed mechanisms, and clinical data on laser transmyocardial revascularization.

Lasers

Since the inception of transmyocardial revascularization (TMR), LASER (Light amplification by stimulated emission of radiation) has been used as the energy source. The effects of laser on the tissue depend upon the laser wavelength, frequency, pulse energy, pulse duration, as well as the photonic absorption and scattering by the target tissue. Three types of lasers have been employed: two infrared lasers (Holmium YAG (Ho:YAG) and carbon dioxide (CO_2)) and one ultraviolet laser (excimer). The technical details are presented in Table 8.1. The major clinical trials have been conducted using the infrared Ho:YAG and CO_2 lasers, which rely on thermal ablation to create channels in the myocardium. The tissue absorbs energy from the infrared laser and reaches a supervibrational state. This breaks the molecular bonds. Molecular fragments thus formed dissipate as gas. The resultant increase in the volume leads to an acoustic shock in surrounding region. Excimer lasers are cold lasers and operate in the deep ultraviolet spectrum. They depend on molecular bond dissociation for tissue ablation [3].

CO_2 depends on total energy over time, power per unit area, as well as duration of exposure for effect. In contrast, Ho:YAG laser depends on pulse duration, pulse energy, total energy per unit time, pulse energy/pulse

J.S. Shah • J.J. Wykrzykowska • R.J. Laham (✉)
Cardiovascular Division, Beth Israel Deaconess Medical Center and Harvard Medical School, Boston, MA, USA
e-mail: rlaham@bidmc.harvard.edu

G.W. Barsness and D.R. Holmes Jr. (eds.), *Coronary Artery Disease*,
DOI 10.1007/978-1-84628-712-1_8,

Table 8.1 Types of Lasers used in clinical and pre-clinical trials

	Ho:YAG	CO_2	Excimer
Spectrum	Infrared	Infrared	Ultraviolet
Mechanism	Pulsed thermal ablation	Continuous thermal ablation	Molecular dissociation
Fiber optic	Yes	No	
Lateral damage	Yes	No	No
Power (W)	40	850	
Pulses	20–30	1	
Energy/pulse (J)	2	25–30	
Wavelength (μm)	2.10–2.15	10.6	

duration, and pulse energy/unit area for its effects. Fisher performed histological studies to differentiate the channels made by these two laser sources. Though there was more acute damage by Ho:YAG laser, at 6 weeks the channels created by both sources look similar. It is widely believed, however, that neither source offers a distinct clinical advantage over the other [4].

Technique

TMR is a surgical procedure performed under epidural anesthesia (to prevent coronary spasm) or as an adjunct to coronary arterial bypass graft (CABG). Optimal exposure is obtained by placing the patient in the left lateral decubitus position. Anterior or anterolateral left thoracotomy incision is made in the fourth or fifth intercostal space to expose the anterior and lateral wall, respectively. Muscles are retracted and the pericardium is opened and folded back. The laser probe is placed directly on the epicardial surface and fired until the probe enters the ventricular cavity. The presence of bubbles on transesophageal echocardiography (TEE) or pulsatile spurts of blood indicate entry into the ventricular cavity and hence completion of the channel. Hemostasis of the pulsatile flow is achieved by manual pressure. A total of 25–40 channels are made each 1 cm apart in the left ventricle. Chest tube drains are placed at the completion of the procedure. Some operators recommend placing intercostal blocks under direct vision. These intercostal blocks keep the patient pain free, thereby preventing extremes of autonomic changes and may affect postoperative outcomes. The incision is then closed and patient observed in the intensive care unit. Most patients are extubated the same day and maintained on a nitroglycerin drip. If the chest tube drains less than 100 cm^3 over the first 6 h, the drain is removed. Ambulation is begun on the first postoperative day. Most patients are discharged on postoperative day 3 or 4 [5, 6]. Thoracoscopic as well as robotically assisted TMR has also been reported [7, 8]. Thoracoscopic TMR is performed under general anesthesia via a thoracoscopic ports in the (a) fifth intercostal space along midaxillary line (b) fifth intercostal space in the midclavicular line, and (c) fourth intercostal space in the midclavicular line. Standard Metzenbaum scissors are used to open the pericardium, which is then held by endoscopic graspers. Hand-held laser piece is then introduced via the two midclavicular ports to create channels in the anterior and lateral walls and hemostasis is achieved by direct pressure through the incisions. Quick postoperative recovery using this technique has been reported by Horvath [8].

Complications

Up to 30% of the patients undergoing TMR will have complications related to the procedure. Initial studies found a 30 day mortality of up to 20%, however, mortality of only 1–5% has been reported in the randomized trials [9, 10]. This improvement has been attributed to exclusion of patients who are clinically unstable and postponing their procedure after clinical stabilization at least 2 weeks after CABG [9]. Other complications of the procedure include atrial (10%) and ventricular arrhythmias (12%), pericardial effusion with or without tamponade (6%), and postoperative heart failure (4–29%). In a study by Wehberg et al., the intensive care unit time and length of stay were shorter in CABG plus TMR group compared to CABG only group (2.1 ± 0.2 days vs 1.6 ± 0.2 days, and 8.2 ± 0.4 days vs 7.1 ± 0.6 days). The 30 day readmission rate was lower in CABG + TMR group (7.8% vs 2.8%) [11]. The risk of procedural complications is related to underlying patient characteristics as described below. In the largest database study among 173 centers, Peterson et al. reported a 30 day mortality of 6.4% after TMR in 3,717 patients. The rate of renal failure was 4.8% and that of stroke was 0.8% in this patient group [12]. However, it needs to be noted that the reporting to this database was voluntary and hence bias-prone.

Mechanism of Action

Open Channel Hypothesis

TMR was envisioned as a means of creating sinusoids to promote direct perfusion of the myocardium by oxygenated blood from the left ventricular cavity, in effect recreating patterns identified in the reptilian heart [1]. This original channel hypothesis was challenged by numerous experimental and autopsy results demonstrating that the channels created fill up with necrotic debris very early in the postoperative period and hence do not remain patent. In the long term, scar formation takes place in these channels, with no histological evidence of persistent communications with the ventricular cavity [13].

Angiogenesis

Further insight into the potential mechanism of effect was proposed by histological evidence of angiogenesis associated with areas of laser injury. Hardy et al. first noted an increase in neovascularization in the region of the channels [14]. Subsequent studies have confirmed these findings [15–17]. With immunohistochemical staining, the presence of CD31 and factor VIII antibody has been demonstrated thereby confirming the presence of endothelial linings. As much as a threefold increase in the new blood vessels in ischemic regions (near the channels) has been noted in TMR patients compared to controls [18]. Histochemical analysis has confirmed increased expression of transforming growth factor Beta and basic fibroblast growth factor in the tissue surrounding TMR channels. A twofold increase in vascular endothelial growth factor mRNA in patients undergoing TMR has also been noted [19]. Some studies have shown similar degrees of neovascularization independent of the method of channel formation. Mechanical needle or power drill injury has been associated with a similar degree of angiogenesis as laser injury [20]. This suggests that both laser and mechanical injuries induce specific stimulation of vascular growth. Importantly, however, laser injury is not a more potent angiogenic stimulant than mechanical injury. However, other studies have failed to confirm similar outcomes with mechanical channel formation [21]. Thus, angiogenesis may be a specific or a nonspecific response to damage induced by laser energy. Regardless of the specificity, the finding of increased neovascularization has been consistent across multiple studies. More importantly, not only have the preclinical and clinical studies demonstrated an improvement in the quality of life and exercise tolerance, but also an objective increase in myocardial function and perfusion on stress echocardiography [22], positron emission tomography [23], and magnetic resonance imaging [24]. While quality of life improvement may be due, at least in part, to a powerful placebo effect (discussed elsewhere in this text) [25], the sensitive imaging techniques suggest a physiologic therapeutic effect of TMR in enhancing neovascularization.

Myocardial Denervation

A third hypothesis suggests that TMR leads to damage to the epicardial sympathetic nerves and may have antianginal effects. Loss of tyrosine hydroxylase, a neural-specific enzyme, and decreased uptake of Positron Emission Tomography (PET) tracer C11 hydroxyephedrine have been documented, thereby lending some credence to this hypothesis [26, 27]. Denervation, however, is difficult to demonstrate given the dual innervation of the heart by both sympathetic and parasympathetic systems. Some studies have noted no change in the reflex response to epicardial or intracoronary bradykinin after TMR in dogs with sinoaortic denervation and vagotomy [28]. In addition, other studies documented reinnervation of the sympathetic fibers in the chronic phase post TMR [29]. Hence, myocardial denervation as the sole mechanism for the antianginal effect of TMR is unlikely.

Microscopy (Fig. 8.1, Table 8.2)

Histochemical analysis performed on autopsy specimens shows very early loss of myocardial channel patency, especially after Ho:YAG laser use [13]. The hypothesis of channel endothelialization has also been refuted based on lack of histopathological evidence. The channels are lined by necrotic myocardial debris. At necropsy, scar formation is visible at intermediate- and long-term follow-up in the region of the created channels [16, 30]. However, in the adjacent viable myocardium, a significant increase in the capillary

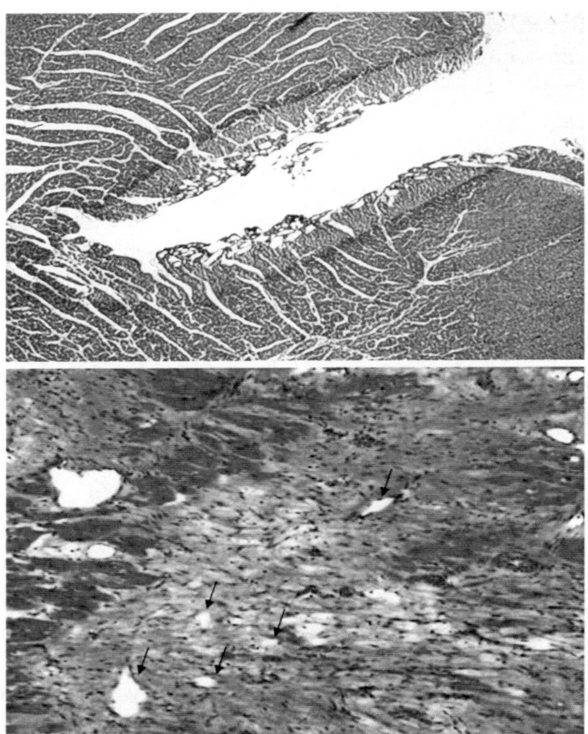

Fig. 8.1 Histology in laser myocardial revascularization: *top*: laser channel within days of procedure. Channel eventually close negating the perfusion via channel hypothesis. *Bottom*: weeks after procedure, channel is replaced by fibrous tissue with neovascularization (*arrows*) in scar and surrounding areas

Table 8.2 Possible mechanisms of Laser myocardial revascularization with early and late histopathologic findings

Early:
Laser channels filled with granulocytes, thrombocytes, fibrinous network, detritus
Laser channels surrounded by severe myocardial necrosis
Infiltrating lymphocytes and macrophages surrounding the laser channels
Channels were filled with RBC or fibrinous network
No connections between laser channels and the ventricular cavity
Late
Cicatricial tissue
Perichannel scarring
Positive staining for CD31 and factor VIII
Increased capillary vascular density
RBC visualized in neovessels

vascular density is observed compared to the non-laser-treated myocardium [16, 18, 29, 31]. Histochemical analysis has demonstrated increases in VEGF mRNA, as well as an increase in the expression of transforming growth factor beta (TGF-β) and basic fibroblast growth factor (bFGF) [19]. A similar degree of neovascularization, however, has been observed after needle injury and may be nonspecific [20] to the laser effect.

Patient Selection

The eligibility criteria used for patient selection among various trials are remarkably similar with only minor variations. These randomized trials have included patients who were not suitable candidates for percutaneous intervention (PCI) or CABG but were considered eligible for TMR. The inclusion criteria were: anginal class (CCS) ≥2 not amenable to medical therapy, ejection fraction 20–25%, and ischemic territory comprising 20% of the left ventricle. Patients with myocardial infarction within 3 weeks, left ventricular thrombus, aortic valve disease, known cancer, or retinopathy were excluded. The criteria for ineligibility for PCI in the trials to date included chronic total occlusion with unfavorable morphologic features (ostial location, long-gap segment, major branch at occlusion), multiple restenosis, diffuse disease, and severely degenerated saphenous vein grafts [9, 32]. With advances in percutaneous techniques such as greater success in opening chronic total occlusions, these patients would likely have been eligible for PCI and excluded from the TMR trials. Ineligibility for CABG was determined based on presence of poor targets, lack of suitable conduits, and severe comorbidities such as very low forced expiratory volume on pulmonary function testing, metastatic cancer, or severely calcified aorta [33, 34]. Studies have reported poor outcome in patients with the following conditions, thereby making them poor candidates and at high risk for complications after TMR [35, 36]. These criteria include: recent MI, unstable angina within the last 7 days, depressed EF<35%, ischemic region in the intraventricular septum, diabetes, body mass index<25 kg/m^2, poor vascularity from native or graft vessels, and severe mitral regurgitation

Considering these broad exclusion criteria, the actual number of patients clinically eligible for the procedure was questioned. In a study to evaluate the proportion of patients eligible for TMR, Mukherjee et al. evaluated charts and cine angiograms from 500 consecutive patients undergoing angiography over a

5 month period. Of the 500 patients, 2.2% were considered candidates for TMR, 3.4% for percutaneous TMR, and 1% for a combined TMR and CABG procedure. The eligibility for the different modalities was not mutually exclusive. With 1,713,000 cardiac catheterizations performed in 1996 in the USA, the number of patients clinically and angiographically eligible for these procedures annually based on the FDA approved indications are: 37,000 for TMR, 58,000 for percutaneous TMR and 17,000 for CABG+TMR [37]. The most important result of this study, however, was the increased morbidity, worsening angina, and poor outcomes observed in the group of patients treated medically.

Evidence of Clinical Efficacy of TMR

The efficacy of TMR has been assessed by multiple diverse modalities: patient symptoms and quality of life, functional capacity, cardiac disease-related hospitalization, cardiovascular mortality, and a variety of imaging modalities, including sestamibi and thallium nuclear studies, positron emission tomography, stress echocardiography, and magnetic resonance imaging. All these studies included patients with at least class II or III angina who were not candidates for traditional revascularization (see below). Here, we discuss the studies evaluating objective end points such as cardiac mortality and cardiac-related hospitalization, followed by those assessing evidence of ischemia by myocardial perfusion studies and functional capacity. Finally, we discuss studies using patient symptoms and quality of life as end points to assess the efficacy of TMR.

Cardiac Mortality and Cardiac-Related Hospitalization

Several short- and intermediate-term mortality and hospitalization-related studies were published in the late 1990s. Frazier et al., reported in 1999 their experience among 192 patients randomized to TMR or continuing medical management for unrevascularizable CAD [9]. There was a significant difference in the two groups with regard to the number of hospitalizations (2% for TMR vs 69% for medical therapy, $p<0.001$) but no difference in the survival at 1 year follow-up (85% for TMR vs 79%, for medical therapy $p=0.5$) (Table 8.3). Aaberge et al. reported their findings of the late follow-up of the Norwegian Randomized trial with CO_2 laser in which 100 eligible patients were block-randomized 1:1 between November 1995 and January 1998 to achieve either continued optimal medical treatment alone or in combination with TMR in a non-crossover design [40, 41, 47]. Baseline patient characteristics in terms of their demographics, clinical status, as well as medication use were similar in the two groups. The mortality rate was 24% in the control group compared to 22% in the TMR group at 5 years ($p=$NS). At 32 months there were 53 admissions for unstable angina in the TMR group compared to 95 in the control group ($p=0.047$). There was no difference in the hospitalization rates for acute myocardial infarction (AMI) (8 in TMR group vs 12 in medical therapy group) or congestive heart failure (CHF) (19 in TMR group vs 11 in medical therapy group) (Table 8.3). A similar decrease in the cardiac-related hospitalization rate was reported by Horvath et al [48]. In eight centers, 200 patients with severe angina refractory to medical therapy, reversible ischemia documented by a radionuclide myocardial perfusion scan, and contraindications to PCI or CABG or transplant, underwent TMR. The authors reported a substantial decrease in the number of hospitalizations from 2.5 ± 2 before the procedure to 0.4 ± 0.6 after the procedure [48]. Allen et al. reported significantly greater freedom from cardiac-related rehospitalization (61% vs 33%, $p<0.001$) at 12 months in their multicenter, randomized study of 275 patients with class IV angina with unrevascularizable CAD [32]. However, the survival estimates among the 32 TMR patients compared to 143 controls (84% vs 89% $p=0.23$) were similar (Table 8.3). Schofield et al. reported the British experience in 188 unrevascularizable patients with refractory angina randomly assigned to TMR plus medical treatment or medical management alone [10]. Survival at 12 months was 89% (83–96%) in the TMR group and 96% (92–100) in the medical-management group ($p=0.14$). Thus, the data on hospitalizations and survival seems fairly consistent. The results of these clinical trials and observational studies suggest that TMR does not confer increased survival, however, there is substantial evidence that cardiac-related hospitalizations may decrease in the long term.

Effect on Myocardial Perfusion and LV Ejection Fraction

Multiple studies in animal models as well as humans have been conducted to assess myocardial perfusion prior to, and after TMR, although the results have been inconsistent. Using thallium imaging, Schofield et al. failed to demonstrate any difference in perfusion in 188 patients after a course of CO_2-based TMR [10]. At the end of 12 month follow-up, reversible defect was found in 21% of the TMR patients compared to 22% of the medical. Comparing 94 patients who underwent TMR with 94 similar controls on medical management, Burns et al. showed worsening of perfusion during stress in the region of TMR at 3 and 6 months after the procedure [49]. Allen et al. also assessed computer-quantified changes in perfusion between base line and 12 months in their multicenter, randomized trial (Table 8.3) [38]. There were no significant differences between the TMR group and the medical-therapy group with respect to changes in ischemia (–0.9 vs –0.6, $p=0.9$), defects in perfusion at rest (1.6 vs 2.2, $p=0.8$), or delayed defects (1.3 vs 0.5, $p=0.8$) [32]. In addition, LV function was unchanged. Similarly, Aaberge et al. found no change in LVEF in the TMR group during long-term follow-up in the Norwegian randomized trial [40].

In contrast to those studies, other nonrandomized studies have suggested an improvement in myocardial perfusion following TMR. Frazier et al. demonstrated improved subendocardial flow in 11 patients treated with TMR using PET scanning [9]. Overall, there was a 20% improvement in myocardial perfusion in the TMR group and 27% worsening in the medical-treatment group ($p=0.002$). In a subgroup of patients from a multicenter study among 200 patients showed even more promising results. PET scans before and after the operations confirmed improved subendocardial versus subepicardial resting perfusion in the laser-treated areas at 12 months (0.96 ± 0.07 vs 1.10 ± 0.04, $p<0.001$, $n=11$) [48]. The discrepancy in results between studies may be attributable to the low sensitivity of thallium nuclear imaging as compared to PET scanning, rendering it less adequate as an outcome measure. Similar problems were encountered in assessing improvement in myocardial perfusion and neovascularization in angiogenesis and myogenesis trials underscoring the need for development and use of imaging modalities with adequate sensitivity (Swartz, Wykrzykowska and Laham, in press).

Magnetic resonance imaging (MRI) is currently accepted as the gold standard for evaluating myocardial perfusion as well as LV systolic function. Laham et al. reported their findings of functional and perfusion MRI at baseline, 1 month and 6 months in a group of 15 patients who underwent Biosense-guided Ho:YAG-based myocardial revascularization [24]. Although there were no changes in nuclear perfusion scans, MRI determined resting radial motion and thickening of the target wall improved significantly during follow-up (wall thickening: baseline, $30.6 \pm 11.7\%$; day 30, $41.2 \pm 13.3\%$ and day 180, $44.2 \pm 11.9\%$, $p=0.01$). The size of the underperfused myocardial area was $14.5 \pm 5.4\%$ at baseline and was reduced to $6.3 \pm 2.8\%$ at 30 days and $7.7 \pm 3.7\%$ at 6 months ($p<0.001$) [24]. These results will require confirmation in a large prospective trial of TMR using MRI to adequately detect perfusion and viability differences between TMR and medically treated groups. Magnetic resonance delayed-enhancement viability assessment prior to the TMR procedure could also facilitate mapping of the injection sites to the areas of scar.

Overall, it is reasonable to infer that differences in the method of assessing ischemia/perfusion may have contributed to the discrepancy in the results of various studies. Further studies using MRI as outcome measures are needed.

Exercise Time

Several studies have assessed exercise tolerance as a marker for improvement in ischemia after TMR. Burkhoff et al. assessed exercise tolerance in a multicenter, randomized clinical trial of 182 patients with unrevascularizable disease [33]. At 12 months, total exercise tolerance increased by a median of 65 s in the TMR group compared with a 46 s decrease in the exercise time in the medication-only group ($p<0{\cdot}0001$, median difference 111 s). Allen et al. also reported better exercise tolerance in the TMR group compared to the control group (exercise tolerance, 5.0 METs [metabolic equivalents] vs 3.9 METs; $p=0.05$) in their multicenter, randomized trial of 275 patients with unrevascularizable disease and class IV angina [32]. Jones et al. reported improvement in exercise tolerance among TMR patients over preoperative values and compared to the control group at 12 months (490 ± 17 s vs 294 ± 12 s., $p=0.0002$) [6]. Schofield et al. also assessed exercise time in their randomized trial of TMR plus medical treatment or medical management alone (Table 8.3) [10]. Mean treadmill exercise time increased by 40 s (95% CI, 15–94 s) in the TMR group compared to the medical management group at 12 months ($p=0.152$). Overall, published studies have consistently documented significant improvement in the exercise capacity of patients undergoing TMR. These improvements in the time of exercise, as well as improvements in symptoms and quality of life described below, however, maybe attributable in large part to failure to properly blind the studies comparing TMR and medical therapy, and the potent placebo effect of the procedure [25]. As illustrated in Table 8.3 the majority of the trials were non-blinded.

Symptoms and Quality of Life

Multiple studies have documented subjective improvement in patients undergoing TMR. In addition, symptomatic improvement has translated into significant improvement in the quality of life, as well as a decrease in the consumption of antianginal medications.

In their randomized trial among 192 unrevascularizable patients Frazier et al., reported 72% of the TMR patients improved by at least two Canadian Cardiovascular Society (CCS) classes compared with 13% of the control group ($p<0.001$) over a 12 month duration [9]. Quality of life as measured by the standardized SF-36 questionnaire, demonstrated that the patients undergoing TMR had a greater improvement in their quality of life than patients in the medical-treatment group (38% vs 6% improvement) as compared with base line at 3 months ($p<0.001$). The difference was sustained at 6 and 12 months ($p=0.01$ and $p<0.001$, respectively). On individual components of the Seattle Angina Questionnaire, TMR was associated with a significantly better result than medical treatment [9]. Burkhoff et al. reported the results of the multicenter, randomized clinical trial (ATLANTIC) in 182 patients with unrevascularizable disease [33]. There was a substantial improvement in the angina score among 47.8% of the treatment group compared to 14.3% of the control group ($p<0.001$). During the follow-up period, scores of each quality-of-life index in the Seattle angina questionnaire rose significantly more in the TMR group than in the medication-only group ($p<0.001$) [33]. In their multicenter trial among 200 patients, Horvath et al. reported a substantial decrease in the angina class compared to preoperative level sustained for up to 12 months ($p<0.001$). They reported complete relief of angina over an average 10 ± 3 months of follow-up. There was a decrease in the angina class of ≥2 in 73% of the patients compared to baseline. Allen et al. reported similar results in a prospective, randomized study at 18 centers, among 275 patients with medically refractory class IV angina. At 1 year of follow-up, 76% of the TMR group had an improvement in angina symptoms compared to 32% in the control group ($p<0.001$). This corresponded to higher quality-of-life scores in the TMR group ($p=0.003$) [48]. Jones et al. randomized 86 similar patients to TMR or medical management [6]. At 12 month follow-up, there was a significant improvement in the angina class among patients undergoing TMR compared with the control group (3.77 ± 0.07 vs 1.71 ± 0.2, $p<0.0001$). Spertus et al. reported the results of their multicenter, randomized trial in 197 patients [43]. By intention to treat analysis, 44% of the TMR group and 21% of the control group had their angina eliminated at 12 month follow-up (difference = 23%; 95% confidence interval [CI], 11–34%). Concordant results were noted in physical activities as well as quality of life. However, the authors point out that of the 99 patients assigned to medical therapy, 59 (60%) subsequently underwent TMR. An efficacy analysis that excluded patients who crossed over from the medical treatment to TMR suggested even greater treatment benefit [43]. Schofield et al. reported a decrease in the CCS angina score by two classes in 25% of the TMR and 4% of the medical management group at 12 months ($p<0.001$) among their 188 patient randomly assigned to TMR or medical management (Table 8.3) [10].

There are a limited number of studies reporting symptom-related outcomes at longer than 12 month follow-up period. The longest follow-up data comes from Aaberge et al., the Norwegian Randomized trial (Table 8.3). In 24% of the TMR group and 3% of the control group, there was ≥2 NYHA class angina improvement ($p=0.001$) at 43 months [41]. They also reported significant improvement in the physical subscales of the SF 36 in patients undergoing TMR [40]. Similar long-term outcomes were reported in an obser-

Table 8.3 Summary of clinical trials of TMR to-date

Trial	Type of trial	Number of patients	+/–CABG	Change in angina class	EF change	Change in exercise duration	Change in perfusion	Change in quality of life	Change in survival
Burkhoff et al. 1999 [33]	Prospective randomized non-blinded	182	No	Yes	Small decrease	Yes	No	Yes	No
Schofiled et al. 1999 [10]	Prospective randomized non-blinded	188	No	Yes	–	Yes	No	Yes	No
Allen et al. 1999 and 2004 [32, 38]	Prospective randomized non-blinded	275	No	Yes		Yes	No	Yes	No at 1 year (less hospitalizations for cardiac causes) but Yes at 5 years
Frazier et al. 1999 [9]	Prospective randomized non-blinded	192	No	Yes	–	–	Yes (R-R Thalium)	Yes	No
Stone et al. 2002 [39]	Prospective randomized blinded (placebo-controlled)	141 (failed chronic total occlusion PCI)	No	No	–	No	–	–	No
Aaberge et al. 2000 and 2002 [40, 41]	Prospective randomized non-blinded	100	No	Yes	No	No	–	–	No
Horvath et al. 2001 [42]	Non-randomized prospective	78	No	Yes	–	–	–	Yes	–
Spertus et al. 2000 [43]	Prospective randomized (intention to treat)	99	No	Yes	–	–	–	Yes	–
Van der Sloot et al. 2004 [44]	Prospective randomized (non-blinded)	30	No	Yes	No	Yes	No	Yes	–
Allen et al. 2004 [38]	Prospective randomized blinded	218	Yes	Yes	–	–	–	–	No
Frazier et al. 2004 [45]	Prospective randomized blinded	44	Yes	Yes	–	–	–	–	Yes (approached statistical significance)
Oesterle et al. 2000 [46]	Prospective randomized non-blinded (percutaneous)	221	No	Yes	–	Yes	–	–	No

vational study by Horvath et al. In this group of patients, the average angina class decreased from 3.7 ± 0.4 pre-TMR to 1.5 ± 1 at 1 year and 1.6 ± 1 ($p = 0.0001$) at 5 years of follow-up. There was a significant decrease in the number of patients in class IV angina. Preoperatively, 76% had class IV angina symptoms, and 24% had class III symptoms, but at follow-up, 81% of patients had class II or better symptoms, with 17% having complete resolution of anginal symptoms. The 3 year Seattle angina questionnaire scores showed an average improvement of 170% (CI 150–250%, $p < 0.001$) over the baseline results.

Thus, there is substantial evidence for significant improvement in symptomatology as well as quality of life after TMR, particularly in patients with class III/IV angina. These positive results are sustained at long-term follow-up. One can speculate that this translates into the decreased cardiac-related hospitalization rate that has been reported.

Percutaneous TMR (Fig. 8.2)

The goal of PTMR is to create a similar tissue effect as TMR by creating partial thickness channels by photoacoustic laser energy via the endomyocardium. It also eliminates the need for thoracotomy or general anesthesia and possibly reduces the perioperative risk of TMR. It also has the advantage of accessing the septum as well as the posterior wall, which is inaccessible by the standard TMR approach.

Systems available include: Biosense/Johnson and Johnson, Cardiogenesis and Eclipse.

The energy used for all three is Ho: YAG laser. The details of the systems are described in Table 8.4.

Technique

Femoral arterial access is obtained. Ventriculography and coronary arteriography are performed to define the target areas. A guiding catheter is loaded onto the 6F diagnostic catheter and introduced into the left ventricle. The diagnostic catheter is then exchanged for the laser catheter. The laser catheter exits out of the guiding catheter and the optical fiber is positioned near the endocardium of interest. Good contact of the optical fiber is confirmed and laser is fired. A laser pulse is delivered 100–150 ms after the QRS with two bursts to create each channel. The optical fiber is then retracted and repositioned under fluoroscopy. Up to 20 channels are created in one region with a spacing of 1 channel/cm^2. A post-procedure echocardiogram is generally performed to rule out perforation or tamponade.

Patient Selection

Patients who are at high risk for general anesthesia required for open TMR would be ideal for the percutaneous TMR (PTMR) procedure. Predominant ischemia in the septal region would also favor the use of PTMR over TMR. As this procedure gets more refined, it would be favored over TMR as it could be used in a larger number of patients. However, patients with target area wall thickness <8 mm and with aortic stenosis would still have to be excluded due to high risk of mortality and morbidity.

Clinical Efficacy

Several trials have evaluated this technique. Most prominent among these was the single blinded trial among 141 patients with class III or IV angina who failed treatment with PCI, and who were prospectively randomized at 17 medical centers to PTMR plus maximal medical therapy (MMT) ($n = 71$) or MMT alone ($n = 70$). Blinding was achieved through heavy sedation, dark goggles, and the concurrent performance of angiography in all patients. At 6 months, the angina class improved by two or more classes in 49% of the PTMR patients compared to 37% in those assigned to MMT ($p = 0.33$). The improvement in exercise duration at 6 months was 64 s with PTMR versus 52 s with MMT ($p = 0.73$). There were no differences in the 6-months rates of death (8.6% vs 8.8%), myocardial infarction (4.3% vs 2.9%), or need for revascularization (4.3% vs 5.9%) in the PTMR and MMT groups, respectively ($p = \text{NS}$). These findings are congruent with the findings of the DIRECT study. DIRECT was a randomized, blinded study of PTMR in 298 no-option patients treated with the Johnson & Johnson (Warren, New Jersey) Ho:YAG laser with electromechanical map guidance. Patients were divided into low dose, high dose, and no laser treatment. There was no difference in the incidence of death, stroke, myocardial

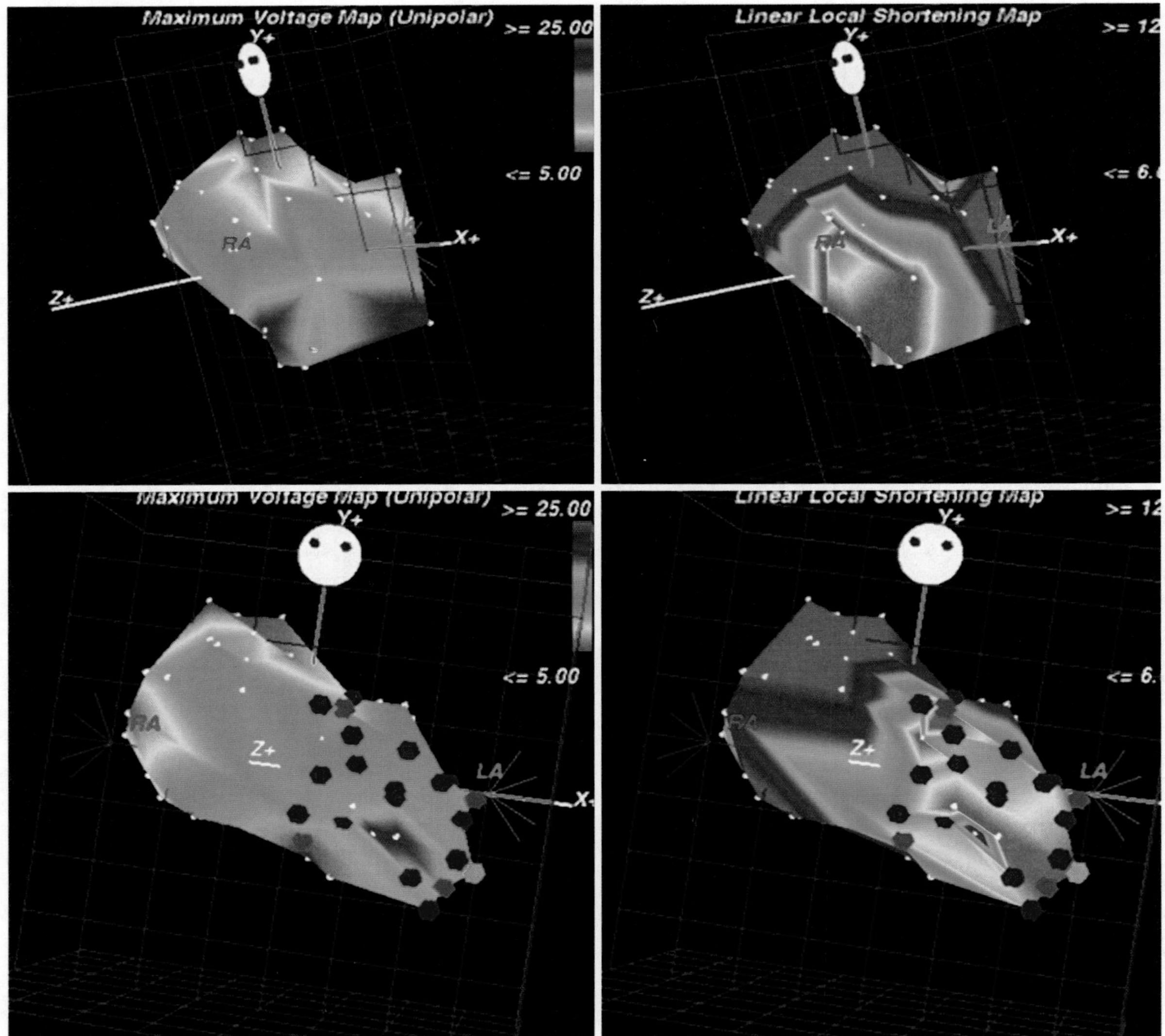

Fig. 8.2 Percuteneous laser myocardial revascularization using the Biosense NOGA mapping system with electrical (unipolar voltage maps, *left*) and mechanical (linear local shortening, *right*) maps. Location of catheter tip and mapping is performed by triangulation using three magnets placed under the patients and the strength of the magnetic field at catheter tip. Electrical maps show preserved voltage (viable tissue) with mechanical maps showing reduced local shortening (ischemic in *red*) myocardium. *Bottom panel* shows laser channels (*brown dots*) placed in area of reduced motion but preserved voltage

infarction, or coronary revascularization. In the intermediate-term follow-up, there was no change in the exercise time, SPECT score, angina symptoms, or quality of life [50].

In the Potential Angina Class Improvement From Intramyocardial Channels trial (PACIFIC trial), 221 unrevascularizable patients were randomized into Ho:YAG laser-based PTMR using the Cardiogenesis system [46]. The angina status at 6 months was improved by two or more classes in 46% of patients randomized to PTMR and in 6% of those treated conservatively ($p<0.001$), and the exercise duration increased correspondingly [46]. In a randomized trial of 325 no-option patients, in whom the Eclipse system was used, patients assigned to PTMR had an 85 s improvement in exercise time from baseline at 6 months post-procedure. This was compared with a 58 s decline among control subjects ($p<0.0001$). Angina improved

Table 8.4 Types of catheter based laser systems. Catheter based systems are no approved for clinical use. The only approved systems are the Carbon dioxide laser (Novadaq, Fl) and Sologrip III/Peal Lasers (Cardiogenesis, CA) Transmyocardial Laser Revascularization systems (epicardial)

	Biosense	Cardiogenesis	Eclipse
Guidance	Nonfluoroscopic	Fluoroscopic	Fluoroscopic
LV mapping	Yes	No	No
Laser catheter	7F shaft, 8F tip	6F laser, 9F aligning catheter	8.3F preformed
Energy	2 J/pulse X1	2 J/pulse X 4	0.7 J/pulse X3
Delivery	Single fiber 300 mcm	Single fiber 330 mcm	Multiple fibers
		1.75 mm lens	No lens

by two or more classes in 55% versus 31% of patients at 12 months, respectively, treated with PTMR and medications alone ($p<0.001$) [51]. A relatively smaller, randomized trial, the Blinded Evaluation of Laser Intervention Electively for Angina Pectoris study, using Eclipse-based PTMR compared with a blinded sham procedure in 82 no-option patients, provided results somewhat discordant with other experiences. Compared with the sham control group, PTMR resulted in a greater relief of angina at 6 months (≥2 class improvement in 41% vs 13%, $p=0.004$). The total exercise duration at 6 months increased by just 10 s in the PTMR arm and 7 s in the sham arm (p=NS). This suggested that the laser's photo-acoustic effect may reduce some patient's pain perception by denervation, without relieving ischemia or improving perfusion [52].

Conclusions and Future Directions

A preponderance of trials to date show symptomatic benefit from both TMR and PTMR techniques, particularly in patients with class IV angina. The objective assessment of increased perfusion in the infarct area will require studies with appropriate outcome measures such as delayed enhancement and dobutamine MRI or newer PET and Single Photon Emission Computed Tomography (SPECT) imaging modalities. It is not surprising that a mortality benefit is not detectable after TMR or percutaneous TMR (PTMR) given that percutaneous revascularization is not felt to offer mortality benefit in patients like these with preserved left ventricular function. The population of patients eligible for this procedure needs to be better defined as it may have changed significantly since the first trials of this technology in the late 1990s. For instance, patients with chronic totally occluded arteries until recently were considered "no-option" candidates. This has changed with the improved outcomes of chronic total occlusion recanalization [39]. A subset of these patients, however, might benefit from a combination approach of epicardial vessel revascularization in combination with percutaneous myocardial revascularization and/or possibly other angiogenic therapies. In addition percutaneous approach to the procedure will allow for blinded and properly controlled trials to be performed in the future that will eliminate confounding from the potent placebo effect in this "no-option" patient population.

References

1. Mirhoseini M, Cayton MM. Revascularization of the heart by laser. J Microsurg. 1981;2(4):253–60.
2. Horvath KA. Transmyocardial laser revascularization. Curr Treat Options Cardiovasc Med. 2004;6(1):53–9.
3. Jansen ED, Frenz M, Kadipasaoglu KA, et al. Laser-tissue interaction during transmyocardial laser revascularization. Ann Thorac Surg. 1997;63(3):640–7.
4. Fisher PE, Khomoto T, DeRosa CM, Spotnitz HM, Smith CR, Burkhoff D. Histologic analysis of transmyocardial channels: comparison of CO_2 and holmium:YAG lasers. Ann Thorac Surg. 1997;64(2):466–72.
5. Jones JW, Richman BW, Crigger NA, Baldwin JC. Technique of transmyocardial revascularization: avoiding complications in high-risk patients. J Cardiovasc Surg (Torino). 2001;42(3):353–7.
6. Jones JW, Schmidt SE, Richman BW, et al. Holmium:YAG laser transmyocardial revascularization relieves angina and improves functional status. Ann Thorac Surg. 1999;67(6):1596–601, discussion 601–2.
7. Izutani H, Gill IS, Svanidze O. Robotically assisted endoscopic transmyocardial laser revascularization. Can J Cardiol. 2004;20(9):907–9.
8. Horvath KA. Thoracoscopic transmyocardial laser revascularization. Ann Thorac Surg. 1998;65(5):1439–41.
9. Frazier OH, March RJ, Horvath KA. Transmyocardial revascularization with a carbon dioxide laser in patients with end-stage coronary artery disease. N Engl J Med. 1999;341(14):1021–8.
10. Schofield PM, Sharples LD, Caine N, et al. Transmyocardial laser revascularisation in patients with refractory angina: a randomised controlled trial. Lancet. 1999;353(9152):519–24.

11. Wehberg KE, Julian JS, Todd 3rd JC, Ogburn N, Klopp E, Buchness M. Improved patient outcomes when transmyocardial revascularization is used as adjunctive revascularization. Heart Surg Forum. 2003;6(5):328–30.
12. Peterson ED, Kaul P, Kaczmarek RG, et al. From controlled trials to clinical practice: monitoring transmyocardial revascularization use and outcomes. J Am Coll Cardiol. 2003; 42(9):1611–6.
13. Gassler N, Wintzer HO, Stubbe HM, Wullbrand A, Helmchen U. Transmyocardial laser revascularization. Histological features in human nonresponder myocardium. Circulation. 1997;95(2):371–5.
14. Hardy RI, Bove KE, James FW, Kaplan S, Goldman L. A histologic study of laser-induced transmyocardial channels. Lasers Surg Med. 1987;6(6):563–73.
15. Pelletier MP, Giaid A, Sivaraman S, et al. Angiogenesis and growth factor expression in a model of transmyocardial revascularization. Ann Thorac Surg. 1998;66(1):12–8.
16. Kohmoto T, DeRosa CM, Yamamoto N, et al. Evidence of vascular growth associated with laser treatment of normal canine myocardium. Ann Thorac Surg. 1998;65(5):1360–7.
17. Yamamoto N, Kohmoto T, Gu A, DeRosa C, Smith CR, Burkhoff D. Angiogenesis is enhanced in ischemic canine myocardium by transmyocardial laser revascularization. J Am Coll Cardiol. 1998;31(6):1426–33.
18. Domkowski PW, Biswas SS, Steenbergen C, Lowe JE. Histological evidence of angiogenesis 9 months after transmyocardial laser revascularization. Circulation. 2001;103(3):469–71.
19. Horvath KA, Chiu E, Maun DC, et al. Up-regulation of vascular endothelial growth factor mRNA and angiogenesis after transmyocardial laser revascularization. Ann Thorac Surg. 1999;68(3):825–9.
20. Chu VF, Giaid A, Kuang JQ, et al. Thoracic surgery directors association award. Angiogenesis in transmyocardial revascularization: comparison of laser versus mechanical punctures. Ann Thorac Surg. 1999;68(2):301–7, discussion 7–8.
21. Horvath KA, Belkind N, Wu I, et al. Functional comparison of transmyocardial revascularization by mechanical and laser means. Ann Thorac Surg. 2001;72(6):1997–2002.
22. Donovan CL, Landolfo KP, Lowe JE, Clements F, Coleman RB, Ryan T. Improvement in inducible ischemia during dobutamine stress echocardiography after transmyocardial laser revascularization in patients with refractory angina pectoris. J Am Coll Cardiol. 1997;30(3):607–12.
23. Frazier OHCD, Kadipasaoglu KA, Pehlivanoglu S, Lindenmeir M, Barasch E, Conger JL, et al. Myocardial revascularization with laser. Preliminary findings. Circulation. 1995;92(9 Suppl):II58–65.
24. Laham RJ, Simons M, Pearlman JD, Ho KK, Baim DS. Magnetic resonance imaging demonstrates improved regional systolic wall motion and thickening and myocardial perfusion of myocardial territories treated by laser myocardial revascularization. J Am Coll Cardiol. 2002; 39(1):1–8.
25. Rana JS, Mannam A, Donnell-Fink L, Gervino EV, Sellke FW, Laham RJ. Longevity of the placebo effect in the therapeutic angiogenesis and laser myocardial revascularization trials in patients with coronary heart disease. Am J Cardiol. 2005;95(12):1456–9.
26. Kwong KF, Kanellopoulos GK, Nickols JC, et al. Transmyocardial laser treatment denervates canine myocardium. J Thorac Cardiovasc Surg. 1997;114(6):883–9, discussion 9–90.
27. Al-Sheikh T, Allen KB, Straka SP, et al. Cardiac sympathetic denervation after transmyocardial laser revascularization. Circulation. 1999;100(2):135–40.
28. Minisi AJ, Topaz O, Quinn MS, Mohanty LB. Cardiac nociceptive reflexes after transmyocardial laser revascularization: implications for the neural hypothesis of angina relief. J Thorac Cardiovasc Surg. 2001;122(4):712–9.
29. Hughes GC, Lowe JE, Kypson AP, et al. Neovascularization after transmyocardial laser revascularization in a model of chronic ischemia. Ann Thorac Surg. 1998;66(6):2029–36.
30. Cherian SM, Bobryshev YV, Liang H, et al. Ultrastructural and immunohistochemical analysis of early myocardial changes following transmyocardial laser revascularization. J Card Surg. 2000;15(5):341–6.
31. Mack CA, Magovern CJ, Hahn RT, et al. Channel patency and neovascularization after transmyocardial revascularization using an excimer laser: results and comparisons to nonlased channels. Circulation. 1997;96(9 Suppl): II-65–9.
32. Allen KB, Dowling RD, Fudge TL, et al. Comparison of transmyocardial revascularization with medical therapy in patients with refractory angina. N Engl J Med. 1999;341(14): 1029–36.
33. Burkhoff D, Schmidt S, Schulman SP, et al. Transmyocardial laser revascularisation compared with continued medical therapy for treatment of refractory angina pectoris: a prospective randomised trial. ATLANTIC investigators. Angina treatments-lasers and normal therapies in comparison. Lancet. 1999;354(9182):885–90.
34. Burkhoff D, Wesley MN, Resar JR, Lansing AM. Factors correlating with risk of mortality after transmyocardial revascularization. J Am Coll Cardiol. 1999;34(1):55–61.
35. Guleserian KJ, Maniar HS, Camillo CJ, Bailey MS, Damiano Jr RJ, Moon MR. Quality of life and survival after transmyocardial laser revascularization with the holmium:YAG laser. Ann Thorac Surg. 2003;75(6):1842–7, discussion 7–8.
36. Krabatsch T, Petzina R, Hausmann H, Koster A, Hetzer R. Factors influencing results and outcome after transmyocardial laser revascularization. Ann Thorac Surg. 2002; 73(6):1888–92.
37. Mukherjee D, Bhatt DL, Roe MT, Patel V, Ellis SG. Direct myocardial revascularization and angiogenesis – how many patients might be eligible? Am J Cardiol. 1999;84(5):598–600, A8.
38. Allen KB, Dowling RD, Schuch DR, et al. Adjunctive transmyocardial revascularization: five-year follow-up of a prospective, randomized trial. Ann Thorac Surg. 2004; 78(2):458–65, discussion 465.
39. Stone GW, Teirstein PS, Rubenstein R, et al. A prospective, multicenter, randomized trial of percutaneous transmyocardial laser revascularization in patients with nonrecanalizable chronic total occlusions. J Am Coll Cardiol. 2002;39(10): 1581–7.
40. Aaberge L, Nordstrand K, Dragsund M, et al. Transmyocardial revascularization with CO_2 laser in patients with refractory angina pectoris clinical results from the Norwegian randomized trial. J Am Coll Cardiol. 2000;35(5):1170–7.
41. Aaberge L, Rootwelt K, Blomhoff S, Saatvedt K, Abdelnoor M, Forfang K. Continued symptomatic improvement three

to five years after transmyocardial revascularization with CO(2) laser: a late clinical follow-up of the Norwegian randomized trial with transmyocardial revascularization. J Am Coll Cardiol. 2002;39(10):1588–93.

42. Horvath KA, Aranki SF, Cohn LH, et al. Sustained angina relief 5 years after transmyocardial laser revascularization with a CO(2) laser. Circulation. 2001;104(12 Suppl 1): I81–4.
43. Spertus JA, Jones PG, Coen M, et al. Transmyocardial CO(2) laser revascularization improves symptoms, function, and quality of life: 12-month results from a randomized controlled trial. Am J Med. 2001;111(5):341–8.
44. van der Sloot JAHM, Tukkie R, Verberne HJ, van der Meulen J, van Eck-Smit BL, van Gemert MJ, et al. Transmyocardial revascularization using an XeCl excimer laser: results of a randomized trial. Ann Thorac Surg. 2004; 78(3):875–81.
45. Frazier OH, Tuzun E, Eichstadt H, et al. Transmyocardial laser revascularization as an adjunct to coronary artery bypass grafting: a randomized, multicenter study with 4-year follow-up. Tex Heart Inst J. 2004;31(3):231–9.
46. Oesterle SN, Sanborn TA, Ali N, et al. Percutaneous transmyocardial laser revascularisation for severe angina: the PACIFIC randomised trial. Potential class improvement from intramyocardial channels. Lancet. 2000;356(9243):1705–10.
47. Aaberge L, Aakhus S, Nordstrand K, Abdelnoor M, Ihlen H, Forfang K. Myocardial performance after transmyocardial revascularization with CO(2)laser. A dobutamine stress echocardiographic study. Eur J Echocardiogr. 2001;2(3):187–96.
48. Horvath KA, Cohn LH, Cooley DA, et al. Transmyocardial laser revascularization: results of a multicenter trial with transmyocardial laser revascularization used as sole therapy for end-stage coronary artery disease. J Thorac Cardiovasc Surg. 1997;113(4):645–53, discussion 653–4.
49. Burns SM, Brown S, White CA, Tait S, Sharples L, Schofield PM. Quantitative analysis of myocardial perfusion changes with transmyocardial laser revascularization. Am J Cardiol. 2001;87(7):861–7.
50. Leon MB, Kornowski R, Downey WE, et al. A blinded, randomized, placebo-controlled trial of percutaneous laser myocardial revascularization to improve angina symptoms in patients with severe coronary disease. J Am Coll Cardiol. 2005;46(10):1812–9.
51. Whitlow PL, DeMaio Jr SJ, Perin EC, et al. One-year results of percutaneous myocardial revascularization for refractory angina pectoris. Am J Cardiol. 2003;91(11):1342–6.
52. Salem M, Rotevatn S, Stavnes S, Brekke M, Vollset SE, Nordrehaug JE. Usefulness and safety of percutaneous myocardial laser revascularization for refractory angina pectoris. Am J Cardiol. 2004;93(9):1086–91.

Invasive and Device Management of Refractory Angina

9

E. Marc Jolicoeur, Gregory W. Barsness, and Martial G. Bourassa

Introduction

Within the last 20 years, aggressive coronary revascularization and medical therapies have enabled the emergence of a large population of symptomatic patients who have exhausted all therapeutic options. Paradoxically, only one new anti-angina medication has been approved by the USA Food and Drug administration during the same period. New therapeutic options are needed. Classically, anti-angina medications reduce myocardial oxygen demand by reducing heart rate, left ventricular contractility or left ventricular wall tension. Similarly, coronary revascularization increases myocardial oxygen supply by improving coronary blood flow. Invasive interventions in general and devices in particular propose novel solutions to modulate myocardial ischemia and pain transmission in patients with refractory angina.

E.M. Jolicoeur (✉)
Montreal Heart Institute, Université de Montréal, Montreal, QC, Canada
e-mail: marc.jolicoeur@icm-mhi.org

G.W. Barsness
Mayo Clinic College of Medicine, Rochester, MN, USA

M.G. Bourassa
Montreal Heart Institute, Université de Montréal, Montreal, QC, Canada

The Unrevascularizable Patient

The concept of the "unrevascularizable" patient is complex. A patient may not be amenable to percutaneous coronary intervention (PCI) or coronary artery bypass surgery (CABG) because of severe comorbidities or impracticable coronary anatomy. One important lesson learned from the therapeutic angiogenesis trials performed in the 1990s is that the state of being unfit for revascularization may be temporary and must be reassessed periodically by a competent heart team [1]. As novel technologies emerge, the risk–benefit ratio may be altered in favor of revascularization. A recent example is the use of retrograde recanalization of chronic total occlusion (CTO), a technique that allows high recanalization rates in selected cases [2]. Likewise, patients previously labelled as "no-option" or "unrevascularizable" can suddenly become suitable for revascularization because of their changing medical condition. In some cases, symptomatic exacerbations may be explained by disease progression in previously unaffected coronary beds. In selected cases, these new or progressing coronary lesions may be amenable to revascularization. Independent groups have observed revascularization rates up to 30% at 5 years in cohorts of unrevascularizable patients [3–5].

Chronic Total Occlusion Percutaneous Coronary Interventions

A coronary artery is said to be chronically occluded when its flow is completely obstructed for a period longer than 3 months [6]. Chronic total occlusions (CTOs) are frequent in patients with symptomatic

G.W. Barsness and D.R. Holmes Jr. (eds.), *Coronary Artery Disease*,
DOI 10.1007/978-1-84628-712-1_9, © Springer-Verlag London Limited 2012

angina. In contemporary series, CTOs were seen in nearly 30% of diagnostic coronary angiograms [7]. Because of higher procedural risk and reduced likelihood of success, coronary intervention is infrequently performed to treat these lesions. Most often, patients with a CTO are either treated medically or sent to CABG surgery [8]. Still, a successful CTO recanalization by PCI offers potential benefits such as left ventricular function improvement [9, 10] and improved survival [11, 12].

No less than 10 observational studies have described the association between CTO intervention and outcomes in the stent era [11, 13–21]. These retrospective CTO studies significantly diverged in terms of the populations studied. This heterogeneity makes it difficult to fully appreciate the consequence of a CTO recanalization on cardiovascular outcomes. Still, it is reasonable to believe that in selected populations, a successful CTO recanalization could reduce angina. In the prospective Total Occlusion Angioplasty Study–Società Italiana di Cardiologia Invasiva (TOAST-GISE), successful PCI of a CTO was associated with increased freedom from angina at 12 months (88.7% versus 75.0%; $p=0.008$) [18]. In a recent pooled analysis of 6 observational studies, successful CTO recanalization was associated with a striking reduction in residual or recurrent angina when compared to failed CTO recanalization (OR 0.45, 95% CI 0.30–0.67). Interestingly, in the same pooled analysis, successful CTO recanalization was not associated with a reduction in myocardial infarction or major adverse cardiovascular events. This lack of an associated prognostic benefit with CTO revascularization may be related to differing prognostic effects based on anatomic CTO location. A recent retrospective analysis of patients treated for refractory angina at the Mayo Clinic suggested such a heterogenous impact of CTO location, with an unrevascularized LAD CTO found to confer increased risk for poor long-term survival compared with occlusions in other territories [22]. Ongoing research may further identify high-risk cohorts with greater potential for benefit with CTO revascularization.

While the interest in CTO recanalization is growing, the benefit of a therapeutic strategy of percutaneous revascularization has never been tested in a randomized clinical investigation. Historically, randomized trials in these patients have been difficult to conduct because of variable PCI success rates and a higher likelihood of procedural complications. This situation may change soon with improvements in wire technologies and the introduction of retrograde CTO PCI techniques which are associated with safely achieving revascularization rates above 90% [2, 23]. However, until this direct proof of benefit is available, CTO intervention is likely to remain a procedure performed by only a few specialized interventional cardiologists. Currently, practice guidelines propose reserving CTO intervention to patients remaining symptomatic despite optimal medical therapy and with a large ischemic area in the myocardial segment perfused by an occluded coronary artery [24].

Low-Energy Extracorporeal Shock Wave Therapy

Low-energy extracorporeal shock wave therapy (ESWT) is emerging as an option for the treatment of various ischemic syndromes, including advanced coronary artery disease and peripheral vascular disease. A shock wave is a longitudinal acoustic wave generated from a single brief, high-amplitude pressure pulse that can easily travel through body tissue and be focally converged toward one spot of interest. This property of shock waves makes them ideal to treat conditions where mechanical stress needs to be focally applied, such as the lithotripsy of kidney stones or calcifying tendinitis. During shock wave therapy, two mechanistic phenomena work synergistically to create a local effect: the stress wave, which transmits energy directly to the field, and the cavitation effect, which occurs in situ. In response to an acoustic field, microbubbles in a liquid will naturally oscillate. Cavitation occurs when the intensity of the acoustic field is such that the bubbles collapse. Clinical experience with lithotripsy suggests that shock waves exert a differential effect on resilient and calcified tissues. While high-energy shock wave therapy can fragment stones, it has been shown to cause minimal damage to resilient tissues such as skin and internal organs. Low-energy ESWT for the heart typically utilizes one tenth of the dose used for the kidney lithotripsy.

In the heart, the cavitation effect occurs both inside and outside of the myocytes [25]. At the cellular level, the stress wave and cavitation resulting from a shock wave are thought to induce local shear stress which promotes the expression of proangiogenic factors [26]. In vitro and in vivo experiments have established that

ESWT induces myocytes and endothelial cells to produce nitric oxide (NO) and vascular endothelial growth factor (VEGF) [27–30]. Nishida et al. applied shock waves to cultured human umbilical endothelial cells (HUVEC) and determined that 0.09 mJ/mm^2 was the energy level where VEGF was optimally expressed [30]. Recently, Aicher et al. observed that ESWT enhanced tissue expression of stromal cell-derived factor 1 (SDF-1). In a rat model of chronic hind-limb ischemia, this resulted in a superior recruitment of endothelial progenitor cells in situ [28]. Based on these observations, it has been hypothesized that ESWT mobilizes endothelial progenitor cells and favors angiogenesis. However, this hypothesis could not be validated in a small group of patients with refractory angina treated by ESWT [31]. In a porcine model of chronic ischemic cardiomyopathy, left ventricular ejection fraction and regional blood flow recovered completely in animals subjected to ESWT. By contrast, animals not treated with ESWT in this study suffered progressive ventricular failure with deficient myocardial blood flow [30].

Original clinical investigations originating from Japan and Europe included low-dose shock wave therapy for patients with advanced coronary artery disease not amenable to revascularization. Overall, the clinical experience available to date suggests that ESWT improves myocardial perfusion where it is applied. Globally, less than 100 patients have been recruited into studies of this technology, most of which were case-series or case-control studies [31–38]. Only one randomized controlled trial is available to suggest that ESWT is better than placebo at improving anginal symptoms and at reducing the use of short-acting nitrates [31]. In this trial, ESWT significantly improved the 6-min walk test distance. Most [33, 35, 37, 38] but not all [36] mechanistic studies suggest that ESWT improves myocardial perfusion.

While a limited number of patients have been treated with low-dose cardiac ESWT, the technology appears safe. Early ex vivo studies performed on aortic specimens of healthy subjects have shown that shock waves administered at theoretically destructive levels did not cause macroscopic or histologic damage [39]. What remains unknown is how plaque-laden arterial walls or left ventricular mural thrombi will react to shock wave therapy. Until additional safety information is available, patients with a left ventricular thrombus should not be treated with shock waves. Except for one patient [33], ESWT does not seem to induce myocardial microinjury, as assessed by troponin rise immediately post-therapy [35]. There is a theoretical concern that shock waves may induce malignant ventricular arrhythmias if reaching the heart during myocardial repolarization. To avoid this problem, most systems are ECG-gated to assure a delivery of the impulse on the R wave, during the absolute electrical refractory period.

Unlike most of the interventions presented in this chapter, ESWT is noninvasive. ESWT is therefore an interesting option to treat fragile patients who would not tolerate or accept invasive options. Many questions must be answered before ESWT is ready for clinical use. The optimal number of treatment sessions and the optimal number of shock waves per session remain unknown. As was the case for enhanced external counterpulsation (EECP), the performance of placebo-controlled trials appears challenging since most patients feel compression and pain resulting from the pressure pulse induced by the shock wave [32, 36]. One solution currently used by clinical trialists has been to deliver the shock waves outside the heart field in patients randomized to the control group. As of 2011, at least 5 distinct trials are testing ESWT in various populations with unrevascularizable heart disease [40]. In our present era of evidence-based medicine, there is not enough proof of efficacy to recommend the use of ESWT for the care of patients experiencing refractory angina and myocardial ischemia. Until additional efficacy is available, low-energy shock waves should not be administered to patients outside the context of a properly powered clinical investigation. Still, the apparent safety profile and ease of administration of ESWT are two factors that should accelerate the development of this technology.

Temporary Cardiac Sympathectomy

The stellate ganglion, also known as the cervicothoracic ganglion, is part of a paravertebral trunk that brings sympathetic efferent nerves to thoracic structures, including the heart. Afferent sympathetic fibers originating from the stellate ganglion are primarily noradrenergic neurons. Postganglionic fibers leaving the cervical and thoracic ganglions split into a complex interconnecting network that reaches either the heart or the intrinsic cardiac ganglia. This network is essential for the mediation of cardio-cardiac reflexes. Anatomically, sympathetic afferents are predominant on the left side, which explains the preponderance of left stellate blockade in medical practice.

There is no known nociceptor nerve ending in the heart. Current evidence suggests that the sympathetic nerves are the main afferent pathway transmitting cardiac pain signals to the central nervous system. Sympathetic afferent nerves therefore have a double-sense innervation. The pain signal coming from the heart is brought by sympathetic efferent fibers that converge at cervical and stellate ganglia. These fibers subsequently reach the intermediolateral gray column in the upper thoracic spinal cord, mostly between T2 and T6. Ultimately, the pain signal reaches the central nervous system via spinothalamic tracts.

The left stellate ganglion is an interesting target to control heart pain because an important portion of sympathetic nerves synapse there. The analgesic effect of sympathetectomy has been known since the end of the seventeenth century. The first surgical sympathectomy to treat angina was reported in 1916 by Jonnesco [41]. As early as 1966, Wiener compared stellate ganglion blockade (SGB) to placebo for the control of angina [42]. Alternate routes for temporary sympathectomy have been used, including high thoracic epidural analgesia. The mechanism of action of SGB remains unknown. How a short acting local anesthetic agent can provide prolonged pain relief remains unknown. Reversal of central sensitization and related persistent pain mechanisms have been advanced as potential mechanisms [43]. A substantial placebo effect is possible, as is often the case with invasive interventions used to treat chronic pain disorders [44].

Stellate ganglion blockade has typically been performed for noncardiac sympathetic-mediated pain, such as reflex sympathetic dystrophy. In this setting, meta-analyses have suggested that temporary sympathetic blockade with an analgesic agent was not better than placebo to relieve chronic pain resulting from reflex sympathetic dystrophy and causalgia [45, 46]. The efficacy of temporary cardiac sympathectomy to relieve angina has never been tested against placebo in a randomized trial. This lack of evidence calls into question the legitimacy of this treatment for refractory angina.

Anecdotal reports indicate an incremental improvement in efficacy when left stellate ganglion blockades are repeated. Classically, the first blockade relieves chest pain for 2 to 6 weeks. Subsequent blockade relieves chest pain for up to 4 months [47]. The largest prospective cohort included 59 unrevascularizable patients treated with either left stellate or paravertebral blockade [43]. In this study, 15 ml of 0.5% bupivacaine was used for all blockades. Patients were recruited from a large clinic specializing in the care of refractory angina. Patients with Syndrome X, or microvascular angina, were excluded. On average, left SGB relieved angina for 3.5 weeks (SD ± 3.4 weeks) after the inaugural injection. The overall response rate was 67%, and nearly half of the patients were treated with 4 or more blockades. No serious complication was observed. Of note, no hypotension was observed despite the frequent use of antihypertensive medication in this population. Theoretically, prolonged sympathectomy [48] or even permanent sympathectomy [49] could be envisioned among patients responsive to temporary sympathectomy but with recurrent anginal symptoms.

The left stellate ganglion is readily accessible and blockades are generally done as outpatient procedures. The overall strategy is relatively inexpensive, but repetitive injections are often needed for sustained efficacy. Despite the lack of randomized controlled trials, SGB is still being performed in selected centers. In the largest series reported to date, complication rates ranged from 0.2% to 3%, mostly driven by vertigo, hypotension, frozen shoulder, and local hematoma [43, 50]. Dramatic complications have been reported including cardio-respiratory arrest, esophageal puncture, lock-in syndrome, vertebral artery puncture, and retropharyngeal hematoma [51–57]. Temporary cardiac sympathectomy should be performed by appropriately trained physicians under X-ray or echocardiographic guidance. Patients subjected to temporary cardiac sympathectomy should be enrolled in prospective clinical investigations.

Neuromodulation and Spinal Cord Stimulation

In the cardiac sympathectomy section, we have reviewed the neuroanatomical pathways of cardiac pain transmission. In response to chemical or mechanical stimuli, nociceptive signals are transmitted by afferent sympathetic fibers to the spinal cord. At this level, the afferent sympathetic fibers synapse with

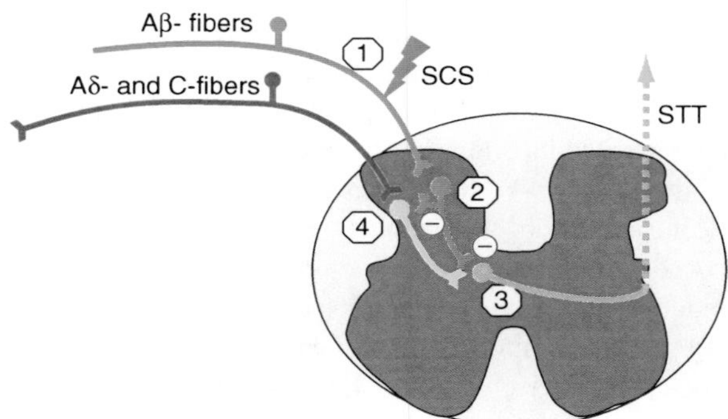

Fig. 9.1 Proposed spinal cord stimulation (SCS) mechanism. (1) Electrical impulses delivered at the spine via the SCS generator activate low-threshold, large diameter Aβ- fibers. (2) Dorsal horn inhibitory GABA-nergic or cholinergic interneurons, through Aβ- fiber synapse activation, (3) release neurotransmitters (e.g., GABA, acetylcholine) to reduce spinal projection neuron excitability in the spinothalamic tract, (4) thereby reducing Aδ and C pain fiber activity. *SCS* spinal cord stimulation, *GABA* gamma-aminobutyric acid, *STT*, spinothalamic tract. (Reproduced with permission: Prager [58])

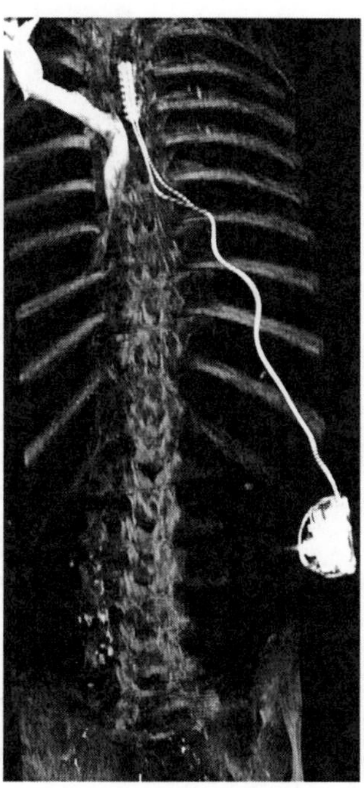

Fig. 9.2 Computed tomographic documentation of spinal cord stimulator placement for chronic pain syndrome. The generator location is noted at the left abdomen, with the subcutaneously tunneled electrode lead seen coursing to the upper thoracic and lower cervical spinal location. In treating chronic refractory angina, electrodes are generally located at the C6-T2 vertebral level. (Reproduced with permission: Zan et al. [61])

second-order sensory neurons in the dorsal horns. As is the case with the stellate ganglia, the dorsal horn is a point of information convergence that is readily accessible and therefore amenable to therapeutic intervention (Fig. 9.1).

In 1965, Melzack and Wall introduced the gate control theory [59], which served as a rationale for the use of neuromodulation to treat cardiac pain syndromes. The contemporary view of the gate control theory assumes that the stimulation of the large afferent non-nociceptive A-alpha and A-beta fibers by spinal cord stimulation (SCS) can stop the transmission of the nociceptive impulse in the small afferent A-delta and C fibers to the central nervous system.

Transmission of nociceptive signals in the spinal cord is modulated by descending inhibitory pathways coming from central regulatory centers such as the sensory cortex, the hypothalamic region, and the periaqueductal gray region. At the dorsal horn level, imbalance between afferent transmission and central modulation can result in an appropriate passage of lower threshold pain signals. The effect of the descending inhibitory pathways on the dorsal horn varies according to the local chemical environment. SCS is thought to alter the dorsal horn neurochemistry, which subsequently affects the pain signal transmission. SCS has been shown to promote the release of γ-Aminobutyric acid (GABA) at the spinal level. GABA counteracts the effect of the descending inhibitory pathways which normally favor the passage of nociceptive signals to the brain [60]. Conversely, other local factors such as glutamate and β-endorphin can decrease the effect of GABA on descending inhibitory pathways.

Neuromodulation of the anginal signal can be performed either with transcutaneous electrical nerve stimulation (TENS) or SCS. TENS is now infrequently used in patients with refractory angina because of electrode-related skin irritation. Spinal cord stimulation is performed with a minimally invasive epidural electrode positioned at the C6-T2 vertebrae level, under local anesthesia (Fig. 9.2). The pulse generator connects to the epidural electrode by a subcutaneous extension. The pulse generator is entirely subcutaneously implantable, most frequently in the upper left abdominal region. From the pulse generator, stimulation parameters can be optimized for each patient by adjusting the amplitude (V), the pulse width (μs), and the frequency (Hz). Some groups

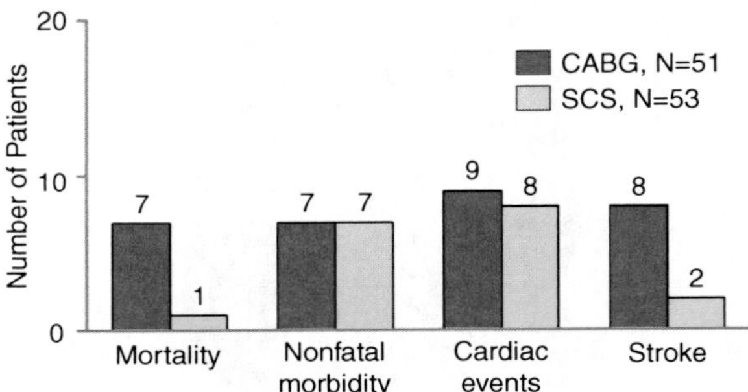

Fig. 9.3 Six-month major adverse cardiac events among 104 patients randomized to spinal cord stimulation (SCS) or coronary artery bypass grafting (*CABG*) in the Electrical Stimulation versus Coronary Artery Bypass Surgery in Severe Angina Pectoris (*ESPY*) study. All patients had symptomatic coronary artery disease and were felt to be at increased risk for CABG (cerebrovascular disease, unfavorable coronary arterial anatomy, diabetes mellitus, left ventricular ejection fraction < 40%, peripheral arterial disease, prior CABG, and/or renal dysfunction) but unsuitable for percutaneous coronary intervention. Angina relief was significant and similar between groups (data not shown). Overall 6-month events were not significantly different between groups ($p = 0.08$), although mortality and cerebrovascular morbidity were significantly less among those subjects randomized to SCS ($p = 0.02$ and $p = 0.03$, respectively). (Modified from: Mannheimer et al. 12 [67])

have recommended using TENS before the actual pulse generator implantation to screen for patients likely to respond to SCS.

In a series of small randomized controlled trials, SCS has been compared to medical therapy, enhanced external counterpulsation (EECP), and even CABG surgery [62–66] (Fig. 9.3 and Table 9.1). These studies have been systematically reviewed in two distinct meta-analyses [74, 75]. Overall, the quality of available trials varied considerably. When looking exclusively at randomized controlled trials (7 trials, 270 patients), SCS was associated with an improved total exercise time compared to no spinal cord stimulation (standardized mean difference = 0.76, 95% CI = 0.07–1.46, $p = 0.03$) [74]. SCS was also associated with an improved quality of life (standardized mean difference = 0.83, 95% CI = 0.32–1.34, $p = 0.001$). Complementary evidence also suggests that SCS may be equally effective in the subgroup of patients with cardiac Syndrome X [76, 77]. SCS might be associated with a significant placebo effect, although the persistent beneficial SCS effect seen in several series beyond 1 year argues against this as the primary mode of action [62, 78].

In registries, SCS has been associated with fewer anginal attacks, reduced nitrate consumption, and improved quality of life. Registries may provide important efficacy information in a real-world environment. In the Prospective Italian Registry of SCS for Angina Pectoris, 73% of the patients treated with SCS experienced improvement in their anginal symptoms (≥50% reduction of weekly angina episodes) [79]. Interestingly, 80% improved more than one Canadian Cardiovascular Society (CCS) class, and 42% improved more than two CCS classes. While impressive, similar figures have been observed in the past in the placebo arms of controlled trials testing new invasive technology for refractory angina [80, 81]. In this registry, none of the factors measured at baseline could be used to discriminate SCS responders from nonresponders. In the European Angina Registry Link (EARL) study, all refractory angina patients referred for SCS over a 3-year period were prospectively followed [78, 82]. Ten European sites participated in the study. Of the 235 patients referred for SCS, 121 were actually treated with the permanent device after being deemed responsive to temporary SCS or transcutaneous electric nerve stimulation (TENS). On average, patients were followed up for 12.1 months. Implanted patients reported fewer angina attacks and reduced short-acting nitrate consumption. Before SCS, 71.9% of the patients experienced daily anginal episodes, as compared to only 25.6% twelve months later. Impressively, quality of life significantly improved in every single aspect captured by the Short Form 36 (SF-36) and the Seattle Angina Questionnaire (SAQ). Of note, only patients with complete follow-up were included in the efficacy analysis. This may have led to an overestimation of efficacy, as nonresponders may have been more likely to drop out.

The antianginal effect of SCS is not completely understood. In addition to pain modulation as described above, it has been proposed that SCS could relieve angina by actually reducing myocardial ischemia. During ambulatory ECG monitoring, de Jongste et al. observed a significant reduction in median total ST-segment depression after SCS (27.9 mm × min [IQR: 1.9 to 278.2] before SCS vs. 0 mm × min [0 to 70.2] after SCS, $p < 0.03$). When present, ischemic episodes were also shorter in duration (20.6 min [IQR: 1.7 to 155.4] before SCS vs. 0 min [IQR: 0 to 48.3] after SCS, $p < 0.03$) [83]. The reduction in ischemic burden measured by ambulatory monitoring has been

Table 9.1 Selected contemporary devices studies in refractory angina

Study, year	Study design, (n) Investigational device	Specifications	Key inclusion criteria	Principal findings	Comments
Extracorporeal shock wave therapy					
Fukumoto et al.2005 [32]	Case-series, (n=9) Modulith SLC, (Storz Medical)	3 sessions/w, 200 shoots/spot at 0.09 mJ/mm^2 for 20–40 spots a session	Angina despite optimal medical therapy, unrevascularizable CAD by consensus[a]	ESWT associated with improved CCS angina class and short-acting nitrates use; these effects persisted for 1 year. No acute or long-term side effects reported	Patients with left ventricle thrombus, diabetic retinopathy, or recent malignant tumor were excluded from the trial. ESWT improved the myocardial perfusion focally where it was applied. Paradoxically, myocardial perfusion tended to deteriorate in untreated area. Exercise tolerance was not improved by ESWT
Gutersohn et al. 2006 [37]	Case-control, (n=34) Modified Minilith, (Storz Medical)	Cases: ESWT 3 x 1800 impulses at 0.1 mJ/mm^2 Controls: PMLR using the Axcis laser system	End-stage CAD	ESWT associated with improved myocardial perfusion measured by SPECT in 70% of the patients. PMLR did not improve myocardial perfusion	Abstract. Unlike PMLR, ESWT could be performed on every patient enrolled in the study
Khattab et al. 2007 [33]	Case-series, (n=10) Modulith SLC, (Storz Medical)	9 sessions in 3 cycles over 3 m	CCS III or IV despite optimal medical therapy, unrevascularizable CAD on a recent angiogram	ESWT associated with improved angina and myocardial ischemia in 6 out of 8 patients. Therapy discontinued in two patients because of pain and troponin elevation	One death observed 4 weeks after therapy. Myocardial ischemia was assessed by Tc [68] SPECT perfusion scans
Wang et al. 2010 [36]	Case-series, (n=9) Modulith SLC, (Storz Medical)	9 sessions in 3 cycles over 3 m. Each ischemic region treated at 9 points at 0.09 mJ/mm^2	Unstable refractory angina despite optimal medical therapy and recent PCI	ESWT associated with improved CCS angina class and short-acting nitrates use. Myocardial perfusion index measured by stress echo not improved in response to ESWT. No acute or long-term side effects reported	Because patients with unstable angina were enrolled, this case-series may be confounded by the regression to the mean (nadir) bias
Vasyuk et al. 2010 [35]	Case-series, (n=24) Cardiospect, (Medispect)	9 sessions in 3 cycles over 3 m, 100 shocks per spot at 0.09 mJ/mm^2	Chronic stable ischemic heart failure with LVEF<40%, no planned revascularization	ESWT associated with a modest improvement in LVEF at 3 and 6 months after therapy. Clinically, ESWT improved both the NYHA and the CCS classes. No troponin rises were measured after therapy	Patients received optimal medical therapy for CHF. ESWT targeted at hibernating/ischemic segments detected by stress echocardiography. Four patients died during the 6 months follow-up
Faber et al. 2010 [38]	Case-series, (n=16)	9 sessions, over 9w, 500 shocks per session	CCS III or IV angina despite optimal medical therapy, unrevascularizable CAD	ESWT associated with improved angina CCS class 14 patients. Regional myocardial blood flow measured by NH3-PET scan improved significantly in the targeted LV region	

(continued)

Table 9.1 (continued)

Study, year	Study design, (n) Investigational device	Specifications	Key inclusion criteria	Principal findings	Comments
Kikuchi et al. 2010 [31]	Double-blind cross-over RCT, (n=8) Modulith SLC, (Storz Medical)	200 shoots/spot at 0.09 mJ/mm^2 for 40–60 spots a session vs. sham ESWT	Angina despite optimal medical therapy, unrevascularizable CAD by consensus[a]	ESWT better than sham at improving CCS angina class and short-acting nitrates use. ESWT improved 6MWT. No acute or long-term side effects reported	The wash-out period between cross-over may have been inappropriately short (3 m) for patients initially treated with ESWT; beneficial effect persisting over 1 y have been seen in previous study. Statistical design not appropriate for cross-over trial. Exercise tolerance may have been underestimated because of the high prevalence of peripheral arterial disease in the study population
Temporary cardiac sympathectomy					
Moore et al. 2005 [43]	Prospective cohort, (n=59) Left stellate or paravertebral blockade	Single or repetitive paravertebral injections of 15 ml of 0.5% bupivacaine	Unrevascularizable CAD by consensus[a]. Patients with syndrome X excluded	The pain relief lasted on average 3.5 w (SD 3.4w) after the first blockade. The overall response rate was 67% with left stellate and 52% with paravertebral blockade	A two-week pain relief was used as a cut-off to define responders eligible for additional blockade. 52% patients underwent ≥ 4 treatment cycles. Overnight hospital stay was never required because of a complication
Spinal cord stimulation					
De Jongste et al. 1994 [62]	Open-label RCT, (n=17) SCS vs. medical therapy	SCS 1 h, 3 times/d for 8 w, 210 ms pulse width, 85 cycle/s, intensity set to paresthesia threshold	CCS III or IV angina despite optimal medical therapy, unrevascularizable CAD	SCS better than medical therapy at improving treadmill exercise duration and quality of life	After 8 weeks, patients initially randomized to medical therapy were cross-over to SCS and followed up for 1 y. SCS was associated with a persistent beneficial effect. Two patients had electrode dislodgement requiring intervention
Hautvast et al. 1998 [64]	Open label RCT, (n=25) Itrel, (Medtronic)	SCS 1 h, 3 times/d + on demand vs. medical therapy	CCS III or IV angina despite optimal medical therapy, unrevascularizable CAD	SCS better than medical therapy at improving treadmill exercise duration and time to angina	SCS was associated with a reduced ischemic burden on 48-h electrocardiogram and with an improved perception in quality of life

ESBY 1998 [67]	Open label RCT, (n=104) Itrel, (Medtronic)	SCS 2 h, 4 times/d vs. CABG	Patients with a symptomatic indication for CABG but unsuitable for complete revascularization by PCI	No differences between SCS and CABG with respect to angina frequency and short-acting nitrates consumption. Both treatments associated with long-lasting quality-of-life improvment [69]	Patients randomized to CABG had a better exercise capacity with lesser ST-segment depression on comparable workloads. Seven deaths occurred in the CABG group compared to 1 in the SCS group. Fifteen patients not available for follow-up
Jessurun et al. 1999 [70]	Cross-over RCT, (n=24)	SCS 1 h, 3 times/d+on demand vs. SCS discontinuation	Patients with angina chronically treated with SCS (>3 years)	SCS withdrawal did not significantly increase the frequency of ischemic events or the total ischemic burden	Study underpowered to detect clinically relevant differences. Study suggests however that SCS can be safely withdrawn after long-term administration
SPiRiT 2006 [66]	Open label RCT, (n=68)	SCS 1 h, 3 times/d vs. PMLR (Holmium: YAG laser)	CCS III despite optimal medical therapy, unrevascularizable CAD by consensus[a]. Reversible myocardial ischemia	SCS did not significantly improve the total exercise time compared to PMLR at 12 months	A numerically greater proportion of patients treated with SCS improved of at least two CCS angina class at 3 months (37% vs. 15%, p=0.07)
Eddicks et al. 2007 [63]	Cross-over RCT, (n=12) Itrell and synergy, (Medtronic)	4 consecutive treatments, each lasting 4 w: A) conventional 3 x 2 h/d, B) conventional 24 h/d, C) subliminal 3 x 2 h/d, D) Sham 0.1 mV 24 h/d	CCS III or IV angina despite optimal medical therapy, unrevascularizable CAD	Walking distance on the 6MWT did not significantly differ between treatment arm A, B, and C, but sham (0.1 V) was inferior. A greater number of patients treated with sham stimulation experienced angina	Pilot study. Treatment allocation and concealment not specified. No wash-out observed between treatments. Trial critically underpowered to detect statistical difference between conventional and subliminal spinal cord stimulation
SCS-ITA 2011 [65]	RCT, single-blind, 3-arms , (n=25)	Conventional SCS vs. subliminal SCS vs. sham	Reversible myocardial ischemia, unrevascularizable CAD	At 1 month, Conventional SCS was better than placebo but not than subliminal SCS at reducing angina episodes. Similar results were observed for nitrate consumption and CCS class	Partial cross-over design, as patients randomized to sham were switched to either paresthesic of subliminal SCS after 1 m. Trial critically underpowered to detect efficacy difference between subliminal and conventional SCS

(continued)

Table 9.1 (continued)

Study, year	Study design, (n) Investigational device	Specifications	Key inclusion criteria	Principal findings	Comments
Coronary sinus occlusion					
Banai et al. 2007 [71]	Case-series, (n = 15), Reducer, (Neovasc)	Stainless steel balloon-expandable stent implanted into the coronary sinus	CCS III or IV angina despite optimal medical therapy, unrevascularizable CAD, reversible myocardial ischemia, LVEF > 30%	No device-related major adverse cardiac events were noted at 6 months. Twelve out of the 14 treated patients improved their angina of at least one CCS class	Stress-induced ST-segment depression was reduced in 8 of the 9 subjects tested. Myocardial ischemia quantified by dobutamine echocardiography was significantly reduced compared to baseline
Percutaneous in situ coronary venous arterializations					
Oesterle et al. 2003 [72]	Case-series, (n = 11) TransVascular system	Self-expanding noncovered stent + venous occlusion with customized device	CCS III or IV angina, unrevascularizable CAD	Procedure performed in only 6 of the 11 selected cases. Among attempted subjects, 2 procedural deaths,and 2 tamponades occurred	
Percutaneous myocardial cryotreatment					
Gallo et al. 2009 [73]	Case-series, (n = 20) Freezor catheter, (Cryocath technologies)	10 IM Cryoapplications (at − 50 °C for 2 min), in one area of ischemic myocardium	CCS III or IV angina despite optimal medical therapy, unrevascularizable CAD, reversible myocardial ischemia, LVEF > 40%	Procedure successful in 16 patients; 3 procedural complication occurred, including one pericardial tamponade, one pericardial effusion, and one VT episode	16 patients improved their angina symptoms at 6 m. The total exercise time and the quality of life improved significantly compared to baseline. There was no improvement in myocardial ischemia quantified by 99 m dipyridamole SPECT

[a]Both the cardiologist and the cardiac surgeon had to agree that revascularization was not possible

6MWT 6 minutes walk test, *CABG* coronary artery bypass graft, *CAD* coronary artery disease, *CCS* Canadian Cardiovascular Society, *CHF* congestive heart failure, *D* day, *ESWT* extracorporeal shock wave therapy, *H* hour, *IM* intramyocardial, *LV* left ventricle, *LVEF* left ventricle ejection fraction, *M* month, *min* minutes, *mJ* milli-joules, *NYHA* New-York Heart Association, *PCI* percutaneous coronary intervention, *PET* positron emission tomography, *PMLR* percutaneous myocardial laser revascularization, *RCT* randomized controlled trial, *SCS* spinal cord stimulation, *SD* standard deviation, *SPECT* single photon emission computed tomography, *VT* ventricular tachycardia, *W* weeks validated by an independent group [82]. The mechanism for myocardial ischemia reduction is not known but could involve changes in myocardial blood flow. In response to SCS, Hautvast et al. observed a reduction in the perfusion gradient between ischemic and nonischemic myocardial segments [84]. Because total myocardial perfusion remained identical before and after SCS, Hautvast et al. hypothesized that SCS modulates a redistribution of blood flow toward underperfused myocardial segments. It has been hypothesized from earlier TENS studies that a sympathicolytic effect resulting from spinal cord stimulation could indirectly reduce myocardial ischemia [85, 86]. The association between SCS and reduction of myocardial ischemia, however, has not been consistent [87–89]. Additionally, all studies suggesting an anti-ischemic effect of SCS were small and uncontrolled. For these reasons, SCS should not be claimed to reduce myocardial ischemia until larger clinical investigations are available.

A limited number of trials have assessed healthcare utilization associated with SCS. Of the two studies available, one study, published in 1998, compared SCS to coronary artery bypass graft (CABG) surgery (Fig. 9.3) [67, 90] while the other compared SCS to myocardial laser revascularization (in 2006) [91]. Compared to CABG, SCS proved to be less expensive, mostly because of the initial cost associated with the surgery. Interestingly, fewer hospitalization days due to cardiac events were recorded among patients recruited in the SCS group [90].

It is difficult to get a precise safety estimate for SCS, as clinical trials, registries, and case-reports present discordant views. One original safety concern has been that SCS could conceal pain signals and therefore mask the symptoms of life-threatening conditions, such as myocardial infarction. This concern did not appear to be warranted as similar rates of death and myocardial infarction have been observed among SCS and medically treated patients [82, 92, 93]. Spinal lead migration has been reported to occur in 7.8% of treated patients [74]. Lead infection seems a rare occurrence, with an incidence of around 1%. In the Prospective Italian registry, no life-threatening or serious adverse events were observed. Pulse generator site infection was observed in nearly 6% of patients [82]. Based on the hypothesis that SCS acts partly through a sympatholytic effect, a rebound phenomenon would theoretically be possible upon SCS discontinuation. Conceptually, this rebound phenomenon would be somehow similar to the reflex tachycardia seen after β-blocker cessation in clinical practice [94]. Jessurum et al. sought to assess this possibility in 24 patients with refractory angina responsive to SCS after crossing them over to no SCS [70]. Upon SCS discontinuation, neither the symptoms nor the aerobic capacity were altered.

Coronary Sinus Occlusion

Before CABG was technically possible, Beck and Leighninger used to perform a surgical narrowing of the coronary sinus to treat the disabling angina of patients with advanced coronary artery disease [95]. The coronary sinus is the main venous structure that drains blood away from the heart. By occluding this conduit, Beck and Leighninger sought to redistribute blood already in the coronary system into relatively underperfused, ischemic territories. In their series, 9 out of 10 patients were back at work and relatively free of pain after surgery. More than 50 years after the first Beck-1 surgeries, the concept of coronary sinus reduction has been updated with a percutaneous endoluminal device that mimics the narrowing obtained by surgery. The Reducer (Neovasc Medical, Canada) is a stainless steel, balloon-expandable, hourglass-shaped device that creates a controlled narrowing of the coronary sinus (Fig. 9.4). The device is implantable by a percutaneous transvenous approach (Fig. 9.5). The coronary sinus Reducer appears to reverse the pathophysiology of advanced coronary artery disease. In the healthy myocardium, subepicardial vessels will constrict in response to stress to ensure adequate perfusion of the more vulnerable subendocardium. In patients with critical coronary stenosis, this compensatory mechanism appears dysfunctional [96]. Likewise, the augmentation in left ventricular end-diastolic pressure seen with advanced CAD further compromises the endocardial blood perfusion [97]. The hourglass shape of the coronary sinus reducer creates a functional stenosis which increases upstream coronary sinus pressure (Figs. 9.4 and 9.5). Increased upstream pressure induces a regional capillary pressure imbalance which is thought to force a redistribution of antegrade blood flow toward regions of lesser resistance.

In 2007, the first-in-man experience with this device was reported in 15 patients with refractory angina in India and Germany [71]. In a single-arm safety and

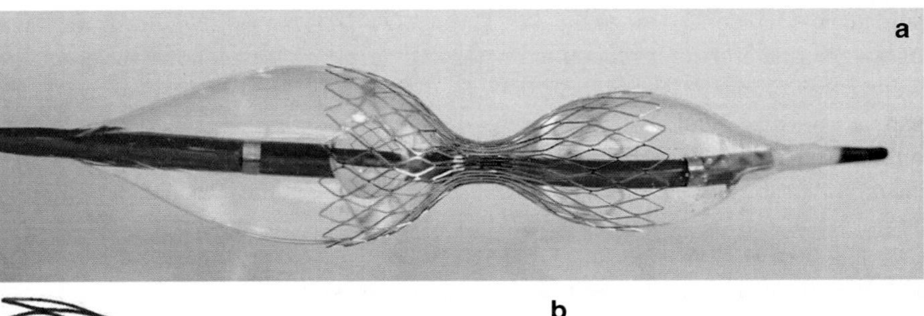

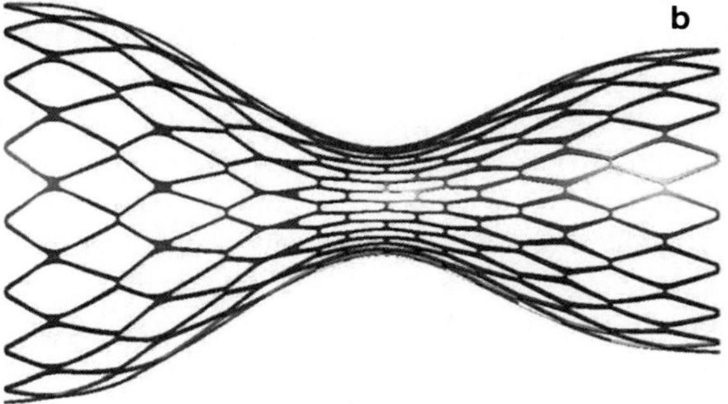

Fig. 9.4 The Coronary Sinus Reducer stent (Neovasc Medical, Inc., Vancouver, Canada), a stainless steel, balloon expandable stent (**a**) on, and (**b**) off of the delivery balloon. The stent is 3 mm at the midportion and can reach diameters of 7–13 mm at the ends to approximate the coronary sinus caliber when inflated at 2–4 atmospheres of balloon pressure.

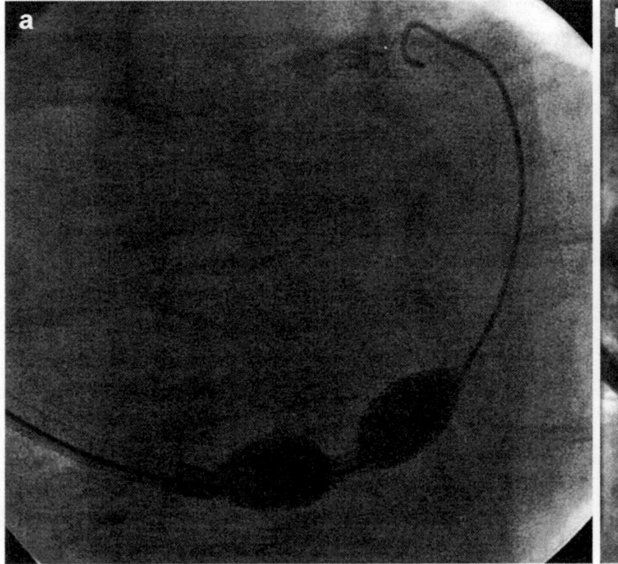

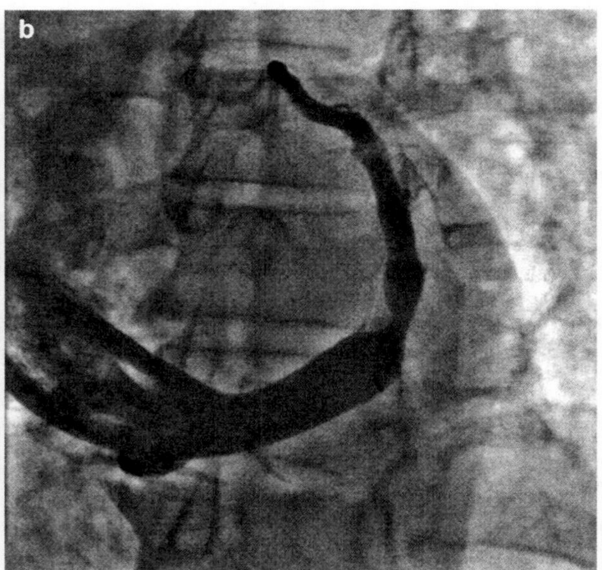

Fig. 9.5 Percutaneous delivery of the Coronary Sinus Reducer stent at the proximal coronary sinus. (**a**) Inflation of the contrast-filled delivery balloon at the proximal coronary sinus. (**b**) Postimplantation retrograde angiography demonstrating induced coronary sinus narrowing. (Reproduced with permission: Banai et al. [71])

feasibility study, the Reducer was shown to improve symptoms in 12 of 15 patients (average CCS score 3.07 at baseline vs. 1.64 at follow-up, $p<0.0001$). Improvement in symptoms correlated with a reduction in myocardial infarction quantified by dobutamine echocardiography and by thallium single-photon emission computed tomography. No procedure-related adverse events were noted. Results of the long-term surveillance program were reported in 2009 and suggested sustained safety and efficacy. At 3 years, no death or myocardial infarction was recorded. Computed tomography angiography revealed that all Reducers were patent. Most importantly, the improvement in angina observed early in the study was maintained throughout the long-term follow-up.

The upcoming international Coronary Sinus Reducer for Treatment of Refractory Angina (COSIRA) trial should bring additional efficacy and safety information to light on this device [98].

Percutaneous Coronary Bypasses and Sinus Retroperfusion Technologies

This section describes concepts not currently available for the clinical treatment of unrevascularizable patients. Still, catheter-based coronary bypass and coronary vein retroperfusion technologies are revolutionary in principle. CABG classically links the aorta or one of its branches to a coronary artery. Several variations of the classical CABG have been proposed over the years. In the late 1970s, Hockberg et al. developed an experimental model whereby a saphenous vein was interposed between the aorta and the left anterior descending coronary vein. The resulting arteriovenous fistula was intended to retroperfuse oxygenated blood into the left ventricle. In Hockberg's model, the retroperfused blood was sufficient to prevent myocardial infarction despite permanent left anterior descending artery ligation [99]. These experiments and others opened the door for the use of the cardiac venous system to retroperfuse oxygenated blood into ischemic myocardial tissues. The concept of cardiac retroperfusion never gained wide acceptance among cardiovascular surgeons. This could change with the recent developments of minimally invasive, catheter-based bypass techniques.

In 2001, Oesterle et al, reported the first-in-man case of percutaneous in situ coronary venous arterialization (PICVA) [100], whereby a fistula is constructed between the left anterior descending coronary artery and its companion vein. During PICVA, arterial blood is shunted away from a diseased artery into a coronary vein. By permanently blocking the venous drainage beyond the fistula insertion point, the shunted arterial blood is forced backward through the venules and subsequently into the microcirculation where it feeds the ischemic myocardium. Poor results were seen with PICVA in a phase I trial [72] (Table 9.1). Of the 11 patients attempted, 6 could not be implanted with the system, mostly because of impractical anatomical variations such as vessel cross-over or unexpected artery–vein distance. Of the 5 implanted patients, two experienced dramatic procedural complications resulting in death. Both patients displayed major epicardial hemorrhage. Of the remaining 3 cases, one required urgent pericardial drainage due to an anterior interventricular vein perforation. Only one patient maintained PICVA patency beyond one month.

A proposed variation of PICVA is percutaneous in situ coronary bypass (PICAB). Oesterle et al. suggested that PICAB could eventually replace classical CABG surgery [100]. In PICAB, the coronary vein is used as the bypass conduit. To achieve this, two fistulas are constructed between the coronary artery and its companion vein; one proximal to the coronary artery occlusion, and one distal. With these communications, oxygenated blood transits across the coronary vein and goes back into the coronary artery, distal to the stenosis. Technically, the coronary vein must be occluded above and below the fistula entry points to avoid contamination of the oxygen-rich arterial blood with poorly oxygenated venous blood. While appealing, proof-of-concept experiments using PICAB have not been reported to date.

Another interesting concept is direct ventricle-to-coronary artery bypass (VCAB), where the ventricle serves as a source of oxygenated blood. The concept of ventricular sourcing has been described since the mid 1950s [101] and surgical proofs of principle have been performed [68]. In normal coronary arteries, most of the blood flows in during ventricular diastole. When a significant epicardial stenosis is present, diastolic inflow is compromised and ischemia occurs. With VCAB, the left ventricle pushes oxygenated blood into the coronary artery during ventricular systole. The artery therefore serves as a reservoir from which oxygenated blood will flow during the next diastole. The concept of ventricle-to-coronary artery bypass has never been tested among unrevascularizable patients, but it could be easily adapted to this population. As part of the phase I European ADVANTAGE trial, twelve patients undergoing traditional bypass surgery were concomitantly treated with the VSTENT (Percardia), a catheter-based, ePTFE-covered, heparin-coated surgically implantable VACB system that connects the floor of the coronary artery to the left ventricular cavity. In the ADVANTAGE trial, the VSTENT was successfully implanted in 11 patients [102]. One patient could not be implanted because of an arterial rupture. VSTENTs were shown to be angiographically patent early after surgery in 8 of the 11 patients. Subsequent physiologic studies revealed that despite the predominantly systolic inflow, the vessel supplied by the VSTENT had a flow reserve similar to what was seen in vessels supplied by conventional bypass conduits [103]. At 2- to 6-month follow-up, the VSTENT stayed patent in 5 patients, but a significant in-stent stenosis was present in 4 of those 5. These results illustrate a certain potential of VCAB in selected patients with refractory angina. The concept appears especially appealing for unrevascularizable patients lacking graft material and for patients with heavily calcified (porcelain) aorta. An interesting variation of VCAB has been proposed whereby the left ventricle is connected to a coronary vein, instead of an artery. As was the case with the PICVA, the blood is retroperfused into the microcirculation. In its current format, the intervention is entirely percutaneous and could therefore help patients not amenable to revascularization with traditional methods. Conclusive proof-of-concept experiments in large mammals have set the ground for future clinical developments [104].

Future Directions: The Challenges of Developing New Devices to Treat Angina

The development of new devices to treat refractory angina is difficult. New technologies can be revolutionary in principle, but may not translate into clinically viable options, most often because of safety concerns. A concrete example of this challenge is demonstrated by percutaneous myocardial cryotreatment [73], a technology felt capable of inducing myocardial neovascularization. Among 20 treated patients, 3 major device-related complications occurred, including one pericardial tamponade and one episode of ventricular tachycardia. Similar safety concerns occurred with percutaneous in situ coronary venous arterialization (PICVA) [72, 100].

Beyond safety considerations, device trials run the risk of being confounded by many biases. For instance, it may be impossible to compare a device to a placebo or to a sham intervention when the device itself acts through a physical action felt by the patient. A classical example has been enhanced external counterpulsation (EECP) among patients with refractory angina, where lower extremity compression is an obvious mechanism of action felt by the patient [105, 106]. Another example previously discussed in this chapter is spinal cord stimulation, during which the induction of chest paresthesia is thought to be necessary to relieve cardiac pain. Interestingly, one group of investigators has reported functional improvement with spinal cord stimulation at intensities below the paresthesia threshold [80]. Using a subliminal electrical stimulation protocol, placebo-controlled trials are technically possible. Whether subliminal electrical stimulation is as effective as conventional paresthesic cord stimulation is being questioned [65]. Still, it may be impossible to conduct blinded or placebo-controlled trials in some cases, and clinical trialists must be imaginative in order to minimize these limitations.

The carry-over effect is another bias that potentially confounds trials testing temporary devices, especially when a cross-over design is used. A carry-over effect occurs when the benefit of an investigational treatment persists beyond its period of use. When a carry-over effect is suspected, a wash-out period should be observed before actually crossing patients over from one group to the other. To some extent, a carry-over effect has been reported with low-energy extracorporeal shock wave therapy, stellate blockade, and spinal cord stimulation [63, 107]. For obvious reasons, cross-over designs should be avoided for devices with a permanent effect.

Innovation in trial design is a key component of future device development. Under the US Food and Drug Administration mandate to use the least burdensome appropriate means of evaluating effectiveness of devices, the Center for Devices and Radiological Health (CDRH), and the Center for Biologics Evaluation and Research (CBER) recently launched a guidance document promoting the use of Bayesian statistics in medical device trials [108]. Known since the mideighteenth century, Bayesian statistics start with a prior probability of a given hypothesis before the latest evidence has been observed and calculates a posterior probability of the hypothesis after this evidence is considered [109]. Bayesian statistics allow learning and adaptation as evidence accumulates. In selected situations, Bayesian statistics are an appealing alternative to the frequency statistics classically used in clinical trials. Bayesian statistics offer a flexibility that frequency statistics do not have, especially for small phase I and II trials, as is often the case with investigational devices.

Bayesian statistics work best when good prior efficacy evidence is available. When good prior information is available, Bayesian assumptions in trial design can be a less burdensome method to assess a new device. There are recent examples of cardiovascular device trials that used Bayesian statistics [110–112]. Unlike drugs which have a systemic effect, devices typically exert their action locally, which in turn allow for predictable evolution. This claim is especially true when a slightly modified, new generation of an old device is being investigated.

Unrevascularizable patients are notoriously difficult to recruit into clinical trials. Bayesian trial design can therefore offer strategic advantages when investigating new devices and therapies for this population. A concrete example is the Bayesian sequential design with adaptive randomization. In this type of trial, the probability that a patient is randomized to a given treatment arm is set by the efficacy measured in patients previously enrolled in the trial. The aim of the adaptive design is to improve the efficacy and safety of the trial as it progresses, by changing the rules by which one determines how participants are allocated to the different treatment arms [113]. When used properly, adaptive design can lead to smaller and more ethical trials. Other claimed advantages of Bayesian statistics are the possibility to move seamlessly from a phase I to a phase II to a phase III trial [114], the potential to closely monitor possibly hazardous devices without compromising statistical power [115, 116], and the ability to borrow statistical power from previous clinical investigations, therefore reducing the number of subjects needed to reach a statistically sound conclusion in a trial [117]. Clearly, the place of Bayesian statistics in new device development should grow in the years to come, clearing the way for rapid improvements in our refractory angina treatment armamentarium.

References

1. Jolicoeur EM, Ohman EM, Temple R, et al. Clinical and research issues regarding chronic advanced coronary artery disease part II: trial design, outcomes, and regulatory issues. Am Heart J. 2008;155(3):435–44.
2. Rathore S, Katoh O, Matsuo H, et al. Retrograde percutaneous recanalization of chronic total occlusion of the coronary arteries: procedural outcomes and predictors of success in contemporary practice. Circ Cardiovasc Interv. 2009;2(2):124–32.
3. Jax TW, Peters AJ, Khattab AA, Heintzen MP, Schoebel FC. Percutaneous coronary revascularization in patients with formerly "refractory angina pectoris in end-stage coronary artery disease" - not "end-stage" after all. BMC Cardiovasc Disord. 2009;9:42.
4. Horvath KA, Aranki SF, Cohn LH, et al. Sustained Angina Relief 5 Years After Transmyocardial Laser Revascularization With a CO2 Laser. Circulation. 2001;104(12 Suppl 1):I81–4.
5. Henry TD, Satran D, Johnson R. Natural history of patients with refractory angina. J Am Coll Cardiol. 2006;47:231.
6. Stone GW. Percutaneous recanalization of chronically occluded coronary arteries: a consensus document: part I. 2005.
7. Srinivas VS, Brooks MM, Detre KM, et al. Contemporary percutaneous coronary intervention versus balloon angioplasty for multivessel coronary artery disease: a comparison of the National Heart, Lung and Blood Institute Dynamic Registry and the Bypass Angioplasty Revascularization Investigation (BARI) study. Circulation. 2002;106(13):1627–33.
8. Abbott JD, Kip KE, Vlachos HA, et al. Recent trends in the percutaneous treatment of chronic total coronary occlusions. Am J Cardiol. 2006;97(12):1691–6.
9. Dzavik V, Carere RG, Mancini GB, et al. Predictors of improvement in left ventricular function after percutaneous revascularization of occluded coronary arteries: a report from the Total Occlusion Study of Canada (TOSCA). Am Heart J. 2001;142(2):301–8.
10. Sirnes PA, Myreng Y, Molstad P, Bonarjee V, Golf S. Improvement in left ventricular ejection fraction and wall motion after successful recanalization of chronic coronary occlusions. Eur Heart J. 1998;19(2):273–81.
11. Safley DM, House JA, Marso SP, Grantham JA, Rutherford BD. Improvement in survival following successful percutaneous coronary intervention of coronary chronic total occlusions: variability by target vessel. JACC Cardiovasc Interv. 2008;1(3):295–302.
12. Joyal D, Afilalo J, Rinfret S. Effectiveness of recanalization of chronic total occlusions: a systematic review and meta-analysis. Am Heart J. 2010;160(1):179–87.
13. Aziz S, Stables RH, Grayson AD, Perry RA, Ramsdale DR. Percutaneous coronary intervention for chronic total occlusions: improved survival for patients with successful revascularization compared to a failed procedure. Catheter Cardiovasc Interv. 2007;70(1):15–20.
14. de Labriolle A, Bonello L, Roy P, et al. Comparison of safety, efficacy, and outcome of successful versus unsuccessful percutaneous coronary intervention in "True" chronic total occlusions. Am J Cardiol. 2008;102(9):1175–81.
15. Drozd J, Wojcik J, Opalinska E, Zapolski T, Widomska-Czekajska T. Percutaneous angioplasty of chronically occluded coronary arteries: long-term clinical follow-up. Kardiol Pol. 2006;64(7):667–73.
16. Hoye A, van Domburg RT, Sonnenschein K, Serruys PW. Percutaneous coronary intervention for chronic total occlusions: the Thoraxcenter experience 1992–2002. Eur Heart J. 2005;26(24):2630–6.
17. Noguchi T, Miyazaki MS, Morii I, Daikoku S, Goto Y, Nonogi H. Percutaneous transluminal coronary angioplasty of chronic total occlusions. Determinants of primary success and long-term clinical outcome. Catheter Cardiovasc Interv. 2000;49(3):258–64.

18. Olivari Z, Rubartelli P, Piscione F, et al. Immediate results and one-year clinical outcome after percutaneous coronary interventions in chronic total occlusions: data from a multicenter, prospective, observational study (TOAST-GISE). J Am Coll Cardiol. 2003;41(10):1672–8.
19. Prasad A, Rihal CS, Lennon RJ, Wiste HJ, Singh M, Holmes Jr DR. Trends in outcomes after percutaneous coronary intervention for chronic total occlusions: a 25-year experience from the Mayo Clinic. J Am Coll Cardiol. 2007;49(15):1611–8.
20. Suero JA, Marso SP, Jones PG, et al. Procedural outcomes and long-term survival among patients undergoing percutaneous coronary intervention of a chronic total occlusion in native coronary arteries: a 20-year experience. J Am Coll Cardiol. 2001;38(2):409–14.
21. Valenti R, Migliorini A. Signorini U et al. Eur Heart J: Impact of complete revascularization with percutaneous coronary intervention on survival in patients with at least one chronic total occlusion; 2008.
22. Barsoum M, Ford M, Rihal C, et al. Angiographic and Clinical Outcome of Chronic Total Occlusion with Intractable Angian on Enhanced External Counterpulsation: An Institutional Case Series Review. Catheterization and Cardiovascular Intervention. 2010; 75(S2):S77.
23. Thompson CA, Jayne JE, Robb JF, et al. Retrograde Techniques and the Impact of Operator Volume on Percutaneous Intervention for Coronary Chronic Total Occlusions: An Early U.S. Experience. Journal of the American College of Cardiology: Cardiovascular Interventions. 2009;2(9): 834–42.
24. Patel MR, Dehmer GJ, Hirshfeld JW, Smith PK, Spertus JA. ACCF/SCAI/STS/AATS/AHA/ASNC 2009 Appropriateness Criteria for Coronary Revascularization: a report by the American College of Cardiology Foundation Appropriateness Criteria Task Force, Society for Cardiovascular Angiography and Interventions, Society of Thoracic Surgeons, American Association for Thoracic Surgery, American Heart Association, and the American Society of Nuclear Cardiology Endorsed by the American Society of Echocardiography, the Heart Failure Society of America, and the Society of Cardiovascular Computed Tomography. J Am Coll Cardiol. 2009;53(6): 530–53.
25. Apfel RE. Acoustic cavitation: a possible consequence of biomedical uses of ultrasound. Br J Cancer Suppl. 1982;5: 140–6.
26. Maisonhaute E, Prado C, White PC, Compton RG. Surface acoustic cavitation understood via nanosecond electrochemistry. Part III: Shear stress in ultrasonic cleaning. Ultrason Sonochem. 2002;9(6):297–303.
27. Mariotto S, Cavalieri E, Amelio E, et al. Extracorporeal shock waves: from lithotripsy to anti-inflammatory action by NO production. Nitric Oxide. 2005;12(2):89–96.
28. Aicher A, Heeschen C, Sasaki K, Urbich C, Zeiher AM, Dimmeler S. Low-energy shock wave for enhancing recruitment of endothelial progenitor cells: a new modality to increase efficacy of cell therapy in chronic hind limb ischemia. Circulation. 2006;114(25):2823–30.
29. Oi K, Fukumoto Y, Ito K, et al. Extracorporeal shock wave therapy ameliorates hindlimb ischemia in rabbits. Tohoku J Exp Med. 2008;214(2):151–8.
30. Nishida T, Shimokawa H, Oi K, et al. Extracorporeal cardiac shock wave therapy markedly ameliorates ischemia-induced myocardial dysfunction in pigs in vivo. Circulation. 2004;110(19):3055–61.
31. Kikuchi Y, Ito K, Ito Y, et al. Double-blind and placebo-controlled study of the effectiveness and safety of extracorporeal cardiac shock wave therapy for severe angina pectoris. Circ J. 2010;74(3):589–91.
32. Fukumoto Y, Ito A, Uwatoku T, et al. Extracorporeal cardiac shock wave therapy ameliorates myocardial ischemia in patients with severe coronary artery disease. Coron Artery Dis. 2006;17(1):63–70.
33. Khattab AA, Brodersen B, Schuermann-Kuchenbrandt D, et al. Extracorporeal cardiac shock wave therapy: first experience in the everyday practice for treatment of chronic refractory angina pectoris. Int J Cardiol. 2007;121(1): 84–5.
34. Prinz C, Lindner O, Bitter T, et al. Extracorporeal cardiac shock wave therapy ameliorates clinical symptoms and improves regional myocardial blood flow in a patient with severe coronary artery disease and refractory angina. Case Report Med. 2009;2009:639594.
35. Vasyuk YA, Hadzegova AB, Shkolnik EL, et al. Initial clinical experience with extracorporeal shock wave therapy in treatment of ischemic heart failure. Congest Heart Fail. 2010;16(5):226–30.
36. Wang Y, Guo T, Cai HY, et al. Cardiac shock wave therapy reduces angina and improves myocardial function in patients with refractory coronary artery disease. Clin Cardiol. 2010;33(11):693–9.
37. Gutersohn A, Caspari GH, Marlinghaus E. Haude M. Presented at World Congress of Cardiology: Comparison of Cardiac Shock Wave Therapy and Percutaneous Myocardial Laser Revascularization Therapy in Endstage CAD Patients with Refractory Angina; 2006.
38. Faber L, Linder O, Prinz C, et al. Echo-Guided Extracorporeal Shock Wave Therapy for Refractory Angina Improves Myocardial Blood Flow as Assessed by PET Imaging. J Am Coll Cardiol. 2011;55(A120):E1125.
39. Belcaro G, Nicolaides AN, Marlinghaus EH, et al. Shock waves in vascular diseases: an in-vitro study. Angiology. 1998;49(10):777–88.
40. http://clinicaltrials.gov/ct2/results?term=extracorporeal+shock+wave+therapy+heart. 14-1-2011. Ref Type: Online Source
41. Jonnesco T. Angine de poitrine guérie par la résection du sympatique dans la maladie de Basedow, l'épilepsie, l'idiotie, et du glaucome. Bull Acad Med Paris. 2011;84:93–102.
42. Wiener L, Cox JW. Influence of stellate ganglion block on angina pectoris and the post-exercise electrocardiogram. Am J Med Sci. 1966;252(3):289–95.
43. Moore R, Groves D, Hammond C, Leach A, Chester MR. Temporary sympathectomy in the treatment of chronic refractory angina. J Pain Symptom Manage. 2005;30(2): 183–91.
44. Cobb LA, Thomas GI, Dillard DH, Merendino KA, Bruce RA. An evaluation of internal-mammary-artery ligation by a double-blind technic. N Engl J Med. 1959;260(22):1115–8.
45. Schott GD. Interrupting the sympathetic outflow in causalgia and reflex sympathetic dystrophy. BMJ. 1998; 316(7134):792–3.

46. Jadad AR, Carroll D, Glynn CJ, McQuay HJ. Intravenous regional sympathetic blockade for pain relief in reflex sympathetic dystrophy: a systematic review and a randomized, double-blind crossover study. J Pain Symptom Manage. 1995;10(1):13–20.
47. Chester M, Hammond C, Leach A. Long-term benefits of stellate ganglion block in severe chronic refractory angina. Pain. 2000;87(1):103–5.
48. Gramling-Babb P, Miller MJ, Reeves ST, Roy RC, Zile MR. Treatment of medically and surgically refractory angina pectoris with high thoracic epidural analgesia: initial clinical experience. Am Heart J. 1997;133(6):648–55.
49. Forouzanfar T, van KM, Weber WE. Radiofrequency lesions of the stellate ganglion in chronic pain syndromes: retrospective analysis of clinical efficacy in 86 patients. Clin J Pain. 2000;16(2):164–8.
50. Wulf H, Maier C. Complications and side effects of stellate ganglion blockade. Results of a questionnaire survey. Anaesthesist. 1992;41(3):146–51.
51. Chan CW, Chalkiadis GA. A case of sympathetically mediated headache treated with stellate ganglion blockade. Pain Med. 2010;11(8):1294–8.
52. Chaturvedi A, Dash H. Locked-in syndrome during stellate ganglion block. Indian J Anaesth. 2010;54(4):324–6.
53. Huntoon MA. The vertebral artery is unlikely to be the sole source of vascular complications occurring during stellate ganglion block. Pain Pract. 2010;10(1):25–30.
54. Narouze S, Vydyanathan A, Patel N. Ultrasound-guided stellate ganglion block successfully prevented esophageal puncture. Pain Physician. 2007;10(6):747–52.
55. Varela C, Palacio F, Reina MA, Lopez A, Benito-Leon J. Horner's syndrome secondary to epidural anesthesia. Neurologia. 2007;22(3):196–200.
56. Higa K, Hirata K, Hirota K, Nitahara K, Shono S. Retropharyngeal hematoma after stellate ganglion block: analysis of 27 patients reported in the literature. Anesthesiology. 2006;105(6):1238–45.
57. Masuda A, Fujiki A. Sinus arrest after right stellate ganglion block. Anesth Analg. 1994;79(3):607.
58. Prager JP. What does the mechanism of spinal cord stimulation tell us about complex regional pain syndrome? Pain Medicine. 2010;11(8):1278–83.
59. Melzack R, Wall PD. Pain mechanisms: a new theory. Science. 1965;150(699):971–9.
60. Crick SJ, Sheppard MN, Anderson RH. Nerve Supply of the Heart. In: ter Host GJ, editor. The nervous system and the heart. Humana Press ed. 2000.
61. Zan E, Kurt KN, Yousem DM, Christo PJ. Spinal cord stimulators: typical positioning and postsurgical complications. Am J Roentgenol. 2011;196(2):437–45.
62. de Jongste MJ, Hautvast RW, Hillege HL, Lie KI. Efficacy of spinal cord stimulation as adjuvant therapy for intractable angina pectoris: a prospective, randomized clinical study. Working group on neurocardiology. J Am Coll Cardiol. 1994;23(7):1592–7.
63. Eddicks S, Maier-Hauff K, Schenk M, Muller A, Baumann G, Theres H. Thoracic spinal cord stimulation improves functional status and relieves symptoms in patients with refractory angina pectoris: the first placebo-controlled randomised study. Heart. 2007;93(5):585–90.
64. Hautvast RW, Dejongste MJ, Staal MJ, van Gilst WH, Lie KI. Spinal cord stimulation in chronic intractable angina pectoris: a randomized, controlled efficacy study. Am Heart J. 1998;136(6):1114–20.
65. Lanza GA, Grimaldi R, Greco S, et al. Spinal cord stimulation for the treatment of refractory angina pectoris: a multicenter randomized single-blind study (the SCS-ITA trial). Pain. 2011;152(1):45–52.
66. McNab D, Khan SN, Sharples LD, et al. An open label, single-centre, randomized trial of spinal cord stimulation vs. percutaneous myocardial laser revascularization in patients with refractory angina pectoris: the SPiRiT trial. Eur Heart J. 2006;27(9):1048–53.
67. Mannheimer C, Eliasson T, Augustinsson LE, Blomstrand C, Emanuelsson H, Larsson S, et al. Electrical stimulation versus coronary artery bypass surgery in severe angina pectoris: the ESBY study. Circulation. 1998;97(12):1157–63.
68. Emery RW, Eales F, Van Meter CHJ, Knudson MB, Solien EE, Tweden KS. Ventriculocoronary artery bypass results using a mesh-tipped device in a porcine model. Ann Thorac Surg. 2001;72(3):S1004–8.
69. Ekre O, Eliasson T, Norrsell H, Wahrborg P, Mannheimer C. Long-term effects of spinal cord stimulation and coronary artery bypass grafting on quality of life and survival in the ESBY study. Eur Heart J. 2002;23(24):1938–45.
70. Jessurun GA, DeJongste MJ, Hautvast RW, et al. Clinical follow-up after cessation of chronic electrical neuromodulation in patients with severe coronary artery disease: a prospective randomized controlled study on putative involvement of sympathetic activity. Pacing Clin Electrophysiol. 1999;22(10):1432–9.
71. Banai S, Ben MS, Parikh KH, et al. Coronary sinus reducer stent for the treatment of chronic refractory angina pectoris: a prospective, open-label, multicenter, safety feasibility first-in-man study. J Am Coll Cardiol. 2007;49(17):1783–9.
72. Oesterle SN, Reifart N, Hayase M, et al. Catheter-based coronary bypass: a development update. Catheter Cardiovasc Interv. 2003;58(2):212–8.
73. Gallo R, Fefer P, Freeman M, et al. A first-in-man study of percutaneous myocardial cryotreatment in nonrevascularizable patients with refractory angina. Catheter Cardiovasc Interv. 2009;74(3):387–94.
74. Taylor RS, De VJ, Buchser E, Dejongste MJ. Spinal cord stimulation in the treatment of refractory angina: systematic review and meta-analysis of randomised controlled trials. BMC Cardiovasc Disord. 2009;9:13.
75. Borjesson M, Andrell P, Lundberg D, Mannheimer C. Spinal cord stimulation in severe angina pectoris–a systematic review based on the Swedish Council on Technology assessment in health care report on long-standing pain. Pain. 2008;140(3):501–8.
76. Sestito A, Lanza GA, Le PD, et al. Spinal cord stimulation normalizes abnormal cortical pain processing in patients with cardiac syndrome X. Pain. 2008;139(1):82–9.
77. Lanza GA, Sestito A, Sgueglia GA, et al. Effect of spinal cord stimulation on spontaneous and stress-induced angina and 'ischemia-like' ST-segment depression in patients with cardiac syndrome X. Eur Heart J. 2005;26(10):983–9.
78. Andrell P, Yu W, Gersbach P, et al. Long-term effects of spinal cord stimulation on angina symptoms and quality of life in patients with refractory angina pectoris–results from the

European Angina Registry Link Study (EARL). Heart. 2010;96(14):1132–6.
79. Di PF, Lanza GA, Zuin G, et al. Immediate and long-term clinical outcome after spinal cord stimulation for refractory stable angina pectoris. Am J Cardiol. 2003;91(8):951–5.
80. Hrobjartsson A, Gotzsche PC. Is the placebo powerless? An analysis of clinical trials comparing placebo with no treatment. N Engl J Med. 2001;344(21):1594–602.
81. Leon MB, Kornowski R, Downey WE, et al. A blinded, randomized, placebo-controlled trial of percutaneous laser myocardial revascularization to improve angina symptoms in patients with severe coronary disease. J Am Coll Cardiol. 2005;46(10):1812–9.
82. Di PF, Zuin G, Giada F, et al. Long-term effects of spinal cord stimulation on myocardial ischemia and heart rate variability: results of a 48-hour ambulatory electrocardiographic monitoring. Ital Heart J. 2001;2(9):690–5.
83. de Jongste MJ, Haaksma J, Hautvast RW, et al. Effects of spinal cord stimulation on myocardial ischaemia during daily life in patients with severe coronary artery disease. A prospective ambulatory electrocardiographic study. Br Heart J. 1994;71(5):413–8.
84. Hautvast RW, Blanksma PK, Dejongste MJ, et al. Effect of spinal cord stimulation on myocardial blood flow assessed by positron emission tomography in patients with refractory angina pectoris. Am J Cardiol. 1996;77(7):462–7.
85. Chauhan A, Mullins PA, Thuraisingham SI, Taylor G, Petch MC, Schofield PM. Effect of transcutaneous electrical nerve stimulation on coronary blood flow. Circulation. 1994;89(2):694–702.
86. Remme WJ, Kruyssen DA, Look MP, Bootsma M, de Leeuw PW. Systemic and cardiac neuroendocrine activation and severity of myocardial ischemia in humans. J Am Coll Cardiol. 1994;23(1):82–91.
87. De LC, Mannheimer C, Habets A, et al. Effect of spinal cord stimulation on regional myocardial perfusion assessed by positron emission tomography. Am J Cardiol. 1992;69(14):1143–9.
88. Fricke E, Eckert S, Dongas A, et al. Myocardial perfusion after one year of spinal cord stimulation in patients with refractory angina. Nuklearmedizin. 2009;48(3):104–9.
89. Kingma Jr JG, Linderoth B, Ardell JL, Armour JA, Dejongste MJ, Foreman RD. Neuromodulation therapy does not influence blood flow distribution or left-ventricular dynamics during acute myocardial ischemia. Auton Neurosci. 2001;91(1–2):47–54.
90. Andrell P, Ekre O, Eliasson T, et al. Cost-effectiveness of spinal cord stimulation versus coronary artery bypass grafting in patients with severe angina pectoris–long-term results from the ESBY study. Cardiology. 2003;99(1):20–4.
91. Dyer MT, Goldsmith KA, Khan SN, et al. Clinical and cost-effectiveness analysis of an open label, single-centre, randomised trial of spinal cord stimulation (SCS) versus percutaneous myocardial laser revascularisation (PMR) in patients with refractory angina pectoris: the SPiRiT trial. Trials. 2008;9:40.
92. Andersen C, Hole P, Oxhoj H. Does pain relief with spinal cord stimulation for angina conceal myocardial infarction? Br Heart J. 1994;71(5):419–21.
93. Kim MC, Kini A, Sharma SK. Refractory angina pectoris: mechanism and therapeutic options. J Am Coll Cardiol. 2002;39(6):923–34.
94. Anselmino M, Ravera L, De LA, et al. Spinal cord stimulation and 30-minute heart rate variability in refractory angina patients. Pacing Clin Electrophysiol. 2009; 32(1):37–42.
95. Beck CS, Stanton E. Revascularization of heart by graft of systemic artery into coronary sinus. J Am Med Assoc. 1948;137(5):436–42.
96. Camici PG, Crea F. Coronary microvascular dysfunction. N Engl J Med. 2007;356(8):830–40.
97. Ido A, Hasebe N, Matsuhashi H, Kikuchi K. Coronary sinus occlusion enhances coronary collateral flow and reduces subendocardial ischemia. Am J Physiol Heart Circ Physiol. 2001;280(3):H1361–7.
98. http://clinicaltrials.gov/ct2/show/NCT01205893?term=COSIRA&rank=1. 13-2-2011. Ref Type: Online Source
99. Hochberg MS, Roberts WC, Morrow AG, Austen WG. Selective arterialization of the coronary venous system. Encouraging long-term flow evaluation utilizing radioactive microspheres. J Thorac Cardiovasc Surg. 1979;77(1): 1–12.
100. Oesterle SN, Reifart N, Hauptmann E, Hayase M, Yeung AC. Percutaneous in situ coronary venous arterialization: report of the first human catheter-based coronary artery bypass. Circulation. 2001;103(21):2539–43.
101. Goldman A, Greenstone SM, Preuss FS, Strauss SH, Chang ES. Experimental methods for producing a collateral circulation to the heart directly from the left ventricular. J Thorac Surg. 1956;31(3):364–74.
102. Vicol C, Reichart B, Eifert S, et al. First clinical experience with the VSTENT: a device for direct left ventricle-to-coronary artery bypass. Ann Thorac Surg. 2005;79(2): 573–9.
103. Boekstegers P, Raake P, Hinkel R, et al. Hemodynamic and vascular effects of ventricular sourcing by stent-based ventricle to coronary artery bypass in patients with multivessel disease undergoing coronary artery bypass surgery. Circulation. 2005;112(9 Suppl):I304–10.
104. Raake P, Hinkel R, Kupatt C, et al. Percutaneous approach to a stent-based ventricle to coronary vein bypass (venous VPASS): comparison to catheter-based selective pressure-regulated retro-infusion of the coronary vein. Eur Heart J. 2005;26(12):1228–34.
105. Arora RR, Chou TM, Jain D, et al. The multicenter study of enhanced external counterpulsation (MUST-EECP): effect of EECP on exercise-induced myocardial ischemia and anginal episodes. J Am Coll Cardiol. 1999;33(7): 1833–40.
106. Barsness G, Feldman AM, Holmes Jr DR, Holubkov R, Kelsey SF, Kennard ED. The International EECP Patient Registry (IEPR): design, methods, baseline characteristics, and acute results. Clin Cardiol. 2001;24(6):435–42.
107. Murray S, Collins PD, James MA. An investigation into the 'carry over' effect of neurostimulation in the treatment of angina pectoris. Int J Clin Pract. 2004;58(7): 669–74.
108. Guidance for the Use of Bayesian Statistics in Medical Device Clinical Trials, Center for Biologics Evaluation and Research, and Center for Devices and Radiological Health. http://www.fda.gov/MedicalDevices/DeviceRegulationandGuidance/GuidanceDocuments/ucm071072.htm. 2011. Ref Type: Online Source.

109. Berry DA. Bayesian clinical trials. Nat Rev Drug Discov. 2006;5(1):27–36.
110. Holmes DR, Reddy VY, Turi ZG, et al. Percutaneous closure of the left atrial appendage versus warfarin therapy for prevention of stroke in patients with atrial fibrillation: a randomised non-inferiority trial. Lancet. 2009;374(9689):534–42.
111. Holmes Jr DR, Teirstein P, Satler L, et al. Sirolimus-eluting stents vs vascular brachytherapy for instent restenosis within bare-metal stents: the SISR randomized trial. JAMA. 2006;295(11):1264–73.
112. Wilber DJ, Pappone C, Neuzil P, et al. Comparison of antiarrhythmic drug therapy and radiofrequency catheter ablation in patients with paroxysmal atrial fibrillation: a randomized controlled trial. JAMA. 2010;303(4):333–40.
113. Berry DA, Eick SG. Adaptive assignment versus balanced randomization in clinical trials: a decision analysis. Stat Med. 1995;14(3):231–46.
114. Inoue LY, Thall PF, Berry DA. Seamlessly expanding a randomized phase II trial to phase III. Biometrics. 2002;58(4):823–31.
115. Dmitrienko A, Wang MD. Bayesian predictive approach to interim monitoring in clinical trials. Stat Med. 2006; 25(13):2178–95.
116. Berry DA. Bayesian statistics and the efficiency and ethics of clinical trials. Stat Sci. 2004;19(1):175–87.
117. Cornfield J. The Bayesian outlook and its application. Biometrics. 1969;25(4):617–57.

Cardiac Transplantation for Ischemic Heart Disease

10

Robroy H. Mac Iver, Edwin C. McGee Jr., and Patrick M. McCarthy

Introduction

According to recent data by the American Heart Association, Coronary Artery Disease (CAD) has a prevalence of 6.9% in the US population [1]. In 2002, 494,382 people died in the USA from the effects of CAD with a cost that reached 142.1 billion dollars in 2005 [1]. It is well established that patients with evidence of myocardial viability and target vessels for revascularization live longer with surgical revascularization as opposed to medical management especially if they have severe left ventricular dysfunction [2]. However, patients who reach end-stage ischemic cardiomyopathy without evidence of viability do not benefit from revascularization [2]. This chapter discusses transplantation as treatment for these patients with end-stage ischemic cardiomyopathy.

History

In 1912 the pioneering cardiologist James B. Herrick (Fig. 10.1) foreshadowed the first one hundred years of treatment for CAD stating that "hope for the damaged myocardium lies in the direction of securing a supply of blood so as to restore as far as possible its functional integrity" [3]. Indeed this philosophy, not replacement, has served as the basis for procedural treatment of CAD for the last 50 years.

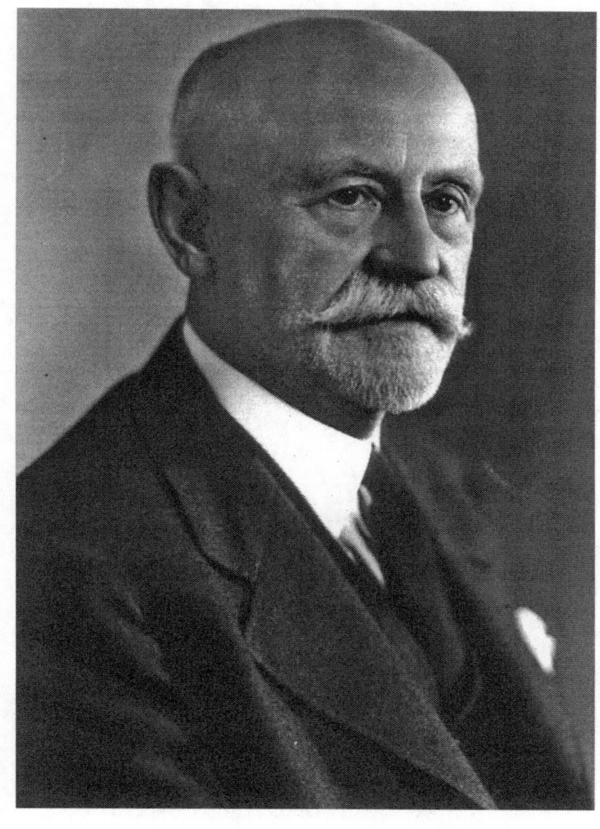

Fig. 10.1 The cardiologist James B. Herrick. (Courtesy of the National Library of Medicine)

Carrel and Guthrie at the University of Chicago first began experiments with heart transplantation in 1905 [4]. The first cardiac transplant in an animal was a heterotopic transplant where a puppy's heart was

R.H. Mac Iver • E.C. McGee Jr. (✉) • P.M. McCarthy
Division of Cardiothoracic Surgery, Bluhm Cardiovascular Institute, Northwestern Memorial Hospital, Northwestern University's Feinberg School of Medicine,
Chicago, IL, USA
e-mail: emcgee@nmh.org

G.W. Barsness and D.R. Holmes Jr. (eds.), *Coronary Artery Disease*,
DOI 10.1007/978-1-84628-712-1_10,

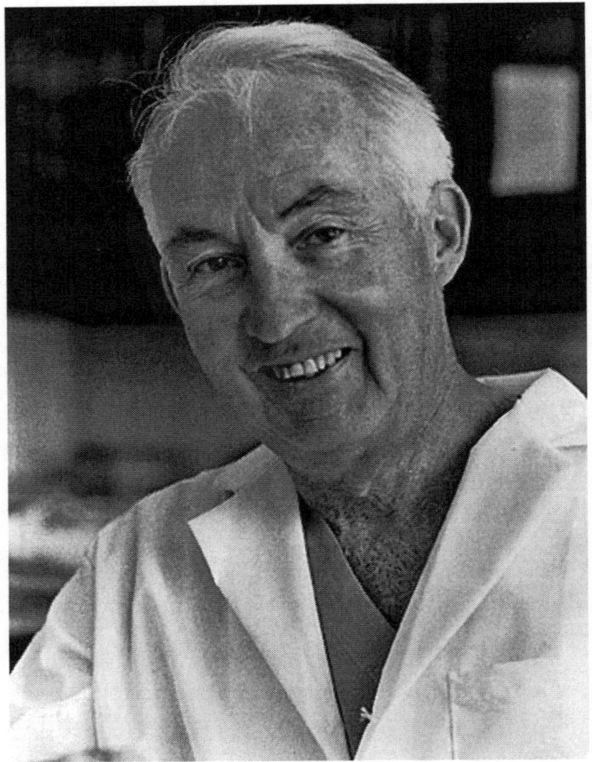

Fig. 10.2 The "Father" of cardiac transplant, Norman Shumway. (Used with permission from the Office of Communication and Public Affairs, Stanford University School of Medicine)

anastomosed to the carotid and jugular vessels of an adult dog [4]. Norman Shumway (Fig. 10.2) and his team at Stanford would perfect the technique of atrial preservation improving the results in dogs to a point where a human transplant was deemed possible.

Utilizing the technique of Shumway and Lower, the first human transplant was performed in 1967 by Dr. Christiaan Barnard in South Africa [5]. Over the subsequent year 102 transplants throughout the world were performed with universally dismal results. Shumway summarized the situation by stating that "suddenly heart transplants were being done in places where one would hesitate to have his atrial septal defect closed" [6]. Again, Shumway and his group at Stanford through dedicated work in the lab were able to perfect not only the anastomotic technique, but also the postoperative management in order to improve results. In 1973 the group at Stanford led by Shumway reported 29 patients transplanted with an overall actuarial survival rate of 49% at 6 months, 37% at 18 months, and 30% at 2 years [7]. By 1984 there were approximately 10 cardiac transplant programs in the USA [8]. Cyclosporine was introduced in 1983 and by 1985 the worldwide registry reported a survival rate at 1 year of 80% and at 4 years of 70% [9]. Today, survival rates continue to improve (Fig. 10.3) [10]. Most recent data quote survival rates at 1 and 5 years after heart transplant of 85% and 71%, respectively [10]. Reaching and improving these numbers requires a full understanding of recipient and donor selection, operative decision making, and postoperative management.

Patient Selection for Transplantation

Ideally patient selection for heart transplantation would be clear. Due to the multiple medical and surgical treatments available and the ever changing status of the patient's heart, the decision though is often a difficult one.

Determining function of the patient is often a moving target as both objective signs and subjective symptomatology can vary with changes in medical management and risk factor modification. It is important to create objective data in ranking acuity of possible recipients [11] (Table 10.1).

Objectifying the data prevents overexuberance in listing patients for transplant. Overuse of heart transplant is detrimental because the transplanted heart will often only achieve 60–70% of predicted values for maximal exercise capacity [12, 13]. It has also been shown that long-term mortality benefits are not as substantial for patients considered low or medium risk while on the waiting list [14]. In data collected in 889 patients listed for heart transplant in 1997, there was only a survival benefit found for patients who were considered high risk (where high risk was defined as a 1 year mortality of 51%) [14].

Most risk stratification strategies determining function involve invasive monitoring such as catheterization. There are tools available which stratify patients using noninvasive means [15]. Aminoterminal pro Type B Natriuretic peptide (NT-proBNP) levels have been used by some groups to predict mortality and therefore urgency to transplant [16]. Selection of patients with a high level of NT-proBNP levels (above 5000 pg/mL) corresponded to a mortality rate of 28.4% per year [16]. These levels were thought to be able to discriminate candidates for either left ventricular assist devices or urgent transplantation [16]. Traditionally it

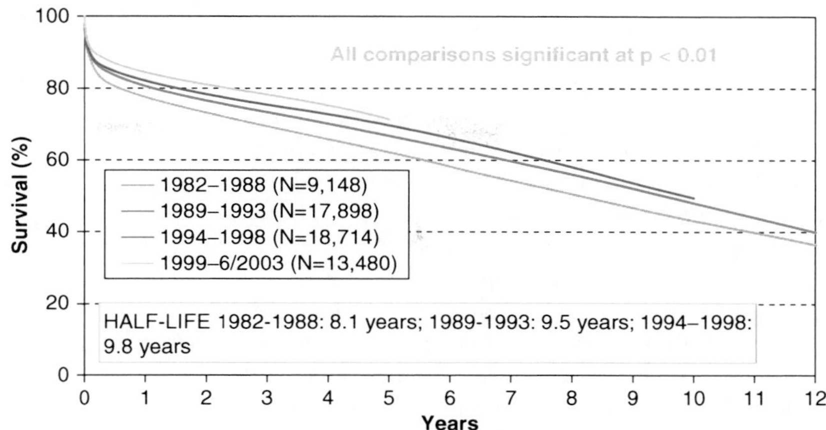

Fig. 10.3 Kaplan-Meier Survival by Era (Transplants: 1/1982 – 6/2003) in adult heart transplant patients. (Reprinted from Taylor et al. [10], Copyright (2005), with permission from International Society for Heart and Lung Transplantation)

Table 10.1 UNOS heart transplantation listing status criteria

Description of UNOS status levels for heart transplant	
Status 1A	Must be an inpatient at a transplant hospital with the following:
	Mechanical circulatory support for acute hemodynamic decompensation that includes either:
	Left or right assist device. May be listed for 30 days once deemed stable
	Total artificial heart
	Intra-aortic balloon pump
	Extracorporeal membrane oxygenator
	Mechanical circulatory support with objective evidence of device-related complications.
	Continuous mechanical ventilation
	Continuous infusion of a single high-dose intravenous inotrope
	Not meeting the above, but approved by the Regional Review Board
Status 1B	Has at least one of the following devices or therapies in place:
	Left and/or right ventricular assist device implanted
	Continuous infusion of intravenous inotropes
	Not meeting the above, but approved by the Regional Review Board
Status 2	Patients who do not meet the criteria for Status 1A or 1B is listed as a Status 2
Status 7	Patients listed as Status 7 is considered temporarily unsuitable to receive a thoracic organ transplant

Reprinted from Semin [11], Copyright (2004), with permission from Elsevier

has been felt that NT-proBNP levels are not valid in patients with renal failure. Recent data from the PRIDE study refutes this belief [17].

Use of peak exercise VO_2 can be used to stratify ambulatory patients awaiting transplant. In a group of patients from University of Pennsylvania with severe left ventricular dysfunction, VO_2 was predictive of mortality. Cardiac transplantation in this study was safely deferred in ambulatory patients when the VO_2 was more than 14 mL/min/kg [18].

The Canadian Cardiovascular Society classification is another noninvasive tool commonly used to assess angina and its morbidity. Although this system is not as useful for predicting severity of coronary artery disease (a study comparing 493 patients was unable to show a significant difference between the four angina class patients and the incidence of single, double, or triple vessel involvement) it remains useful as a tool to compare populations [19].

Once a patient is ranked in the facilities risk stratification system, they must be continually reassessed [20]. Some patients can become "too well" to be a candidate for transplant. Deng et al. reported seven criteria or profiles of a patient they would consider possibly better served by treatments other than transplant. They are: (1) low risk according to the Heart Failure Survival

Score, (2) peak oxygen consumption greater than 14–18 mL/kg/min without other indications, (3) left ventricular ejection fraction less than 20% alone, (4) history of New York Heart Association class III/IV symptoms alone, (5) history of ventricular arrhythmias alone, (6) no previous attempt at comprehensive neurohormonal blockade, and (7) no structured cardiac transplantation center assessment [20].

The last of these criteria is supported by a retrospective observational review performed at the Cleveland Clinic that observed that in 1,174 referrals for cardiac transplant, 588 were reassigned as candidates for either medical therapy or nontransplant surgery. Also of note is that the 3-year survival (82%) of the 217 patients who actually were transplanted was statistically equivalent to the nontransplant operative groups (excluding partial left ventriculectomy patients) [21].

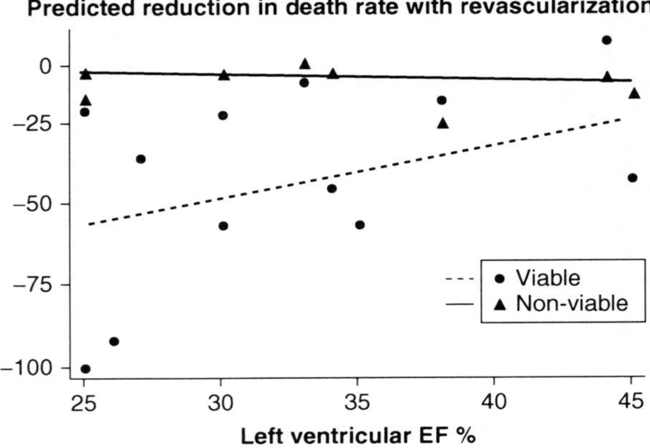

Fig. 10.4 Increasing difference in mortality of patients with viable versus nonviable myocardium. (Reprinted from Allman et al. [2], Copyright (2002), with permission from The American College of Cardiology Foundation)

Surgical Alternatives to Transplant

Surgical treatment for ischemic heart disease needs to be assessed prior to placing a patient on the heart transplant list [22, 23]. "High-risk" conventional surgery has been shown to be a viable alternative to cardiac transplantation in some patient populations [24, 25]. For example, aneurysm repair and reoperative valve replacement can be done on end-stage coronary artery disease patients with acceptable results [26–28].

Most often, it is revascularization that needs to be investigated as an alternative to transplantation. The limiting factor is finding viable tissue to revascularize. In a study of 514 patients with end-stage coronary artery disease and left ventricular ejection fraction between 0.10 and 0.30 undergoing coronary artery bypass, operative mortality rates were 7.1% after revascularization [24]. Left ventricular ejection fraction increased to 0.39 from a mean of 0.24 [24]. The authors concluded that coronary artery bypass grafting can lead to an excellent prognosis for high-risk patients when the myocardium is preoperatively identified as being viable [24].

A meta-analysis performed by Allman et al. strongly suggests that the differentiation of viable from nonviable myocardium could improve outcomes [2, 29, 30]. In Allman's study of 3,088 patients with an average ejection fraction of 32% there was a 79.6% reduction in annual mortality (16% vs. 3.2%) in patients with demonstrated viability preoperatively [2]. The observed improvement in mortality became larger as the ejection fraction of the patient decreased when comparing patients with viable versus nonviable myocardium (See Fig. 10.4).

Kim and Manning wrote in a discussion regarding myocardial viability that 50–75% may be sufficient to provide clinical benefit even without functional improvement after revascularization [31]. They theorized that outcome is due to several factors including prevention or even reversal of adverse remodeling, improved contractile response under stress, prevention of recurrent myocardial ischemia/infarction, and prevention of arrhythmias. This is supported by a study of 135 patients by Samady et al. that noted patients who did not have a significant change in left ventricular function after coronary revascularization did have improvement not only in angina and heart failure scores, but also had similar survival free of cardiac death at a mean follow-up of 32 months to those who did have improvement in left ventricular function [32].

We feel that myocardial viability testing should be a part of every patient's evaluation upon entering a transplant center if they are diagnosed with ischemic cardiomyopathy. If viability is established with targets in patients being considered for transplant the question then becomes when is a patient too sick for revascularization. Or rather, when does the mortality of a revascularization procedure outweigh the mortality of waiting on the transplant list?

The rate of death for staged IA patients has declined while waiting for a transplant from 259/1000 in 1995 to 156/1000 in 2004 [33]. This change is likely from improved medical therapies. This improved mortality changes the algorithm for transplantation. A study by Krakauer et al. followed 9,059 heart transplant candidates 1–2 years after listing to estimate the net benefit achieved from heart transplantation [34]. This study showed a substantial survival benefit only at the highest level of risk. This analysis revealed that there are a high percentage of patients listed and transplanted that may not gain a substantial increase in survival and actually may be harmed. The lack of efficacy of transplant on mortality in these select populations has led some to state that Level 2 patients should not be transplanted. In a study of 7,535 patients listed for transplant between 1999 and 2001 the one-year mortality of patients listed for transplant as Status 2 was no different if the patient was transplanted or not [35].

The correlation between probability of death while awaiting cardiac transplant and probability of receiving a transplant is negative unlike in liver transplantation [34]. This statistic suggests that other factors outside of survival enter into the decision of whom to transplant. The perception exists that the risk to benefit ratios are too high to perform procedures on the end-stage ischemic population. It is therefore difficult to adjust the line where clinicians "throw in the towel" on revascularization and revert to palliation until an organ becomes available. Continual assessment of the state of the art is necessary to balance the necessity of transplant with the option of revascularization.

Exclusion Criteria

Although the heart in isolation may be best treated by transplant, the patient's condition as a whole may not be excluding the patient from being listed for transplantation. The exclusion criteria for heart transplant are decreasing. Advanced age, originally considered a contraindication to transplant, has been shown to be practical in carefully selected patients [36–38]. Morgan et al. compared a subset of patients averaging 67 years of age with a group averaging 48 years of age matched for sex, etiology of heart failure, United Network for Organ Sharing status, and immunosuppression therapy era [38]. They demonstrated no significant difference in overall survival between the groups. Pre-existing patient comorbidities still may preclude transplantation (Table 10.2) [39].

Table 10.2 Risk factors associated with a marked increase in morbidity and mortality after transplant

- Pulmonary Vascular Resistance >6 Wood units, unresponsive to vasodilators
- Pulmonary artery systolic pressure >70 mmHg, unresponsive to treatment
- Active, untreated infection
- Irreversible, severe hepatic disease
- Irreversible, severe renal disease
- Irreversible, severe pulmonary disease
- Age >70 years
- Diabetes mellitus with significant end-organ damage
- Cerebrovascular disease, severe, symptomatic
- Peripheral vascular disease, severe, symptomatic
- Gastrointestinal bleeding, active
- Chronic active hepatitis
- HIV
- Malignancy, recent
- Myocardial infiltrative disease
- Major affective disorder or schizophrenia with poor control
- Substance abuse, active unresolved
- Medical noncompliance

Used with permission by Lippincott, Williams and Wilkins. Adapted from [39]

Assist Devices

A subset of the transplant population will require mechanical assistance prior to their transplant. Currently, mechanical devices mainly function as a safety net to hold patients while they await transplant. It is important to have assist devices available when operating on the end-stage ischemic cardiomyopathy population with low ejection fractions. In a study of low ejection fraction patients undergoing CABG, 51 had an ejection fraction of <20%. Of these 51, 6 used a balloon pump intraoperatively and three needed a left-ventricular assist device [40]. Mechanical assistance allows these patients to be bridged to transplant if it becomes necessary [41–47]. The decision to use a LVAD versus other options such as chronic inotropic therapy is not always a purely medical one. Availability of donors in a particular region and the experience of the LVAD surgical team are all factors [48].

A prospective study of assist devices by Aaronson et al. at the University of Michigan suggested that patients bridged-to-transplantation with an LVAD were more likely to survive to transplantation than those receiving inotropes alone (Fig. 10.5) [49].

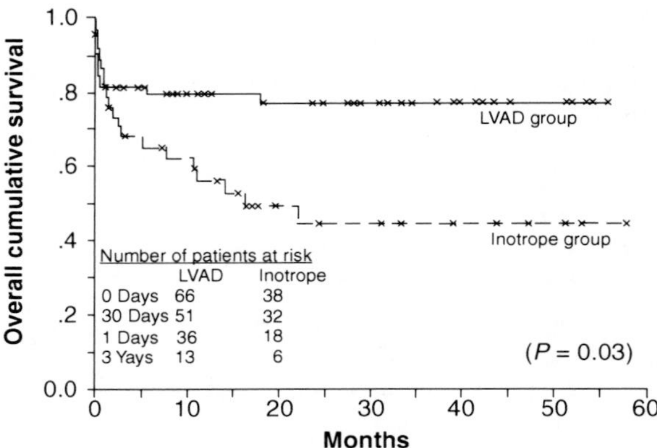

Fig. 10.5 Overall survival from the time of bridging to follow-up: left ventricular assist device (LVAD) group versus inotrope group. (Reprinted from Aaronson et al. [49], Copyright (2002), with permission from The American College of Cardiology Foundation)

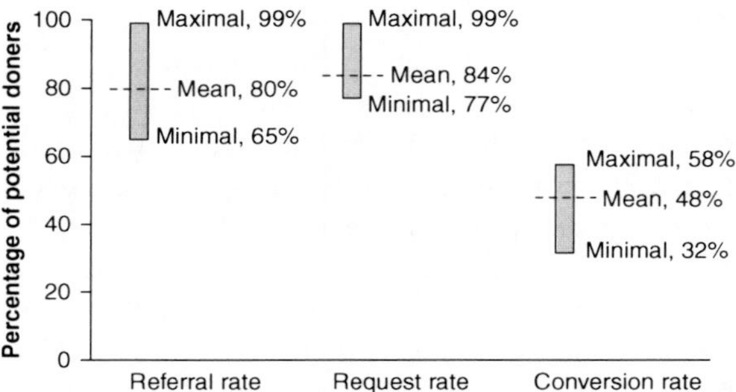

Fig. 10.6 Range of rates of referral, requests, and conversions among the 16 organ-procurement organizations with complete data for 1997 through 1999. (Used with permission from Sheehy et al. [55]. Copyright © 2003 Massachusetts Medical Society. All rights reserved)

Their compilation of data showed that patients who had an LVAD implanted were more likely to be living 3 years later compared to those patients who continued receiving solely inotropes while on the waiting list for transplantation. Copeland et al. also showed an improvement in survival to transplantation by using mechanical assistance. The survival in their historical medical group was 46% which improved to 79% in similar patients treated with a Syncardia Systems Cardiowest™ total artificial heart [42].

Newer devices are under trial that allow for a more miniaturized and simplified design. The inherent design of axial flow pumps, for example, has allowed these devices to be smaller and less complex than pulsatile pumps [50]. There are many pumps available and none are perfect. Each has their own strengths and weaknesses and it is mandatory to individualize the pump to the patient.

Organ Procurement

Organ Shortage

The pool of cardiac transplant candidates is increasing but the pool of donors is static [51]. In North America there were 2,091 cardiac transplants performed in the year 2004 [52]. Of these, 764 were performed secondary to coronary artery disease [52]. The number of heart transplants performed annually in North America has been steadily rising, but it remains a seldom used modality in ischemic heart disease. To put its use in perspective, there were approximately 640,000 patients treated with percutaneous transluminal coronary angioplasty in the year 2002 and 306,000 patients treated with coronary artery bypass grafts in that same year [1]. There are over 112,000 patients awaiting organ transplantation in the United States [53]. The incidence of death while on the waiting list for heart transplantation is about 16% and has remained essentially unchanged over the past decade [54]. The lack of viable organs available in a timely fashion for implant continues to be the Achilles' heel of cardiac transplant.

Legislation and Laws

Legislation such as the 1984 National Organ Transplant Act has helped to increase the amount of donors. The number of potential recipients continues to outpace the rise in donors. The predicted annual number of brain-dead potential organ donors in the USA is between 10,500 and 13,800 [55]. The overall conversion rate (the number of actual donors divided by the number of potential donors) was 42% (Fig. 10.6) [55].

This statistic varies at a regional level. This had led to some territorialism regarding "ownership" of donated organs. The Transplant Act of 1985 stipulated that cadaver donor organs represent a national resource which has helped to decrease geographical turf wars [56]. Incentives such as tax breaks and allowances for lost work have also been made available [57].

Alternate Lists

In an attempt to increase the donor and recipient pool for heart transplant patients, "alternate" lists have been created for donor and recipient candidates otherwise not considered in traditional transplant lists due to diseases such as donor coronary artery disease [58–60]. Laks et al. at UCLA demonstrated that alternate listing did not independently predict early or late mortality [58]. In their group, the only absolute criterion for entering the alternate recipient list was age. In a separate study from the same group, 22 recipients who received donor hearts with mild to moderate coronary artery disease on angiography were shown to have a survival rate of 81.3% at 2 years [59]. Interestingly in this subset of patients freedom from new graft coronary artery disease was 87.5% at 2 years [59]. They concluded that donor hearts with less than mild or moderate plaque in 1 or 2 vessels should be considered for most middle-aged and older recipients who are listed as status 1. The authors also recommended that similar but younger patients be considered for assist devices rather than these "alternate" hearts [59].

Screening angiography has been used to allow older donor hearts previously assumed too diseased with CAD to be added to the alternate donor pool [61]. Age has been found to be a marker of mortality with age 40 appearing to be a cut off value that predicts increased risk of mortality for the recipient [37]. These ages are merely guides though and variables such as hypertension, tobacco use, cocaine abuse, family history of coronary artery disease, and hypercholesterolemia can affect the decision to perform an angiogram. Donor hearts with left ventricular hypertrophy and coronary artery disease are not used as a rule [62].

A partial return to using nonheart beating donors has gained strength because of promising results in renal and hepatic transplantation [63, 64]. Successful cardiac transplants have been performed in hearts retrieved from nonbeating donors in large animal models [65, 66]. Of note, these experiments were done with the aid of heavy pretransplant cardioprotection which may not cross over to practical clinical use.

Donor Selection

Assessing a donor heart for transplant is one of the key components to a successful outcome in heart transplantation. Factors in the assessment of the donor determined in the often used "Crystal City" protocol are age, (>55 years of age should be used selectively), size, Hepatitis B or C status (can be used in selected higher risk patients), left ventricular hypertrophy (donation inadvisable if both ECG shows hypertrophy and echo shows thickness >13 mm), and valvular and congenital abnormalities (often a contraindication although some small defects can be fixed during "benching") [67]. Likely secondary to variability in technique and interpretation by different centers, the use of a single echocardiogram to determine the physiological suitability of a donor is not supported by evidence [67]. The donor yield has been improved by using pulmonary artery catheter measurements to guide decisions [68]. In assessing coronary status, conservative recommendations are for angiography to be performed in male donors >45 years of age and women donors >50 years of age [69]. It has been shown that criteria can be liberalized for recipients with high short-term mortality because of factors such as increased age, prior transplant, or hepatitis C virus-positive status. The visual evaluation of the heart by an experienced surgeon remains one of the best tests of organ suitability.

Organ Matching

Advances in the accuracy and decreased time of processing have allowed HLA typing to gain importance in the matching of organs and recipients. A retrospective analysis of 14,535 cardiac transplants reported to the UNOS registry between 1987 and 1996 strongly supported a positive influence on 3-year survival for both class I HLA-A,B and class II HLA-DR matching [70]. Currently, HLA matching has not gained widespread acceptance given the constraints of organ preservation and recipient acuity.

Organ Preservation

The speed in which the organ is delivered to the recipient remains the key in limiting damage to the donor heart. Preservation solutions continue to vary. Originally the heart was preserved in isotonic saline at 4° Celsius [7]. A retrospective study of all active UNOS heart transplant centers in 1996 revealed 167 different solutions used. Some centers use more than one type of solution [71]. The study was unable to find a consensus regarding the optimal preservation solution. The authors conjectured that short ischemic times may have covered up poorer solution inadequacies. Further understanding of the mechanisms of preservation solutions and new technologies in transporting organs will allow for more flexibility in donor selection [72].

Surgical Technique

Implanting the donated heart has changed little from the anastomotic technique originally described by Shumway and Lower. One of the first modifications was made by Christian Barnard who made the donor right atrial incision from the Inferior Vena Cava (IVC) laterally to the base of the right atrial appendage rather than extending the incision from the IVC proximally to the interatrial septum thereby sparing the sinoatrial node [73]. The Bicaval technique was first described by Cooper and consists of completely excising the recipient right atrium and subsequently performing direct caval anastomoses rather than a right atrial anastomosis [74, 75].

Some groups take this one step further by completely excising both atriums and performing a bicaval anastomosis and two separate pulmonary vein cuff anastomoses [76]. A recent survey of centers performing orthotopic heart transplantation reported that 44% of centers used a combination of more than one technique [77]. In centers that used one technique the majority of the time, 54% used the bicaval technique while 22% used the standard technique [77]. 83% reported reduction of tricuspid valve dysfunction as the reason for changing from the standard to the nonstandard technique [77].

Right heart failure can be a significant source of morbidity after heart transplantation and is often exacerbated by tricuspid regurgitation (TR), which is usually secondary to high recipient pulmonary vascular resistance. As such, some groups now advocate that donor tricuspid annuloplasty be performed with every cardiac transplant [78].

Postoperative Management

Rejection Surveillance

It takes a coordinated multidisciplinary team of nurses, physicians, and paramedical professionals to manage the challenges of the immunosuppressed patient. Improved methods of diagnosing rejection such as use of troponins, biopsies, high-resolution ECG, and MRI have allowed patients to use less amounts of immunosuppresion. The long-term follow-up of function is becoming less invasive which allows closer observation of potential problems within the transplanted organ [79].

The most important technique for follow-up of the graft's status remains the percutaneous transvenous endomyocardial biopsy developed at Stanford in 1973 [80]. The tissue grading of rejection continues to evolve (Table 10.3) [81].

Historically, there have been no reliable serological markers for rejection in heart transplantation. Efforts continue to find a reliable serological method. Studies have been done on B-type natriuretic protein (BNP). High levels after heart transplantation are associated with allograft dysfunction, vasculopathy and are independently predictive of cardiovascular death [82].

Instead of looking at signals that the heart muscle is damaged, some tests are able to measure the immune response to the impending rejection. AlloMap™ has shown promise in some studies performing as a reliable predictor of moderate and severe rejection [83]. Further studies are required though before this method of cardiac monitoring can be used for immunosuppressive maintenance.

Endothelin-1 (ET-1) a vasoconstrictor has been studied as an indicator of acute rejection, post-transplantation ischemic injury, and subsequent development of coronary vasculopathy. A study of 47 heart transplant recipients at 3 months and 2 years after transplant revealed that vascular ET-1 expression was associated with acute rejection while interstitial ET-1 expression was more likely to be associated with post-transplantation ischemic injury and subsequent development of coronary vasculopathy [84].

Imaging such as MRI offers the advantage of reproducibility and comparability and may also offer a method for close surveillance [85, 86]. The reliable prediction of impending rejection by serological means remains a goal of cardiac transplantation.

Changing Immunosuppression

The most important innovation in transplant has been the improvement of immunosuppression. The growth of immunosuppressive options for the patient began

Table 10.3 ISHLT standardized cardiac biopsy grading: acute cellular rejection[a] [81]

2004		1990	
Grade 0 R[b]	No rejection	Grade 0	No rejection
Grade 1 R, mild	Interstitial and/or perivascular infiltrate with up to 1 focus of myocyte damage	Grade 1, mild	
		A – Focal	Focal perivascular and/or interstitial infiltrate without myocyte damage
		B – Diffuse	Diffuse infiltrate without myocyte damage
		Grade 2 moderate (focal)	One focus of infiltrate with associated myocyte damage
Grade 2 R, moderate	Two or more foci of infiltrate with associated myocyte damage	Grade 3, moderate	
		A – Focal	Multifocal infiltrate with myocyte damage
Grade 3 R, severe	Diffuse infiltrate with multifocal myocyte damage ± edema, ± hemorrhage ± vasculitis	B – Diffuse	Diffuse infiltrate with myocyte damage
		Grade 4, severe	Diffuse, polymorphous infiltrate with extensive myocyte damage ± edema, ± hemorrhage + vasculitis

[a]The presence or absence of acute antibody-mediated rejection (AMR) may be recorded as AMR 0 or AMR 1, as required
[b]Where "R" denotes revised grade to avoid confusion with 1990 scheme
Reprinted from Stewart et al. [81]with permission from International Society for Heart and Lung Transplantation

with corticosteroids and now includes calcineurin inhibitors, antimetabolites, and induction agents to name but a few. The future will likely include genetic modifications of both the donor organ and the host to help create a more symbiotic relationship or chimera.

Corticosteroids were one of the first agents used for immunosuppression in 1949 for the treatment of rheumatoid arthritis [87] and foreshadowed the problem immunosuppresion continues to have today; balancing side effects with effective immunosuppresion [88–90]. Side effects include health and cosmetic concerns which decrease compliance especially in the adolescent population. Still used as a method of controlling rejection episodes, today more and more centers are excluding steroids from their daily regimes when possible [91].

Azathioprine (Imuran®) has a long track record and works by decreasing purine synthesis. This drug has largely been replaced by the drug mycophenolate mofetil (MMF)(CellCept®) [81]. Benefits that MMF has include renal protection, possible CAD protection, and improved immunosuppresion [81].

Calcineurin inhibitors are the most significant of the immunosuppressive medications [92]. Cyclosporine (Neoral, Sandimmune) was the first calcineurin inhibitor introduced reducing the transcription of IL-2 in addition to inhibiting IL-3, IL-4, Tumor necrosis factor alpha (TNF-α), and granulocyte macrophage-colony-stimulating factor (GM-CSF) gene activation [92]. A similar medication, Tacrolimus (Prograf®), displays similar patient survival rates and incidences of rejection, nephrotoxicity, diabetes, and infections as cyclosporine, but has a lower incidence of arterial hypertension and hyperlipidemia [93]. Tacrolimus has also been used as rescue therapy from steroid-resistant rejection [93].

Sirolimus (Rapamune®) acts by inhibiting cellular proliferation and migration in response to alloantigens [94]. It can help prevent the proliferation of intimal hyperplasia. In a study of 46 patients with existing allograft vasculopathy treated with sirolimus in addition to a calcineurin antagonists there was a significant reduction in myocardial infarction, requirement for revascularization, and angiographic progression of coronary artery disease [95]. Everolimus (Certican®), a derivative of Rapamycin, has also been shown to reduce the severity and incidence of cardiac-allograft vasculopathy [33].

Polyclonal antibodies such as ALG developed at the University of Minnesota reduce the amount of circulating T cells. The evolution of polyclonal antibodies has been toward gradually "humanizing" the antibody to help prevent adverse first dose effects such as fever, chills, generalized weakness, hypotension, bronchospasm, vomiting, and diarrhea [96].

Although individual patient modifications are a necessity, an example of a modern immunosuppressive regime consists of: (1) FK-506 started POD 1 at a dose of 0.5 mg bid. (2) Methylprednisolone (Solu-Medrol®) 500 mg intraoperatively then three doses every 8 h at 125 mg followed by 20 mg daily of Prednisone which is then tapered as allowable. (3) MMF at a dose of 1 g twice a day. (4) Basiliximab (Simulect®), 20 mg, is given the day of surgery and then postoperative on day four. Further or alternative induction therapy (<2.5–5.0 mg of antithymocyte globulin (Atgam®) per kilogram per day or ≤5 mg of muromonab-CD3 (Orthoclone OKT3®) per day) is also sometimes used for patients at increased risk. Rejection is usually treated with either corticosteroids and/or antibodies dependent on the histologic grade and presence or absence of hemodynamic compromise. In addition to this most centers also put the patients on lipid lowering statin therapy to prevent neointimal hyperplasia and prophylactic trimethoprim-sulfamethoxazole (Bactrim®) and an antifungal for prevention of opportunistic infections. Treatment with intravenous Ganciclovir (Cytovene®) for 14–28 days is done for cytomegalovirus-negative recipients of hearts from cytomegalovirus-positive donors.

Due to these more effective immunosuppressive regimes, acute rejection is now not the leading cause of mortality in transplant patients [97]. A recent analysis by Kirklin et al. of 7,290 patients undergoing cardiac transplantation at 42 different institutions showed the risk of mortality from acute rejection to be decreasing during the decade studied and currently is less than 5% [98]. In this same analysis, the mortality from both malignancy and allograft coronary artery disease has continued to rise during the same period [98].

Improving Results of Heart Transplant

Due to technical and medical innovations, heart transplantation today is the gold standard treatment for end-stage CAD without evidence of viability. Medical management mortality rates continue to be high even with optimal therapy [99]. The ATLAS trial also showed that acute coronary events are frequent and ischemia remains a significant cause of sudden death in patients with medically managed ischemic cardiomyopathy [30].

Today, survival at 1 and 3 year intervals is 85.3 and 77.9%, respectively, for patients with CAD that are treated with heart transplantation [100]. Ischemic heart disease patients can have similar outcomes to other heart disease patients undergoing transplant. Incidence of sudden death in cardiac transplant patients with a history of ischemic heart disease is actually lower in some study groups than in those transplanted for idiopathic cardiomyopathy [101]. In other studies though, a difference in medium and long-term survival has been shown between these groups favoring idiopathic cardiomyopathy [22]. Martinelli et al. also noted a better 5-year actuarial survival rate for dilated cardiomyopathy patients when compared to ischemic cardiomyopathy patients [102]. The two group's differences are likely due to systemic diseases that also progress ischemic heart disease such as diabetes mellitus, hypercholesterolemia, and hypertriglyceridemia.

Transplant Morbidity

Allograft vasculopathy, a manifestation of chronic rejection, and renal failure are significant sources of morbidity for patients who have undergone cardiac transplantation. [103]. In a sample of approximately 70,000 nonrenal solid organ transplant recipients, the risk of developing chronic renal failure in heart transplant recipients was 16% at 10 years post transplant [104]. From annual angiography reports at 1 year after transplant the group at Stanford reported an incidence of moderate-to-severe proximal or midvessel coronary artery disease (defined as 40% or more stenosis in one or more primary or secondary epicardial arteries) to be 15% (54/353) [97].

Angiographic evidence of coronary artery disease occurs in approximately 42% of patients 5 years after transplant 7% of which is severe [105]. The lesions in allograft vasculopathy produce narrowing along the entire length of the coronary tree from the epicardial to intramyocardial segments resulting in a rapid obliteration of third-order vessels [106]. Theories on the mechanism of development of this plague on cardiac grafts include immunological injury, ischemia reperfusion, chronic inflammation, immunosuppressive medications, hyperlipidemia, hypertension, degree of mismatch of major histocompatability complexes, donor atherosclerosis, and viral infections [107]. Traditional symptoms and warning signs of ischemia such as angina are often not experienced by heart transplant patients which adds to the difficulty in diagnosing and treating this population [108]. Intravascular ultrasound is currently the most sensitive imaging technique for early detection of coronary artery disease [109].

Medical management can help allograft vasculopathy. HMG CoA reductase inhibitors have shown a benefit decreasing cardiac allograft vasculopathy and the number of rejection episodes [110]. HMG CoA's mechanism has recently been determined [111]. Perioperative myocardial protection can assist in decreasing incidence of allograft coronary disease as well [112].

Future of Transplant

The shortage of transplantable organs likely will continue. There are two branches in the future of surgical treatment for heart failure. They are either complete mechanical replacement or regeneration at a cellular level either in vivo or as a graft placed into the host after being grown in a lab. Likely the future will involve some combination of these two with machines providing support while the heart is healing at the cellular level [113]. Therapies to promote such cellular growth include gene therapy, transplants of muscle stem cells or cardiac myocytes, and treatment with medication. One agent, the beta-agonist Clenbuterol has been shown to promote physiologic hypertrophy of the heart with subsequent improvement in contraction in patients who have been treated for several months [114].

Research continues to develop methods of growing tissues either in vitro or in vivo for transplant. Xenotransplant continues to evolve. Hyperacute rejection has largely been overcome with using transgenic organisms. It has been shown in vitro that xenogenic transplantation of cardiomyocytes is possible [115]. Delayed xenograft rejection is currently regarded as the major barrier to successful xenotransplantation [116]. The issues of possible spread of viral infections, prions, and ethical concerns will need to be explored in addition to the immunological problems prior to xenotransplant becoming a viable option.

Some hope that myocyte regeneration rather than replacement will be the future of treatment for end-stage ischemic heart disease [117]. It has been shown that at the level of the myocyte, proteins of the cytoskeleton are altered in hypertrophied and failing human hearts. These changes are reversed by the use of an LVAD, suggesting that the cytoskeleton is not the limiting factor in determining full cardiac recovery [118]. Certain cells of the heart may have an extracardiac origin which would support the theory that the heart has the ability to heal [119]. Chimerism of the graft and host appears to hold promise for either providing a mechanism for regeneration or for more effective immunosuppression strategies in the future [120].

Conclusion

Cardiac transplantation continues to be the best long-term option for end-stage ischemic cardiomyopathy. The preoperative evaluation and exhaustion of all other treatment options is essential when managing this population. It appears inevitable that one day the discouraging scarcity of donors will be alleviated by either cultured tissue or engineered machines.

References

1. American Heart Association. Heart Disease and Stroke Statistics – 2005 Update. Dallas, Texas: American Heart Association; 2005.
2. Allman KC, Shaw LJ, Hachamovitch R, Udelson JE. Myocardial viability testing and impact of revascularization on prognosis in patients with coronary artery disease and left ventricular dysfunction: a meta-analysis. J Am Coll Cardiol. 2002;39(7):1151–8.
3. Herrick JB. Landmark article (JAMA 1912). Clinical features of sudden obstruction of the coronary arteries. By James B. Herrick. JAMA. 1983;250(13):1757–65.
4. Ventura HO, Muhammed K. Historical perspectives on cardiac transplantation: the past as prologue to challenges for the 21st century. Curr Opin Cardiol. 2001;16(2):118–23.
5. Barnard CN. The operation. A human cardiac transplant: an interim report of a successful operation performed at Groote Schuur Hospital, Cape Town. S Afr Med J. 1967;41(48): 1271–4.
6. Patterson C, Patterson KB. The history of heart transplantation. Am J Med Sci. 1997;314(3):190–7.
7. DiBardino DJ. The history and development of cardiac transplantation. Tex Heart Inst J. 1999;26(3):198–205.
8. Goodwin JF. Cardiac transplantation. Circulation. 1986; 74(5):913–6.
9. Heimbecker RO. Transplantation: the cyclosporine revolution. Can J Cardiol. 1985;1(6):354–7.
10. Taylor DO, Edwards LB, Boucek MM, et al. Registry of the international society for heart and lung transplantation: twenty-second official adult heart transplant report–2005. J Heart Lung Transplant. 2005;24(8):945–55.
11. Boyle A, Colvin-Adams M. Recipient selection and management. Semin Thorac Cardiovasc Surg. 2004;16(4): 358–63.

12. Mandak JS, Aaronson KD, Mancini DM. Serial assessment of exercise capacity after heart transplantation. J Heart Lung Transplant. 1995;14(3):468–78.
13. Pflugfelder PW, McKenzie FN, Kostuk WJ. Hemodynamic profiles at rest and during supine exercise after orthotopic cardiac transplantation. Am J Cardiol. 1988;61(15): 1328–33.
14. Deng MC, De Meester JM, Smits JM, Heinecke J, Scheld HH. Effect of receiving a heart transplant: analysis of a national cohort entered on to a waiting list, stratified by heart failure severity. Comparative Outcome and Clinical Profiles in Transplantation (COCPIT) Study Group. BMJ. 2000;321(7260):540–5.
15. Aaronson KD, Schwartz JS, Chen TM, Wong KL, Goin JE, Mancini DM. Development and prospective validation of a clinical index to predict survival in ambulatory patients referred for cardiac transplant evaluation. Circulation. 1997;95(12):2660–7.
16. Rothenburger M, Wichter T, Schmid C, et al. Aminoterminal pro type B natriuretic peptide as a predictive and prognostic marker in patients with chronic heart failure. J Heart Lung Transplant. 2004;23(10):1189–97.
17. Anwaruddin S, Lloyd-Jones DM, Baggish A, et al. Renal function, congestive heart failure, and amino-terminal pro-brain natriuretic peptide measurement: results from the ProBNP investigation of Dyspnea in the emergency department (PRIDE) study. J Am Coll Cardiol. 2006;47(1):91–7.
18. Mancini DM, Eisen H, Kussmaul W, Mull R, Edmunds Jr LH, Wilson JR. Value of peak exercise oxygen consumption for optimal timing of cardiac transplantation in ambulatory patients with heart failure. Circulation. 1991;83(3):778–86.
19. Sangareddi V, Chockalingam A, Gnanavelu G, Subramaniam T, Jagannathan V, Elangovan S. Canadian Cardiovascular Society classification of effort angina: an angiographic correlation. Coron Artery Dis. 2004;15(2):111–4.
20. Deng MC, Smits JM, Packer M. Selecting patients for heart transplantation: which patients are too well for transplant? Curr Opin Cardiol. 2002;17(2):137–44.
21. Mahon NG, O'Neill JO, Young JB, et al. Contemporary outcomes of outpatients referred for cardiac transplantation evaluation to a tertiary heart failure center: impact of surgical alternatives. J Card Fail. 2004;10(4):273–8.
22. Aziz T, Burgess M, Rahman AN, Campbell CS, Yonan N. Cardiac transplantation for cardiomyopathy and ischemic heart disease: differences in outcome up to 10 years. J Heart Lung Transplant. 2001;20(5):525–33.
23. Luu M, Stevenson LW, Brunken RC, Drinkwater DM, Schelbert HR, Tillisch JH. Delayed recovery of revascularized myocardium after referral for cardiac transplantation. Am Heart J. 1990;119(3 Pt 1):668–70.
24. Hausmann H, Topp H, Siniawski H, Holz S, Hetzer R. Decision-making in end-stage coronary artery disease: revascularization or heart transplantation? Ann Thorac Surg. 1997;64(5):1296–301. discussion 302.
25. Van Meter Jr CH, Smart FW, Ventura HO, et al. High-risk surgery as an alternative to transplantation. Tex Heart Inst J. 1994;21(4):302–4.
26. Mitre ZV, Cvetanovski V, Hristov N, Petrusevska G. Ischemic dilatative cardiomyopathy and aneurysms of the left ventricular cavity: transplantation vs alternative surgery. Int J Artif Organs. 2002;25(5):401–10.
27. Mitrev Z, Anguseva T, Vasileva A, Hristov N, Risteski P. Transplantation or alternative surgical treatment of patients with ischemic dilative cardiomyopathy and aneurysmatic dilation of the left ventricular cavity. Int J Artif Organs. 2002;25(4):321–6.
28. Sanchez JA, Smith CR, Drusin RE, Reison DS, Malm JR, Rose EA. High-risk reparative surgery. A neglected alternative to heart transplantation. Circulation. 1990;82(5 Suppl):IV302–5.
29. Bonow RO. Myocardial viability and prognosis in patients with ischemic left ventricular dysfunction. J Am Coll Cardiol. 2002;39(7):1159–62.
30. Uretsky BF, Thygesen K, Armstrong PW, et al. Acute coronary findings at autopsy in heart failure patients with sudden death: results from the assessment of treatment with lisinopril and survival (ATLAS) trial. Circulation. 2000;102(6): 611–6.
31. Kim RJ, Manning WJ. Viability assessment by delayed enhancement cardiovascular magnetic resonance: will low-dose dobutamine dull the shine? Circulation. 2004;109(21): 2476–9.
32. Samady H, Elefteriades JA, Abbott BG, Mattera JA, McPherson CA, Wackers FJ. Failure to improve left ventricular function after coronary revascularization for ischemic cardiomyopathy is not associated with worse outcome. Circulation. 1999;100(12):1298–304.
33. Eisen HJ, Tuzcu EM, Dorent R, et al. Everolimus for the prevention of allograft rejection and vasculopathy in cardiac-transplant recipients. N Engl J Med. 2003;349(9): 847–58.
34. Krakauer H, Lin MJ, Bailey RC. Projected survival benefit as criterion for listing and organ allocation in heart transplantation. J Heart Lung Transplant. 2005;24(6):680–9.
35. Jimenez J, Bennett Edwards L, Higgins R, Bauerlein J, Pham S, Mallon S. Should stable UNOS status 2 patients be transplanted? J Heart Lung Transplant. 2005;24(2): 178–83.
36. Demers P, Moffatt S, Oyer PE, Hunt SA, Reitz BA, Robbins RC. Long-term results of heart transplantation in patients older than 60 years. J Thorac Cardiovasc Surg. 2003;126(1):224–31.
37. Gupta D, Piacentino 3rd V, Macha M, et al. Effect of older donor age on risk for mortality after heart transplantation. Ann Thorac Surg. 2004;78(3):890–9.
38. Morgan JA, John R, Weinberg AD, et al. Long-term results of cardiac transplantation in patients 65 years of age and older: a comparative analysis. Ann Thorac Surg. 2003;76(6): 1982–7.
39. Textbook of cardiovascular medicine. Lippincott Williams & Wilkins; Ovid Technologies], 2002. (Accessed at Online version: http://gateway.ovid.com/ovidweb.cgi?T=JS&MODE=ovid&NEWS=n&PAGE=booktext&D=books&SC=00140011&LOGOUT=http://catalog.library.jhu.edu/ Available to US Hopkins Community).
40. Tjan TD, Kondruweit M, Scheld HH, et al. The bad ventricle–revascularization versus transplantation. Thorac Cardiovasc Surg. 2000;48(1):9–14.
41. Castells E, Calbet JM, Saura E, et al. Acute myocardial infarction with cardiogenic shock: treatment with mechanical circulatory assistance and heart transplantation. Transplant Proc. 2003;35(5):1940–1.

42. Copeland JG, Smith RG, Arabia FA, et al. Cardiac replacement with a total artificial heart as a bridge to transplantation. N Engl J Med. 2004;351(9):859–67.
43. Faber C, McCarthy PM, Smedira NG, Young JB, Starling RC, Hoercher KJ. Implantable left ventricular assist device for patients with postinfarction ventricular septal defect. J Thorac Cardiovasc Surg. 2002;124(2):400–1.
44. Grinda JM, Latremouille CH, Chevalier P, et al. Bridge to transplantation with the DeBakey VAD axial pump: a single center report. Eur J Cardiothorac Surg. 2002;22(6):965–70.
45. Morgan JA, Stewart AS, Lee BJ, Oz MC, Naka Y. Role of the Abiomed BVS 5000 device for short-term support and bridge to transplantation. ASAIO J. 2004;50(4):360–3.
46. Navia JL, McCarthy PM, Hoercher KJ, et al. Do left ventricular assist device (LVAD) bridge-to-transplantation outcomes predict the results of permanent LVAD implantation? Ann Thorac Surg. 2002;74(6):2051–62. discussion 62–3.
47. Wang SS, Chu SH, Ko WJ, et al. Ventricular assist as a bridge to heart transplantation. Transplant Proc. 1998;30(7): 3401–2.
48. McCarthy PM. Implantable left ventricular assist device bridge-to-transplantation: natural selection, or is this the natural selection? J Am Coll Cardiol. 2002;39(8):1255–7.
49. Aaronson KD, Eppinger MJ, Dyke DB, Wright S, Pagani FD. Left ventricular assist device therapy improves utilization of donor hearts. J Am Coll Cardiol. 2002;39(8):1247–54.
50. Goldstein DJ, Zucker M, Arroyo L, et al. Safety and feasibility trial of the MicroMed DeBakey ventricular assist device as a bridge to transplantation. J Am Coll Cardiol. 2005;45(6):962–3.
51. Stevenson LW, Warner SL, Steimle AE, et al. The impending crisis awaiting cardiac transplantation. Modeling a solution based on selection. Circulation. 1994;89(1):450–7.
52. Quarterly Report. In: The International Society for Heart and Lung Transplantation; 2004.
53. United Network of Organ Sharing. Accessed at www.unos.org on 19 Nov 2011.
54. Scientific Registry of Transplant Recipients. Accessed at www.ustransplant.org/fastfacts.aspx on 19 Nov 2011.
55. Sheehy E, Conrad SL, Brigham LE, et al. Estimating the number of potential organ donors in the United States. N Engl J Med. 2003;349(7):667–74.
56. Zaontz L. The National Organ Transplantation Act. Bull Am Coll Surg. 1985;70(5):18.
57. Napolitano J. Wisconsin Senate Approves Tax Deduction for Organ Donors. The New York Times;2004.
58. Laks H, Marelli D, Fonarow GC, et al. Use of two recipient lists for adults requiring heart transplantation. J Thorac Cardiovasc Surg. 2003;125(1):49–59.
59. Marelli D, Laks H, Bresson S, et al. Results after transplantation using donor hearts with preexisting coronary artery disease. J Thorac Cardiovasc Surg. 2003;126(3):821–5.
60. Patel J, Kobashigawa JA. Cardiac transplantation: the alternate list and expansion of the donor pool. Curr Opin Cardiol. 2004;19(2):162–5.
61. Hauptman PJ, O'Connor KJ, Wolf RE, McNeil BJ. Angiography of potential cardiac donors. J Am Coll Cardiol. 2001;37(5):1252–8.
62. John R. Donor management and selection for heart transplantation. Semin Thorac Cardiovasc Surg. 2004;16(4): 364–9.
63. Booster MH, Wijnen RM, Vroemen JP, van Hooff JP, Kootstra G. In situ preservation of kidneys from non-heart-beating donors–a proposal for a standardized protocol. Transplantation. 1993;56(3):613–7.
64. Yanaga K, Kakizoe S, Ikeda T, Podesta LG, Demetris AJ, Starzl TE. Procurement of liver allografts from non-heart beating donors. Transplant Proc. 1990;22(1):275–8.
65. Martin J, Sarai K, Yoshitake M, et al. Successful orthotopic pig heart transplantation from non-heart-beating donors. J Heart Lung Transplant. 1999;18(6):597–606.
66. Takagaki M, Hisamochi K, Morimoto T, Bando K, Sano S, Shimizu N. Successful transplantation of cadaver hearts harvested one hour after hypoxic cardiac arrest. J Heart Lung Transplant. 1996;15(5):527–31.
67. Zaroff JG, Rosengard BR, Armstrong WF, et al. Consensus conference report: maximizing use of organs recovered from the cadaver donor: cardiac recommendations, March 28–29, 2001, Crystal City, Va. Circulation. 2002;106(7): 836–41.
68. Wheeldon DR, Potter CD, Oduro A, Wallwork J, Large SR. Transforming the "unacceptable" donor: outcomes from the adoption of a standardized donor management technique. J Heart Lung Transplant. 1995;14(4):734–42.
69. Baldwin JC, Anderson JL, Boucek MM, et al. 24th Bethesda conference: cardiac transplantation. Task Force 2: Donor guidelines. J Am Coll Cardiol. 1993;22(1):15–20.
70. Thompson JS, Thacker 2nd LR, Takemoto S. The influence of conventional and cross-reactive group HLA matching on cardiac transplant outcome: an analysis from the United Network of Organ Sharing Scientific Registry. Transplantation. 2000;69(10):2178–86.
71. Demmy TL, Biddle JS, Bennett LE, Walls JT, Schmaltz RA, Curtis JJ. Organ preservation solutions in heart transplantation–patterns of usage and related survival. Transplantation. 1997;63(2):262–9.
72. Rivard AL, Gallegos RP, Bianco RW, Liao K. The basic science aspect of donor heart preservation: a review. J Extra Corpor Technol. 2004;36(3):269–74.
73. Barnard CN. What we have learned about heart transplants. J Thorac Cardiovasc Surg. 1968;56(4):457–68.
74. Aziz T, Burgess M, Khafagy R, et al. Bicaval and standard techniques in orthotopic heart transplantation: medium-term experience in cardiac performance and survival. J Thorac Cardiovasc Surg. 1999;118(1):115–22.
75. Cooper DK. Experimental development of cardiac transplantation. Br Med J. 1968;4(624):174–81.
76. Liao KK, Bolman 3rd RM. Operative techniques in orthotopic heart transplantation. Semin Thorac Cardiovasc Surg. 2004;16(4):370–7.
77. Aziz TM, Burgess MI, El-Gamel A, et al. Orthotopic cardiac transplantation technique: a survey of current practice. Ann Thorac Surg. 1999;68(4):1242–6.
78. Jeevanandam V, Russell H, Mather P, Furukawa S, Anderson A, Raman J. Donor tricuspid annuloplasty during orthotopic heart transplantation: long-term results of a prospective controlled study. Ann Thorac Surg. 2006;82(6):2089–95. discussion 95.
79. Dandel M, Knollmann FD, Wellnhofer E, Hummel M, Kapell S, Hetzer R. Noninvasive surveillance strategy for early identification of heart transplant recipients with possible coronary stenoses. Transplant Proc. 2003;35(6):2113–6.

80. Billingham ME, Caves PK, Dong Jr E, Shumway NE. The diagnosis of canine orthotopic cardiac allograft rejection by transvenous endomyocardial biopsy. Transplant Proc. 1973;5(1):741–3.
81. Stewart S, Winters GL, Fishbein MC, et al. Revision of the 1990 working formulation for the standardization of nomenclature in the diagnosis of heart rejection. J Heart Lung Transplant. 2005;24(11):1710–20.
82. Mehra MR, Uber PA, Potluri S, Ventura HO, Scott RL, Park MH. Usefulness of an elevated B-type natriuretic peptide to predict allograft failure, cardiac allograft vasculopathy, and survival after heart transplantation. Am J Cardiol. 2004;94(4):454–8.
83. Deng MC, Eisen HJ, Mehra MR, et al. Noninvasive discrimination of rejection in cardiac allograft recipients using gene expression profiling. Am J Transplant. 2006;6(1):150–60.
84. Ferri C, Properzi G, Tomassoni G, et al. Patterns of myocardial endothelin-1 expression and outcome after cardiac transplantation. Circulation. 2002;105(15):1768–71.
85. Bellenger NG, Marcus NJ, Davies C, Yacoub M, Banner NR, Pennell DJ. Left ventricular function and mass after orthotopic heart transplantation: a comparison of cardiovascular magnetic resonance with echocardiography. J Heart Lung Transplant. 2000;19(5):444–52.
86. Marie PY, Angioi M, Carteaux JP, et al. Detection and prediction of acute heart transplant rejection with the myocardial T2 determination provided by a black-blood magnetic resonance imaging sequence. J Am Coll Cardiol. 2001;37(3):825–31.
87. Neeck G. Fifty years of experience with cortisone therapy in the study and treatment of rheumatoid arthritis. Ann N Y Acad Sci. 2002;966:28–38.
88. Chan GL, Gruber SA, Skjei KL, Canafax DM. Principles of immunosuppression. Crit Care Clin. 1990;6(4):841–92.
89. Lan NC, Karin M, Nguyen T, et al. Mechanisms of glucocorticoid hormone action. J Steroid Biochem. 1984;20(1):77–88.
90. Woodley SL, Renlund DG, O'Connell JB, Bristow MR. Immunosuppression following cardiac transplantation. Cardiol Clin. 1990;8(1):83–96.
91. Felkel TO, Smith AL, Reichenspurner HC, et al. Survival and incidence of acute rejection in heart transplant recipients undergoing successful withdrawal from steroid therapy. J Heart Lung Transplant. 2002;21(5):530–9.
92. Cheung A, Menkis AH. Cyclosporine heart transplantation. Transplant Proc. 1998;30(5):1881–4.
93. Taylor DO, Barr ML, Radovancevic B, et al. A randomized, multicenter comparison of tacrolimus and cyclosporine immunosuppressive regimens in cardiac transplantation: decreased hyperlipidemia and hypertension with tacrolimus. J Heart Lung Transplant. 1999;18(4):336–45.
94. Kahan BD, Podbielski J, Napoli KL, Katz SM, Meier-Kriesche HU, Van Buren CT. Immunosuppressive effects and safety of a sirolimus/cyclosporine combination regimen for renal transplantation. Transplantation. 1998;66(8):1040–6.
95. Mancini D, Pinney S, Burkhoff D, et al. Use of rapamycin slows progression of cardiac transplantation vasculopathy. Circulation. 2003;108(1):48–53.
96. Beniaminovitz A, Itescu S, Lietz K, et al. Prevention of rejection in cardiac transplantation by blockade of the interleukin-2 receptor with a monoclonal antibody. N Engl J Med. 2000;342(9):613–9.
97. Keogh AM, Valantine HA, Hunt SA, et al. Impact of proximal or midvessel discrete coronary artery stenoses on survival after heart transplantation. J Heart Lung Transplant. 1992;11(5):892–901.
98. Kirklin JK, Naftel DC, Bourge RC, et al. Evolving trends in risk profiles and causes of death after heart transplantation: a ten-year multi-institutional study. J Thorac Cardiovasc Surg. 2003;125(4):881–90.
99. Pitt B, Zannad F, Remme WJ, et al. The effect of spironolactone on morbidity and mortality in patients with severe heart failure. Randomized Aldactone Evaluation Study Investigators. N Engl J Med. 1999;341(10):709–17.
100. Quarterly Report. The International Society for Heart and Lung Transplantation 2005.
101. Chantranuwat C, Blakey JD, Kobashigawa JA, et al. Sudden, unexpected death in cardiac transplant recipients: an autopsy study. J Heart Lung Transplant. 2004;23(6):683–9.
102. Martinelli L, Rinaldi M, Pederzolli C, et al. Different results of cardiac transplantation in patients with ischemic and dilated cardiomyopathy. Eur J Cardiothorac Surg. 1995;9(11):644–50.
103. Sarris GE, Moore KA, Schroeder JS, et al. Cardiac transplantation: the Stanford experience in the cyclosporine era. J Thorac Cardiovasc Surg. 1994;108(2):240–51. discussion 51–2.
104. Ojo AO, Held PJ, Port FK, et al. Chronic renal failure after transplantation of a nonrenal organ. N Engl J Med. 2003;349(10):931–40.
105. Costanzo MR, Naftel DC, Pritzker MR, et al. Heart transplant coronary artery disease detected by coronary angiography: a multiinstitutional study of preoperative donor and recipient risk factors. Cardiac Transplant Research Database. J Heart Lung Transplant. 1998;17(8):744–53.
106. Lietz K, Miller LW. Current understanding and management of allograft vasculopathy. Semin Thorac Cardiovasc Surg. 2004;16(4):386–94.
107. Russell PS, Chase CM, Winn HJ, Colvin RB. Coronary atherosclerosis in transplanted mouse hearts. I. Time course and immunogenetic and immunopathological considerations. Am J Pathol. 1994;144(2):260–74.
108. Stark RP, McGinn AL, Wilson RF. Chest pain in cardiac-transplant recipients. Evidence of sensory reinnervation after cardiac transplantation. N Engl J Med. 1991;324(25):1791–4.
109. Tsutsui H, Ziada KM, Schoenhagen P, et al. Lumen loss in transplant coronary artery disease is a biphasic process involving early intimal thickening and late constrictive remodeling: results from a 5-year serial intravascular ultrasound study. Circulation. 2001;104(6):653–7.
110. Wenke K, Meiser B, Thiery J, et al. Simvastatin initiated early after heart transplantation: 8-year prospective experience. Circulation. 2003;107(1):93–7.
111. Kwak B, Mulhaupt F, Myit S, Mach F. Statins as a newly recognized type of immunomodulator. Nat Med. 2000;6(12):1399–402.
112. Beyersdorf F. Myocardial and endothelial protection for heart transplantation in the new millenium: lessons learned and future directions. J Heart Lung Transplant. 2004;23(6):657–65.
113. McCarthy PM, Smith WA. Mechanical circulatory support–a long and winding road. Science. 2002;295(5557):998–9.

114. Hon JK, Yacoub MH. Bridge to recovery with the use of left ventricular assist device and clenbuterol. Ann Thorac Surg. 2003;75(6 Suppl):S36–41.
115. Naito H, Nishizaki K, Yoshikawa M, et al. Xenogeneic embryonic stem cell-derived cardiomyocyte transplantation. Transplant Proc. 2004;36(8):2507–8.
116. McGregor CG, Teotia SS, Byrne GW, et al. Cardiac xenotransplantation: progress toward the clinic. Transplantation. 2004;78(11):1569–75.
117. Flugelman MY, Lewis BS. The promise of myocardial repair–towards a better understanding. Eur Heart J. 2004;25(17):1483–5.
118. Aquila LA, McCarthy PM, Smedira NG, Young JB, Moravec CS. Cytoskeletal structure and recovery in single human cardiac myocytes. J Heart Lung Transplant. 2004;23(8):954–63.
119. Fox R. Cell transplants for ischemic myocardium. Circulation. 2002;106(13):e9034.
120. Quaini F, Urbanek K, Beltrami AP, et al. Chimerism of the transplanted heart. N Engl J Med. 2002;346(1):5–15.

Alternative Therapies for Chronic Refractory Coronary Artery Disease

11

Brent A. Bauer

Introduction

Complementary and alternative medicine (CAM) appears to be well embedded into the American culture [1]. This phenomenon, coupled with the explosive growth of the Internet, has provided patients and consumers dramatically increased access to information about a variety of alternative treatments that were relatively unheard of a decade or two ago. Most studies suggest that at least 40% of US adults have used some form of CAM in the past year. Interest in CAM is particularly high in those patients who are facing chronic illnesses, and patients with chronic coronary artery disease (CAD) are no exception. Thus, it is imperative for every physician who deals with patients with chronic CAD to have a basic understanding of CAM and its general risks and benefits. Physicians who have additional familiarity with those CAM therapies specifically targeting CAD will be able to educate their patients and enable them to make informed decisions regarding the use of CAM (Table 11.1).

Definition of CAM

As of yet, there is no universally accepted definition of CAM. Many authors have suggested that "complementary" therapies are things that patients can do in conjunction with conventional care (e.g., practicing meditation while also taking an ACE-inhibitor for hypertension), while "alternative" therapies are those things which patients do in place of conventional care (e.g., using herbs in place of chemotherapy as a cancer treatment). Yet this definition is of limited usefulness since most surveys have shown that the vast majority of CAM users employ CAM therapies in conjunction with usual care; very few patients use CAM exclusively.

Eisenberg et al. [2] published one of the first CAM usage surveys which helped bring the realm of CAM to the attention of conventional medicine. In that survey, CAM was defined largely by what it is not (i.e., health care practices not covered by insurance, not taught in medical schools, and not provided in most hospitals). Interestingly, in the relatively short span of time since that definition was written, the landscape has changed dramatically. In fact, over three fourths of medical schools now offer some form of CAM education in the curriculum [3, 4], many hospitals now offer a wide variety of CAM therapies, and increasingly, insurance coverage for CAM is becoming more widely available.

Some have attempted to define CAM by listing modalities that are considered "CAM" (e.g., acupuncture, herbs, chiropractic, massage therapy, etc.). However, such lists are of limited usefulness as the field is not static. Whereas acupuncture might have been readily identified as a CAM modality 20–30 years ago, the 1994 National Institutes of Health (NIH) Consensus Statement on Acupuncture determined that acupuncture is a validated treatment for postoperative pain and nausea and vomiting associated with chemotherapy [5]. This same consensus statement also identified a num-

B.A. Bauer
Complementary and Integrative Medicine Program,
Mayo Clinic,
Rochester, MN, USA
e-mail: bauer.brent@mayo.edu

G.W. Barsness and D.R. Holmes Jr. (eds.), *Coronary Artery Disease*,
DOI 10.1007/978-1-84628-712-1_11,

Table 11.1 Reported Cardiovascular Effects

	Reported cardiovascular effects	Risks
Chelation	No effect on endothelial vasodilator function[24]	Nausea, vomiting, diarrhea, and headache[30]
	No significant difference in flow mediated vasodilation[26]	Nephrotoxicity
		CHF, renal failure[32]
Acupuncture	Increase in cardiac work capacity[33]	Bruising, rarely bleeding
	Decr. anginal episodes and improved QOL[35]	Drowsiness
	Coronary artery dilatation[39]	
Vitamin C	Decreased risk of peripheral arterial disease in women[51]	GI upset
	Decreased carotid artery atherosclerosis (combined with Vitamin E) in men, not postmenopausal women[52,53]	Renal stones
Vitamin E	Prevention of nonfatal MI[54]	Increase in cardiovascular death and all cause mortality[54]
Soy	Decreased LDL cholesterol, plasma total homocysteine[61]	GI upset
Terminalia	Decrease in post-myocardial infarction angina[64]	None reported
Dan Shen	Inhibition of platelet aggregation	Significant effect on pharmacokinetics of warfarin, resulting in elevated levels of anticoagulation[65,66]
	Possible positive inotropic effects and vasodilation	
Garlic	Protective effect on elastic properties of the aorta in a cohort of elderly patients[67]	GI upset
	Reduced atherosclerosis in femoral and aortic arteries[68]	Increased risk of bleeding
L-arginine	Improved exercise tolerance, quality of life[69,70,71]	GI upset
	No reductions in MI or mortality[72,73,74]	Asthma exacerbation
Quercetin	Reduced risk of coronary heart disease mortality in elderly men[75]	Headaches
Pomegranate	Decreased blood pressure and decreased carotid intima-media thickness[76]	GI upset
		Allergic reactions
Coenzyme Q10	Improved exercise tolerance[77]	GI upset

ber of other problems, (e.g., back pain, neck pain, and other pain syndromes), where acupuncture might also have utility when applied in conjunction with other conventional therapies. While acupuncture may still be considered a CAM modality for some interventions (e.g., as an aid to increasing in vitro fertilization success rates), its use in treating postoperative pain begins to approach that of a conventional therapy based on existing studies. Thus, it is possible for a CAM therapy to "move" from the CAM realm to the mainstream of conventional medicine as increased usage, exposure, and research validate its appropriate role.

Dr. Peter Strauss, former director of the NIH National Center for Complementary and Alternative Medicine (NCCAM) suggested that CAM is "health care practices that are not an integral part of conventional medicine" [6]. This relatively straightforward approach to a complex question may be the best umbrella definition regarding an ever changing realm of therapies and modalities which seem to have become an integral part of the healthcare culture in the United States. Simply recognizing that there are a number of interventions patients are accessing that are neither provided nor overseen by conventional physicians is the first step in helping patients make more informed choices.

Extent of CAM Usage

There have been a number of studies and surveys examining the usage of CAM in the USA and elsewhere. The Eisenberg study of 1993 [2] was really one of the first that brought the issue of CAM usage squarely to the attention of conventional medicine. That survey found that approximately 30% of US adults had used some form of CAM therapy. The survey was repeated 5 years later [7] and at that point usage had grown to 40% of US citizens. This estimate of CAM usage was further validated in two large CDC-NIH surveys of over 30,000 US adults in 2002 and 2007 [1, 8]. Subsequent surveys have looked at specific populations and certain demographic trends have emerged. Generally, CAM users tend to be somewhat younger than nonusers, have higher education levels, and are more likely to be women. Patients with significant illnesses, and especially those not readily treated by conventional means, (e.g., refractory angina, rheumatoid arthritis, cancer, fibromyalgia, etc.) tend to have much higher usage. Richardson et al. [9] surveyed a population of cancer patients and found nearly 80% had used some form of CAM after their diagnosis.

The reasons respondents cite for using CAM are fairly consistent across a number of surveys. Interestingly, most patients who are using CAM do not do so because of dissatisfaction with conventional medicine. As already mentioned, the majority use CAM in conjunction with their conventional care. However, many patients have used CAM because they believed it would give them improved quality of life, boost immunity, enhance their natural ability for healing, and in some cases to gain a sense of control in their medical care. Another clear theme is the fact that many patients are reluctant to discuss the use of CAM with their physicians. In some cases, this nondisclosure was felt to be due to a fear of censure (i.e., patients did not want to be berated by their physician for choosing to use CAM). Others have identified a different set of beliefs among patients regarding certain modalities such as herbs. Patients perceive herbs to be "natural", safe, and therefore, not of interest to their physician.

The NIH surveys done in 2002 [1] and 2007 included over 35,000 US adults and found that approximately 40% have used CAM in the past year. Recognizing that this significant proportion of US adults is using CAM requires all practicing physicians and care providers to take this into account when they encounter patients in the clinical environment. Failure to ask in a nonjudgmental and open fashion regarding a patient's interest in and/or use of CAM may cause the physician or provider to miss important interactions or fail to recognize adverse events arising from the CAM therapy. Yet asking patients about their use of CAM is only the first (albeit, critical) step. The next step is to be able to provide education and guidance regarding the specific therapy. Thus, it is critically important to have a basic understanding of the commonly encountered types of CAM.

NCCAM Domains

In an effort to bring some sense of order to a fairly complex realm, NIH-NCCAM [10] created a five domain approach to the realm of CAM. This includes:

1. *Alternative Medical Systems*

   Alternative medical systems are built upon complete systems of theory and practice. Often, these systems have evolved apart from and earlier than the conventional medical approach used in the United States. Examples of alternative medical systems that have developed in Western cultures include homeopathic medicine and naturopathic medicine. Examples of systems that have developed in non-Western cultures include traditional Chinese medicine and Ayurveda.

2. *Mind–Body Interventions*

   Mind–body medicine uses a variety of techniques designed to enhance the mind's capacity to affect bodily function and symptoms. Some techniques that were considered CAM in the past have become mainstream (for example, patient support groups and cognitive-behavioral therapy). Other mind–body techniques are still considered CAM, including meditation, prayer, mental healing, and therapies that use creative outlets such as art, music, or dance.

3. *Biologically Based Therapies*

   Biologically based therapies in CAM use substances found in nature, such as herbs, foods, and vitamins. Some examples include dietary supplements, herbal products, and the use of other so-called natural but as yet scientifically unproven therapies (for example, using shark cartilage to treat cancer).

4. *Manipulative and Body-Based Methods*

   Manipulative and body-based methods in CAM are based on manipulation and/or movement of one or more parts of the body. Some examples include chiropractic or osteopathic manipulation, and massage.

5. *Energy Therapies*

   Energy therapies involve the use of energy fields. They are of two types:

   Biofield therapies are intended to affect energy fields that purportedly surround and penetrate the human body. The existence of such fields has not yet been scientifically proven. Some forms of energy therapy manipulate biofields by applying pressure and/or manipulating the body by placing the hands in, or through, these fields. Examples include qi gong, Reiki, and Therapeutic Touch.

Bioelectromagnetic-based therapies involve the unconventional use of electromagnetic fields, such as pulsed fields, magnetic fields, or alternating-current or direct-current fields.

This classification system is not perfect but at least provides a framework for considering CAM and organizing an approach to its use by specific patient groups. With regard to CAD, some of the most common CAM therapies fall into the "Biologically based therapies" (e.g., chelation therapy and dietary supplements) and "Alternative Medical Systems" (e.g., acupuncture) classifications.

Chelation

Chelation therapy consists of a series of intravenous infusions of Ethylenediamine Tetraacetic Acid (EDTA), usually combined with a number of other vitamins and antioxidant agents. EDTA is an amino acid complex with a high affinity for divalent and trivalent cations such as lead, magnesium, zinc, iron, and calcium. It is used conventionally for the treatment of lead toxicity and iron overload. Its use as a treatment for CAD and peripheral vascular disease (PVD) began in the 1950s after reports (from small, uncontrolled trials) suggested benefit in patients with angina and peripheral vascular disease (PVD).

A Canadian survey of nearly 6,000 patients who had undergone cardiac catheterization found that 8% had used chelation therapy [11]. This is especially significant when one considers that the annual cost of chelation treatment in Canada is approximately $4,000 [12]. Statistics on use of chelation in the USA are difficult to find, but estimates suggest between 100,000 and 500,000 patients undergo chelation therapy each year in the USA [13, 14].

Chelation Therapy: Theories of Effect

In the 1950s, calcium was believed by many researchers to be the critical component of arterial plaque. EDTA chelation, it was theorized, would remove the calcium, soften the plaque, and allow it to undergo dissolution [15]. By the mid 1970s, as knowledge regarding plaque formation grew, this theoretical mechanism of action was more or less abandoned. A new theory was proposed which claimed that chelation worked by removing calcium from the blood. As calcium was removed from the serum, it would be replaced by calcium taken from the bone. The loss of calcium from the bone would then stimulate parathyroid hormone secretion, which would then promote recalcification of the bone using calcium supplied by "gradual transfer" of calcium from the arterial plaques. This would then soften the plaques and allow them to disintegrate. Again, this theory was gradually abandoned as no evidence for plausibility could be found. By the 1980s, with free radicals taking a more prominent role in the mechanism of plaque creation, proponents then began to claim that EDTA chelation therapy worked by binding iron, thereby making it chemically nonreactive. This would then stop free radical production and thus stop the progression of atheroma formation. Critics have countered that EDTA is too small to bind the entire iron ion, thus leaving it in its catalytically active form. This allows the iron–EDTA complex to catalyze the generation of more hydroxyl radicals, actually increasing the oxidant burden [16]. At this point in time, it is fair to state that a fully defined and plausible mechanism of action of EDTA in the treatment of CAD has not developed.

Chelation Therapy: Clinical Studies

Because there have been very few studies of chelation and CAD, reviewing studies of chelation and peripheral vascular disease may be helpful in deciding on the general role of chelation in vascular disease. One of the earliest reports of chelation being used to treat vascular disease was published in 1956 [17] and reported on an uncontrolled trial of patients with PVD who noted improvement following EDTA treatment. In 1960, Meltzer et al. [18] reported on patients with angina treated with EDTA who noted a subjective benefit (but no objective evidence of improvement was noted). Three years later, Kitchell [19] reviewed the cases of 28 of the patients from Meltzer's 1960 group of EDTA-treated patients and found that all the improvements were temporary and that there was no evidence of an impact on disease progression.

Another study looking at patients with peripheral vascular disease [20] examined the effects of chelation therapy in 153 patients. Outcome measures included walking distance and change in ankle/brachial blood pressure index. This placebo-controlled trial found that both groups improved equally.

Very encouraging results were published in two reviews in 1993 and 1994 [21, 22]. The first, a meta-analysis, showed that 87% of the patients treated with chelation had some measurable improvement. The second, another meta-analysis, this time using unpublished results, also came out with very favorable findings. However, these studies were criticized as having been published in a nonpeer-reviewed journal, created ostensibly as an organ for physicians who perform EDTA chelation [23]. This critique pointed out that many of the studies included in the analyses were retrospective, some showed control outcomes equal to treated patients, and some studies broke blinds and codes prematurely.

In 1994, van Rij et.al. [24] conducted a double-blind randomized trial in 32 patients with intermittent claudication. This study found no benefit. Speculating that it might be difficult to observe significant benefit on variables such as walking distance and peripheral pulse indices in patients with significant established vascular disease, Green et al. [25] chose to look at the effect of chelation therapy on endothelial function. They hypothesized that if chelation benefits biochemical processes that lead to improved vascular function, such changes would likely be noted in improved endothelial function. Eight subjects with CAD received ten chelation treatments over 6 weeks. Forearm blood flow was assessed using plethysmography and graded intrabrachial infusions of acetylcholine and sodium nitroprusside. No effect of chelation on endothelial vasodilator function was noted.

A very rigorous, although small, placebo-controlled, randomized trial involving patients with documented CAD was conducted in Canada between 1996 and 2000 [26]. Patients were recruited from community-based cardiology practices and from cardiac catheterization facilities in Calgary, Canada. Patients were required to be at least 21 years old, to have proven coronary artery disease demonstrated by angiography, or documented myocardiac infarction, and to have had stable angina while taking optimal medical therapy. A qualifying treadmill test had to demonstrate 1 mm downsloping or horizontal ST segment depression.

A total of 3,140 patients were screened and a qualifying treadmill was performed on 171. A total of 84 patients were enrolled in the study with 43 receiving placebo and 41 receiving weight-adjusted EDTA chelation therapy by infusion. The main outcome was exercise time to ischemia (from baseline to 27-week follow-up).

A total of 39 patients from each group completed the full 27-week protocol. The time to ischemia in the control group improved by 54 s, while that in the chelation group improved by 63 s. The difference of 9 s (95% CI, -36–53 s; $P=0.69$) between the groups was not significant. Scores for exercise capacity and quality of life improved in similar fashion in both groups as well. The authors concluded "Based on exercise time to ischemia, exercise capacity, and quality of life measurements, there is no evidence to support a beneficial effect of chelation therapy in patients with ischemic heart disease, stable angina, and a positive treadmill test for ischemia."

The results of another study evaluating the effect of chelation therapy on endothelial function in patients with coronary artery disease were published in 2003 [27]. Forty seven patients who were enrolled in the Program to Assess Alternative Treatment Strategies to Achieve Cardiac Health (PATCH) study participated in this substudy which used high-resolution ultrasound to assess endothelium-dependent brachial artery flow-mediated vasodilation. The primary endpoint was the absolute difference in flow-mediated vasodilation after the 1st and 33 treatments (6 months) of the study groups compared with their baselines. No significant difference in flow-mediated vasodilation between the study groups was noted. The authors concluded that EDTA chelation therapy in combination with vitamins and minerals "does not provide additional benefits on abnormal vasomotor responses in patients with CAD and optimally treated with proven therapies for atherosclerotic risk factors."

A systematic review in 2000 [28] noted the paucity of controlled trials and that many of the studies which reported positive symptomatic improvements typically did not include control groups or objective results. The author noted that the "most striking finding is the almost total lack of convincing evidence for efficacy." He concluded "Given the potential of chelation therapy to cause severe adverse effects, this treatment should now be considered obsolete."

More recently, a Cochrane review [29] reached similar conclusions regarding the quantity and quality of available studies. This review suggested "At present, there is insufficient evidence to decide on the effectiveness or ineffectiveness of chelation therapy in improving clinical outcomes of patients with atherosclerotic cardiovascular disease."

The fact that proponents have continued to challenge the generally negative findings of existing clinical trials suggests that this therapy will remain controversial for the foreseeable future. The question of efficacy may be answered by a large trial currently underway. In August 2002, the National Center for Complementary and Alternative Medicine and the National Heart, Lung, and Blood Institute announced the launch of the Trial to Assess Chelation Therapy (TACT) [30]. This is a placebo-controlled, double-blind study which was designed to involve 2,372 participants age 50 years and older who have suffered a myocardial infarction. Recruitment began in March 2003 and ended in 2010. Patients received 30 weekly intravenous chelation treatments and then ten more treatments on a bimonthly basis over a 28 month period. Final participant data is being collected in 2011 and analysis of results is planned for 2010.

Chelation Therapy: Associated Adverse Events

A number of adverse events and side effects have been reported with chelation therapy. These include abdominal cramps, anorexia, nausea, vomiting, diarrhea, and headache. Also reported are exfoliative dermatitis, fever, chills, fatigue, malaise, thirst, sneezing, and nasal congestion. Muscle cramps are reported not infrequently and back pains, muscle weakness, tremors, tingling, myalgias, and paresthesias have also been documented [31]. The most serious adverse effect is nephrotoxicity, which appears to be dose related. Rapid infusions in particular have caused serious renal damage and a slow infusion is now recommended by proponents.

Grebe and Gregory[32] reported a case of chelation-associated Warfarin resistance in a 64-year-old gentleman whose international normalized ratio (INR) fell from 2.6 the day before chelation therapy to 1.6 the day immediately following. Prabha et al. [33] reported the positive results of a small study of 15 patients with chronic stable angina who underwent chelation therapy. While significant clinical improvements were reported, these could all be attributed to the use of concurrent standard medications, including heparin, beta blockers, and angiotensin converting enzyme inhibitors. What is perhaps more instructive is the number of adverse effects noted. There was a 50% dropout rate due to minor and major adverse drug reactions. These included pain at the injection site (23%), thrombophlebitis (50%), fatigue (23%), tingling and numbness (10%), cramps (10%), nausea/vomiting (10%), and tetany (10%). More serious adverse events included unstable angina (10%), congestive heart failure (13%), hypotension (7%), and symptomatic renal failure (13%). Liver function abnormalities and electrolyte and mineral abnormalities were also common.

Chelation Therapy: Conclusion

Pending definitive results to the contrary from the NIH trial currently underway, the available evidence does not support the use of chelation therapy as an alternative treatment for CAD. The fact that there may be significant risks to its use argues even more strongly for encouraging patients to forego its usage at this time.

Acupuncture

Traditional Chinese Medicine (TCM) has been practiced for at least 3,000 years and is centered on principles of balance exemplified by the concepts of *yin* and *yang* (literally, bright and dark). The philosophy behind *yin* and *yang* encompasses a number of concepts and qualities, (hot and cold, masculine and feminine, etc.). TCM holds that the proper balance of such forces within the individual is necessary for health. A vital force, qi (pronounced "chee") is believed to flow through the body in well-defined channels or "meridians." Qi can be blocked or depleted or be present in excess. Diagnosis of the status of qi involves a comprehensive history and examination of the patient with special attention given to the evaluation of the tongue and pulse. Once a diagnosis is confirmed, a number of interventions may be prescribed, including diet and exercise, herbal compounds, and frequently, acupuncture.

Acupuncture involves the insertion of hair-thin needles into specific points along the meridians. Different points are correlated with specific areas of the body, though not always directly correlated with western anatomical concepts. For example, the Liver Meridian has 14 points. The third point (LV 3) is located on the dorsum of the foot and may be stimulated to address such problems as dizziness, nausea, or insomnia. In TCM, acupuncture is rarely prescribed as an isolated treatment, but is typically provided along with the other interventions mentioned. However, in the USA, acupuncture is frequently provided in isolation. Most studies of acupuncture and CAD have been performed with acupuncture in isolation.

Acupuncture: Clinical Studies in CAD Patients

In 1986, Ballegaard et al. [34] published the first of a series of studies investigating the clinical effects of acupuncture as a treatment for symptomatic CAD. This first study involved 26 patients with stable angina pectoris. Subjects were randomized to either active or sham acupuncture. Sham acupuncture in this study involved inserting needles in a point some distance from the active acupuncture point. Patients who received true acupuncture were noted to have a significant increase in cardiac work capacity but no differences were found for angina frequency or nitroglycerin consumption.

Another study [35] evaluated 49 patients with moderate stable angina who were randomized to genuine or sham acupuncture. Outcomes included exercise tests, angina frequency, and nitroglycerin consumption. Again, subjects receiving true acupuncture appeared to have a significant increase in exercise tolerance, while other outcomes were not significantly different.

A study reported by Richter and colleagues in 1991 [36] evaluated 21 patients with stable effort angina who were randomized in a crossover study to 4 weeks of traditional Chinese acupuncture or placebo tablet treatment. Acupuncture was given three times per week and the medical regimen remained unchanged during the course of the study. The number of anginal attacks per week was reduced in the acupuncture group compared with placebo ($P<0.01$). A quality-of-life questionnaire also showed an improved feeling of well being in the group receiving acupuncture.

Several trials have evaluated potential mechanisms of acupuncture effect. In 1991 [37], Ballegaard and colleagues randomized 33 patients with stable angina pectoris to genuine or sham acupuncture to evaluate effects on skin temperatures and blood flow. Changes in skin temperature correlated significantly with the degree of improvement following either genuine or sham acupuncture. Fourteen patients with no decrease in skin temperature exhibited a significantly better response to acupuncture than 19 patients who showed a decrease in skin temperature. In the former group, there was a 15% immediate improvement in exercise tolerance, a 67% improvement in anginal attack rate, and an 84% improvement in nitroglycerin consumption. A follow-up study in 1993 [38] looking at 23 healthy males further demonstrated a modulatory effect of acupuncture on skin blood flow, heart rate, and blood pressure heart rate product. The authors concluded that "acupuncture has the ability to enhance the regulatory mechanisms of the cardiovascular system" possibly providing a physiological explanation for the use of acupuncture in CAD.

Another study by Ballegaard and colleagues [39] further evaluated the relationship between acupuncture and skin temperature changes in relationship to CAD. Forty nine patients with angina were evaluated. Acupuncture slightly increased exercise tolerance, and decreased nitroglycerin consumption and angina frequency. Those subjects with the greatest response to acupuncture in terms of cardiac parameters also showed a significant rise in local skin temperature in response to acupuncture. Again, the authors postulated that acupuncture may be efficacious in CAD due to hemodynamic alterations.

Yan et al. [40] evaluated the real time effects of acupuncture on patients actively receiving the treatments. Twenty four patients (21 males and 3 females, average age 48.7 years), underwent coronary angiography during acupuncture. A mild dilation effect was observed in all coronary arteries with an average dilation of 8.3%. In a similar fashion, Kurono et al. [41] evaluated the effect of acupuncture using coronary angiography. In patients classified as having Syndrome X, acupuncture was found to produce coronary dilatation that was approximately 70% of that produced by treatment with isosorbide dinitrate.

A study of the effect of acupuncture on heart rate variability (HRV) was reported in 1995 [42]. In this study, the HRV of 20 coronary heart disease patients was determined before and after acupuncture treatment. Findings suggested that acupuncture could improve heart rate variability in coronary heart disease patients.

Effects of LV function have also been studied. Li et al. [43] looked at the use of electro acupuncture (stimulation of the acupuncture needle with a small electrical current) at acupuncture point Neiguan (P6) both in the morning and again in the evening to assess the effect on left ventricular function. Interestingly, acupuncture performed in the morning improved left ventricular function in patients with coronary heart disease, but when performed in the evening, the same acupuncture treatment actually resulted in impairment of left ventricular function.

Twenty two patients with angiographically proven coronary artery disease and 22 normal subjects underwent serial radionuclide angiography to measure LVEF at four different times (at baseline, at 1–15 min, at 16–30 min during acupuncture, and immediately after acupuncture) [44]. One week later, each patient had an identical imaging protocol with acupuncture performed at a dummy point. Results showed that in normal subjects, the mean values of LVEF did not change significantly during or after acupuncture. In contrast, in patients with CAD, the mean values of LVEF in the initial 15 min of acupuncture significantly increased from baseline ($P<0.05$). The increase persisted through the next 15 min of acupuncture and 15 min after acupuncture but became insignificant at 1 week. The authors concluded that acupuncture can temporarily improve LV function in patients with CAD.

In a study evaluating both clinical effects and potential economical impact, 211 patients with CAD were treated with both acupuncture and self-care education, in addition to their established pharmaceutical treatment [45]. In this nonrandomized trial the authors noted a 90% reduction in hospitalization and a 70% reduction in needed surgery. Prior to the intervention, only 8% of subjects were NYHA 0–1. At 1 year, this number increased to 53%, and was 69% after 5 years. Cost savings were estimated at $32,000 (US) per patient over the 5 years.

In 1996 [46], 69 patients with severe angina were treated with acupuncture, Shiatsu, and lifestyle modifications and followed for 2 years. Invasive treatment was postponed in 61% of the patients due to clinical improvement and the annual number of in-hospital days was estimated to have been reduced by 90%. This resulted in an estimated economic savings of $12,000 US dollars for each patient. The authors concluded that combined treatment with acupuncture, Shiatsu, and lifestyle adjustment may be highly cost effective for patients with advanced angina.

Finally, an abstract from the Journal of Traditional Chinese Medicine [47] reports a clinical trial using acupuncture on patients with angina and acute myocardial infarction. A 91% effective rate was found which was claimed to be superior to isosorbide dinitrate and nifedipine ($P<0.01$). However, no details of the study were provided.

Acupuncture: Conclusion

Unfortunately, the majority of studies published to date concerning acupuncture and CAD suffer from significant limitations. Most are small in number, and many are not placebo-controlled or are not blinded. On the other hand, acupuncture is relatively free of significant adverse events. The nearly universal use of disposable needles in the USA has eliminated previous concerns related to hepatitis and other blood-borne infections. While slight bruising at the site of acupuncture is not uncommon, significant bleeding is rare. To be safe, patients with significant coagulopathies are generally counseled to avoid acupuncture.

Thus, while much of the data is suggestive of a possible role for acupuncture in the management of CAD, firm conclusions regarding its proper place in the therapeutic regimen must be deferred until rigorous, large clinical trials are completed. Should your patient decide to try acupuncture, it is fair to tell them that any benefit for CAD is unproven but that the risk of harm is relatively small, provided they work with an experienced practitioner who uses disposable needles.

Herbal Products

Herbs and other natural products appear to have become a permanent part of the American health care landscape. There was a 130% increase in megavitamin use and 380% in herbal product use during the 5 year span of time between Eisenberg's 1993 and 1997 surveys [2, 7]. If one excludes prayer as a CAM modality, the NIH survey in 2002 [1] found that natural products were the most common CAM modality employed by US adults. Since surveys also consistently reveal higher prevalence rates of dietary supplement usage in populations of patients with chronic disabling or life-threatening disease [48], patients with cardiac diseases may be anticipated to be frequent users of supplements. This was borne out in one study which found that 44% of patients referred to a heart failure clinic were using dietary supplements [49]. Because of the limited regulatory environment for dietary supplements in the USA, and because of the narrow therapeutic window for a number of common cardiac medications, knowledge about herb usage in CAD patients may be particularly important.

Dietary Supplements and the Regulatory Environment in the United States

In 1994, Congress passed the Dietary Supplement and Health Education Act (DSHEA) [50] which provides the primary regulatory oversight for the use of herbs in the United States. This act designates dietary supplements as a unique classification, separate from both food and drugs. As such, the usual safeguards associated with both classes of products do not apply to dietary supplements. Of particular note, the act specifically exempts manufacturers from having to prove that their products are either safe or efficacious. This places a significant burden on the consumer who must trust that what they are purchasing is in fact what the label claims. Unfortunately, this has been shown on numerous occasions not to necessarily be reliable. Various consumer groups have analyzed a number of dietary supplement products over the years and found several instances of contamination with heavy metals or pharmaceutical drugs. In many cases, products were found which did not even contain the herb specified on the label. Variable product quality and, in many cases, limited clinical trials, combine to require extracaution when considering the use of herbs in the USA. Fortunately, in 2010, the FDA instituted mandatory Good Manufacturing Practices (GMP's) for all dietary supplements manufactured or sold in the United States. This new rule should improve the quality of products available to US consumers.

Dietary Supplements Used by Patients with CAD

Vitamin C

Proponents claim that supplemental Vitamin C, an antioxidant, may reduce the risk of atherosclerosis. Patients with peripheral arterial disease seem to have both low levels of vitamin C and high levels of C-reactive protein [51] lending plausibility to the hypothesis. Epidemiological studies suggest that, at least in women, vitamin C can decrease the risk of peripheral arterial disease [52]. Other studies have found a beneficial effect on carotid artery atherosclerosis for Vitamin C combined with Vitamin E in both smoking and nonsmoking men (but not postmenopausal women) [53, 54]. Whether Vitamin C has any utility in established CAD is unclear.

Vitamin E

The Cambridge Heart Antioxidant Study [55] evaluated the impact of daily alpha tocopherol supplementation on nonfatal MI and total cardiovascular death in a population of 2,002 patients who had CAD proven by angiography. Median follow-up was 510 days. The results favored treatment for the prevention of nonfatal MI (14 vs. 41 events, $P=0.005$). On the other hand, there was an excess of cardiovascular death in the treatment group (27 vs. 23, $P=0.06$). All-cause mortality was also higher in the treatment group (35% vs. 27%, $P=0.03$).

A subgroup of 1,862 patients from the ATBC trial [56] who had a history of MI was evaluated for the outcomes of nonfatal MI and cardiovascular death. The risk of fatal MI was higher in the group receiving supplements compared with placebo ($P=0.049$) as was the total mortality ($P=0.049$). These differences were most apparent in the beta carotene group ($P=0.007$) and the combined beta carotene/alpha tocopherol group ($P=0.03$). Alpha tocopherol alone had no impact on event rates.

The GISSI trial [57] showed no benefit or risk associated with alpha tocopherol 300 mg daily. Likewise, the Heart Outcomes Prevention Evaluation (HOPE) [58, 59] trial looked at the effects of alpha tocopherol 400 IU per day, ramipril 10 mg daily, the combination or placebo on cardiovascular outcomes in patients who were characterized as high risk. There was no difference in the rate of MI, stroke, or death from cardiovascular causes.

Thus, at this point in time, Vitamin E taken orally doesn't appear to have any effect on atherosclerosis progression or mortality in patients with atherosclerosis. However, recent studies have suggested that alpha-tocopherol may not be the ideal Vitamin E for therapeutic effects, instead suggesting that gamma- and delta-tocopherols may be the forms with the greatest potential health benefits [60, 61]. Whether this different formulation of Vitamin E will prove to be more effective at preventing or treating CAD remains to be determined.

Soy

Tonstad et al. [62] followed a group of 130 men and women on a lipid-lowering diet who were assigned to one of two dosages of isolated soy protein beverage or comparable placebo for 16 weeks. LDL cholesterol and plasma total homocysteine were both significantly lower in the soy groups ($P = 0.01$). HDL and lipoprotein a levels were not affected. The FDA has now approved the use of the health claim, "diets low in saturated fat and cholesterol that include 25 g of soy protein may reduce the risk of heart disease" on soy product labeling [63].

Terminalia

Terminalia arjuna is a botanical frequently used in Ayurvedic medicine as a treatment for angina and heart failure. Two small studies from India suggest that it may be an effective [64, 65] adjunct to conventional therapy for treating postmyocardial infarction angina.

Dan Shen

Dan shen (*Salvia miltiorrhiza*) is an herb commonly included in Traditional Chinese herbal treatments for atherosclerosis-related disorders. Dan shen affects hemostasis via a number of mechanisms, including inhibition of platelet aggregation. Some studies suggest that it may have positive inotropic effects and be vasodilatory as well, though such actions have not been fully validated. It is perhaps most noteworthy in the context of CAD to recognize that it may significantly alter the biochemistry of warfarin, resulting in elevated levels of anticoagulation [66, 67].

Garlic

Low-dose garlic powder (300 mg per day) provided a protective effect on the elastic properties of the aorta in a cohort of elderly patients [68].

Another study, carried out over 4 years and using a higher dose (900 mg per day) resulted in reduced atherosclerosis in femoral and aortic arteries [69].

L-Arginine

Some studies suggest that oral L-arginine results in improved exercise tolerance and quality of life in patients with significant angina [70–72]. However, reductions in MI or mortality have not been observed in large trials of supplemental L-arginine [73–75].

Quercetin

A flavonoid, quercetin is found primarily in fruits and vegetables, particularly in citrus fruits, apples, onions, tea, and red wine. It is one of several flavonoids identified in the Zutphen Elderly Study that appears to reduce risk of coronary heart disease mortality in elderly men [76].

Pomegranate

Consumption of 50 mL per day of concentrated pomegranate juice by subjects with severe but asymptomatic carotid artery disease (70–90% stenosis in the internal carotid arteries) resulted in reductions in both carotid intima-media thickness and blood pressure [77]. The results need to be interpreted in light of the fact that this was a small study ($n = 19$).

Coenzyme Q-10

Though most frequently used by patients with congestive heart failure, at least one trial has evaluated coenzyme Q10 as a treatment for angina [78] suggesting improved exercise tolerance.

Conclusion

Patients with CAD are going to continue to explore the realm of CAM for therapies that provide an alternative to conventional treatment. Whether this is because they fear the discomfort and expense of conventional treatment, or whether it is simply human nature to be curious and wonder if the grass is really greener on the other side of the fence, modalities such as herbs and acupuncture will be a part of the healthcare landscape for the foreseeable future. The clinician's best response is to gain some basic understanding about these treatments, and then maintain an open dialogue with their patients. For example, by always asking about the use of herbs at the same time one inquires about medications, one demonstrates to the patient that supplements really are important and should be discussed openly. From questions about herbs and dietary supplements, it is a natural segue to then ask about any other treatments or therapies the patient is using. Giving examples by saying "Such as acupuncture, yoga or chiropractic" again provides the patient with guidance as to what you would like to know and that it is ok to discuss such issues.

Table 11.2 Herb, dietary supplement, and CAM information on the web

	URL
Databases	
Natural Medicines Comprehensive Database	www.naturaldatabase.com
Natural Standard	www.naturalstandard.com
Herbmed	http://www.herbmed.org
MD Anderson Complementary/Integrative Medicine	www.mdanderson.org/departments/CIMER
Memorial Sloan Cancer Center Integrative Medicine Service Herb and Botanical Information	http://www.mskcc.org/mskcc/html/11570.cfm
MayoClinic.com	www.mayoclinic.com
General information	
NIH	www.healthfinder.gov/
National Center for CAM (NCCAM)	http://nccam.nih.gov
NCI	http://www.cancer.gov/cancerinfo
ACS	www.cancer.org
PubMed	http://www.ncbi.nlm.nih.gov/PubMed
Quackwatch	http://www.quackwatch.org
Herb quality info	
ConsumerLab.com	www.consumerlab.com
Consumer Reports	www.consumerreports.org
United States Pharmacopeia	www.usp.org
Internet info quality	
AMA	www.ama-assn.org/ama/pub/category/1905.html
Health on the Net Foundation	www.hon.ch
Regulatory info	
FDA	http://www.cfsan.fda.gov/~dms/supplmnt.html
FTC	www.ftc.gov

When in fact a patient does express an interest in a CAM modality or relates that they are already using such a therapy, the clinician's task then becomes one of educating the patient to make sure they are supplied with the necessary tools to make an informed decision. Fortunately, there are a number of online resources that can be very helpful. These are included in Table 11.2. Finding one or two of the evidence-based databases and gaining familiarity with them is usually sufficient to address most of the common questions that patients will raise.

By developing a basic understanding of CAM, and in particular, those therapies that patients with CAD might be particularly likely to use, you will be able to discuss with them the pros and cons of such choices. By tapping into online as well as local resources, you can help patients to become educated and therefore be better able to make informed decisions. Until the research matures, CAM will be a somewhat murky part of healthcare in the USA. The American College of Cardiology Foundation (ACCF) Task Force on Clinical Expert Consensus Documents (CECDs) recently published the results of a comprehensive evaluation of the role of CAM in cardiology [79]. While this document provides a broad overview of CAM in regards to cardiovascular medicine and is not specifically focused on the issue of chronic CAD alone, it is nevertheless an excellent resource for those seeking additional evidence-based information. Helping our patients navigate this confusing arena will be an important and ongoing component to providing the best care possible to our patients.

References

1. Barnes P, Powell-Griner E, McFann K, et al. CDC Advance Data Report #343. Complementary and alternative medicine use among adults: United States, 2002. May 27 2004. http://nccam.nih.gov/news/camsurvey.htm. Accessed 15 Jun 2005.
2. Eisenberg DM, Kessler RC, Foster C, et al. Unconventional medicine in the United States. Prevalence, costs, and patterns of use. N Engl J Med. 1993;328:246–52.
3. Wetzel MS, Eisenberg DM, Kaptchuk TJ. Courses involving complementary and alternative medicine at US medical schools. JAMA. 1998;280(9):784–7.
4. Brokaw JJ, Tunnicliff G, Raess BU, et al. The teaching of complementary and alternative medicine in US medical schools: a survey of course directors. Acad Med. 2002;77(9):876–81.
5. Acupuncture. NIH consensus statement 1997 Nov 3–5; 15(5):1–34. http://odp.od.nih.gov/consensus/cons/107/107_statement.htm. Accessed 15 Jun 2005.
6. Straus SE. Complementary and alternative medicine: challenges and opportunities for American medicine. Acad Med. 2000;75(6):572–3.
7. Eisenberg DM, Davis RB, Ettner SL, et al. Trends in alternative medicine use in the United States, 1990–1997: results of a follow-up national survey. JAMA. 1998;280:1569–75.
8. Barnes PM, Bloom B, Nahin RL, Complementary and Alternative medicine use among adults and children: United States 2007 National Health statistics report; No 12. hyattsville, MD National Center for Health Statistics. 2008.
9. Richardson MA, Sanders T, Palmer JL, et al. Complementary/alternative medicine use in a comprehensive cancer center and the implications for oncology. J Clin Oncol. 2000;18(13):2505–14.

10. Anonymous. What is complementary and alternative medicine (CAM)?. 2005. http://nccam.nih.gov/health/whatiscam. Accessed 15 Jun 2005.
11. Quan H, Ghali WA, Verhoef MJ, et al. Use of chelation therapy after coronary angiography. Am J Med. 2001;111:686–91.
12. Anand A, Evans MF. Does chelation therapy work for ischemic heart disease? Can Fam Physician. 2003;49:307–9.
13. Grier MT, Meyers DG. So much writing, so little science: a review of 37 years of literature on edetate sodium chelation therapy. Ann Pharmacother. 1993;27:1504–9.
14. University of Maryland Medical Center, Complementary Medicine Program, Ethylenediaminetetraacetic Acid (EDTA). 2005. http://www.umm.edu/altmed/ConsSupplements/EthylenediaminetetraaceticAcidEDTAcs.html. Accessed 15 Jun 2005.
15. Green S. chelation therapy: unproven claims and unsound. 2005. http://www.quackwatch.org/01QuackeryRelatedTopics/chelation.html. Accessed 15 Jun 2005.
16. McCord JM, Day Jr ED. Superoxide-dependent production of hydroxyl radical catalyzed by iron-EDTA complex. FEBS Lett. 1978;233:1206–8.
17. Clarke NE, Clarke CN, Mosher RE. Treatment of angina pectoris with disodium ethylene diamine tetraacetic acid. Am J Med Sci. 1956;232:654–6.
18. Meltzer LE, Ural E, Kitchell JR. The treatment of coronary artery heart disease with disodium EDTA. In: Seven M, editor. Metal-binding in medicine. Philadelphia: Lippincott; 1960.
19. Kitchell JR. The treatment of coronary artery disease with disodium EDTA: a reappraisal. Am J Cardiol. 1963;11:501–6.
20. Guldager B, Jelnes R, Jorgensen SJ, et al. EDTA treatment of intermittent claudication: a double-blind, placebo-controlled study. J Intern Med. 1992;231:261–7.
21. Chappel L, Stahl J. The correlation between EDTA chelation therapy and improvement in cardiovascular function: a meta-analysis. J Adv Med. 1993;6:139–60.
22. Chappell L, Stahl J, Evans R. EDTA chelation therapy for vascular disease: a meta-analysis using unpublished data. J Adv Med. 1994;7:131–42.
23. Margolis S. Chelation therapy is ineffective for treatment of peripheral vascular disease. Altern Ther Health Med. 1995;1(2):53–7.
24. van Rij AM, Solomon C, Packer SGK, et al. Chelation therapy for intermittent claudication. A double-blind, randomized, controlled trial. Circulation. 1994;90:1194–9.
25. Green DJ, O'Driscoll JG, Maiorana A, et al. Effects of chelation with EDTA and Vitamin B therapy on nitric oxide-related endothelial vasodilator function. Clin Exp Pharmacol Physiol. 1999;26:853–6.
26. Knudtson ML, Wyse DG, Galbraith PD, et al. Chelation therapy for ischemic heart disease: a randomized controlled trial. JAMA. 2002;287:481–6.
27. Anderson TJ, Hubacek J, Wyse DG, et al. Effect of chelation therapy on endothelial function in patients with coronary artery disease: PATCH Substudy. J Am Coll Cardiol. 2003;41:420–5.
28. Ernst E. Chelation therapy for coronary heart disease: an overview of all clinical investigations. Am Heart J. 2000;140:139–41.
29. Villarruz MV, Dans A, Tan F. Cochrane Database Syst Rev. 2002;(4):CD002785. Review. PMID: 12519577.
30. Chelation Therapy Study. 2005. http://nccam.nih.gov/chelation/. Accessed 15 Jun 2005.
31. McKevoy GK, editor. AHFS drug information. Bethesda: American Society of Health-System Pharmacists; 1998.
32. Grebe HB, Gregory PJ. Inhibition of warfarin anticoagulation associated with chelation therapy. Pharmacotherapy. 2002;22(8):1067–9.
33. Prabha A, Shetty M, Thomas J, et al. Chelation therapy for coronary heart disease. Am Heart J. 2002;144(5):E10.
34. Ballegaard S, Jensen G, Pedersen F, et al. Acupuncture in severe, stable angina pectoris: a randomized trial. Acta Med Scand. 1986;220(4):307–13.
35. Ballegaard S, Pedersen F, Pietersen A, et al. Effects of acupuncture in moderate, stable angina pectoris: a controlled study. J Intern Med. 1990;227(1):25–30.
36. Richter A, Herlitz J, Hjalmarson A. Effect of acupuncture in patients with angina pectoris. Eur Heart J. 1991;12(2):175–8.
37. Ballegaard S, Meyer CN, Trojaborg W. Acupuncture in angina pectoris: does acupuncture have a specific effect? J Intern Med. 1991;229(4):357–62.
38. Ballegaard S, Muteki T, Harada H, et al. Modulatory effect of acupuncture on the cardiovascular system: a cross-over study. Acupunct Electrother Res. 1993;18(2):103–15.
39. Ballegaard S, Karpatschoff B, Holck JA, et al. Acupuncture in angina pectoris: do psycho-social and neurophysiological factors relate to the effect? Acupunct Electrother Res. 1995;20(2):101–16.
40. Yan H, Ke Y, Shu B. Angiographic observation of immediate effect of electric pulse stimulation at Zhiyang point on coronary artery. Zhongguo Zhong Xi Yi Jie He Za Zhi. 1998;18(6):330–2, Chinese.
41. Kurono Y, Egawa M, Yano T, et al. The effect of acupuncture on the coronary arteries as evaluated by coronary angiography: a preliminary report. Am J Chin Med. 2002;30(2–3):387–96.
42. Shi X, Wang ZP, Liu KX. Effect of acupuncture on heart rate variability in coronary heart disease patients. Zhongguo Zhong Xi Yi Jie He Za Zhi. 1995;15(9):536–8.
43. Li L, Chen H, Xi Y, et al. Comparative observation on effect of electric acupuncture of neiguan (P 6) at chen time versus xu time on left ventricular function in patients with coronary heart disease. J Tradit Chin Med. 1994;14(4):262–5.
44. Ho FM, Huang PJ, Lo HM, et al. Effect of acupuncture at nei-kuan on left ventricular function in patients with coronary artery disease. Am J Chin Med. 1999;27(2):149–56.
45. Ballegaard S, Johannessen A, Karpatschof B, et al. Addition of acupuncture and self-care education in the treatment of patients with severe angina pectoris may be cost beneficial: an open, prospective study. J Altern Complement Med. 1999;5(5):405–13.
46. Ballegaard S, Norrelund S, Smith DF. Cost-benefit of combined use of acupuncture, Shiatsu and lifestyle adjustment for treatment of patients with severe angina pectoris. Acupunct Electrother Res. 1996;21(3–4):187–97.
47. Meng J. The effects of acupuncture in treatment of coronary heart diseases. J Tradit Chin Med. 2004;24(1):16–9.
48. Hermann DD. Naturoceutical agents in the management of cardiovascular disease. Am J Cardiovasc Drugs. 2002;2(3):173–96.
49. Hermann DD, Kuiper JJ, Shabetai R, et al. Herbal, megavitamin and nutritional supplement use is very common in heart failure patient populations. J Am Coll Cardiol. 1999;33:201A.

50. Dietary Supplement Health and Education Act of 1994 Public Law 103–417 103rd Congress. 2005. http://www.fda.gov/opacom/laws/dshea.html. Accessed 15 Jun 2005.
51. Langlois M, Duprez D, Delanghe J, et al. Serum vitamin C concentration is low in peripheral arterial disease and is associated with inflammation and severity of atherosclerosis. Circulation. 2001;103:1863–8.
52. Klipstein-Grobusch K, den Breeijen J, Grobbee D, et al. Dietary antioxidants and peripheral arterial disease: the Rotterdam Study. Am J Epidemiol. 2001;154:145–9.
53. Salonen JT, Nyyssönen K, Salonen R, et al. Antioxidant Supplementation in Atherosclerosis Prevention (ASAP) study: a randomized trial of the effect of vitamins E and C on 3-year progression of carotid atherosclerosis. J Intern Med. 2000;248:377–86.
54. Salonen R, Nyyssönen K, Kaikkonen J, et al. Six-year effect of vitamin E and vitamin C supplementation on atherosclerosis progression: the Antioxidant Supplementation in Atherosclerosis Prevention (ASAP) study. Circulation. 2003;107:947–53.
55. Stephens NG, Parsons A, Schofield PM, et al. Randomised controlled trial of vitamin E in patients with coronary disease: Cambridge Heart Antioxidant Study (CHAOS). Lancet. 1996;347:781–6.
56. Rapola JM, Virtamo J, Ripatti S, et al. Randomised trial of alpha-tocopherol and beta-carotene supplements on incidence of major coronary events in men with previous myocardial infraction. Lancet. 1997;349:1715–20.
57. Gissi-Prevenzione Investigators. Dietary supplementation with n-3 polyunsaturated fatty acids and vitamin E after myocardial infarction: results of the GISSI Prevenzione trial. Lancet. 1999;354:447–55.
58. Yusuf S, Dagenais G, Pogue J, Bosch J, Sleight P. Vitamin E supplementation and cardiovascular events in high-risk patients. The Heart Outcomes Prevention Evaluation Study Investigators. N Engl J Med. 2000;342:154–60.
59. Yusuf S, Sleight P, Pogue J, Bosch J, Davies R, Dagenais G. Effects of an angiotensin-converting-enzyme inhibitor, ramipril, on cardiovascular events in high-risk patients. The Heart Outcomes Prevention Evaluation Study Investigators. N Engl J Med. 2000;342(3):145–53.
60. Morris M, Evans D, Tangney C, et al. Relation of the tocopherol forms to incident Alzheimer disease and to cognitive change. Am J Clin Nutr. 2005;81:508–14.
61. Wagner KH, Kamal-Eldin A, Elmadfa I. Gamma-tocopherol—an underestimated vitamin? Ann Nutr Metab. 2004;48:169–88.
62. Tonstad S, Smerud K, Hrie L. A comparison of the effects of 2 doses of soy protein or casein on serum lipids, serum lipoproteins and plasma total homocysteine in hypercholesterolemic subjects. Am J Clin Nutr. 2002;76:78–84.
63. Henkel. FDA. Soy: Health claims for soy protein, questions about other components. May-June 2000. Available at: http://vm.cfsan.fda.gov/~dms/fdsoypr.html#health. Accessed 15 Jun 2005.
64. Dwivedi S, Jauhari R. Beneficial effects of Terminalia arjuna in coronary artery disease. Indian Heart J. 1997;49:507–10.
65. Dwivedi S, Agarwal MP. Antianginal and cardioprotective effects of Terminalia arjuna, an indigenous drug, in coronary artery disease. J Assoc Physicians India. 1994;42:287–9.
66. Yu CM et al. Chinese herbs and warfarin potentiation by Danshen. J Intern Med. 1997;241:337–9.
67. Izzat MB, Yim APC, El-Zufari MH. A taste of Chinese medicine! Ann Thorac Surg. 1998;66:941–2.
68. Breithaupt-Grogler K, Ling M, Boudoulas H, et al. Protective effect of chronic garlic intake on elastic properties of aorta in the elderly. Circulation. 1997;96:2649–55.
69. Koscielny J, Klussendorf D, Latza R, et al. The antiatherosclerotic effect of Allium sativum. Atherosclerosis. 1999;144:237–49.
70. Blum A, Porat R, Rosenschein U, et al. Clinical and inflammatory effects of dietary L-arginine in patients with intractable angina pectoris. Am J Cardiol. 1999;15:1488–90.
71. Maxwell AJ, Zapien MP, Pearce GL, et al. Randomized trial of a medical food for the dietary management of chronic, stable angina. J Am Coll Cardiol. 2002;39:37–45.
72. Ceremuzynski L, Chamiec T, Herbaczynska-Cedro K. Effect of supplemental oral L-arginine on exercise capacity in patients with stable angina pectoris. Am J Cardiol. 1997;80:331–3.
73. Oomen CM, van Erk MJ, Feskens E, et al. Arginine intake and risk of coronary heart disease mortality in elderly men. Arterioscler Thromb Vasc Biol. 2000;20:2134–9.
74. Feskens EJM, Oomen CM, Hogendoorn E, et al. Arginine intake and 25-year CHD mortality: the seven countries study (letter). Eur Heart J. 2001;22:611–2.
75. Venho B, Voutilainen S, Valkonen VP, et al. Arginine intake, blood pressure, and the incidence of acute coronary events in men: the Kuopio Ischaemic Heart Disease Risk Factor Study. Am J Clin Nutr. 2002;76:359–64.
76. Hertog MG, Feskens EJ, Hollman PC, et al. Dietary antioxidant flavonoids and risk of coronary heart disease: the Zutphen Elderly Study. Lancet. 1993;342:1007–11.
77. Aviram M, Rosenblat M, Gaitini D, et al. Pomegranate juice consumption for 3 years by patients with carotid artery stenosis reduces common carotid intima-media thickness, blood pressure and LDL oxidation. Clin Nutr. 2004;23:423–33.
78. Kamikawa T, Kobayashi A, Yamashita T, et al. Effects of coenzyme Q10 on exercise tolerance in chronic stable angina pectoris. Am J Cardiol. 1985;56:247–51.
79. Vogel JHK, Bolling SF, Costello RB, Guarneri EM, Krucoff MW, Longhurst JC, et al. Integrating complementary medicine into cardiovascular medicine: a report of the American College of Cardiology Foundation Task Force on Clinical Expert Consensus Documents (Writing Committee to Develop an Expert Consensus Document on Complementary and Integrative Medicine). J Am Coll Cardiol. 2005;46:184–221.

12 Nonspecific Placebo Effects

Piero O. Bonetti

Introduction

Various factors may contribute to clinical improvement in a patient`s condition in response to an intervention. These include: (1) specific effects of the intervention; (2) natural history and regression toward the mean; and (3) nonspecific placebo effects (Fig. 12.1). The natural history of a disease can be highly variable. Symptoms can come and go and, therefore, the natural course of the disease can in itself lead to temporary or permanent improvement or aggravation of the medical condition. Thus, changes in symptoms in connection with the natural course of the disease may be erroneously taken as the result of a specific therapy. Similarly, regression toward the mean can result in wrongly concluding that an effect is due to treatment when it is due to chance. Regression toward the mean is a widespread statistical phenomenon [1]. It means that, left to themselves, things tend to return to normal, whatever that is. Thus, the larger the difference between a selected group and the average population, the larger the effect of regression toward the mean. For example, the more symptomatic a patient, the bigger the chance that his symptoms will improve just because of regression toward the mean, whereby, this improvement may be mistakenly attributed to a specific therapeutic effect. In general terms, "placebo effect" may be defined as "a clinical effect that is unrelated to the specific physicochemical nature of the intervention itself" [2]. However, both the definition of placebo and the question of whether placebo effects really exist are very controversial topics [3, 4]. Based on the classic work by Henry K. Beecher entitled "The Powerful Placebo' it is widely believed that up to one third of all patients may respond to placebo [5]. By analyzing studies of patients with a variety of pain conditions, Beecher claimed that, on average, 35% of patients experienced satisfactory relief of their symptoms by placebo alone. However, two recent studies have questioned the existence of a clinically relevant placebo effect [6, 7]. In their systematic reviews of randomized clinical trials comparing placebo with no treatment, Hróbjartsson and Gøtzsche found no evidence of a generally large effect of placebo on subjective or objective binary or continuous objective outcomes. However, a small benefit on continuous subjective

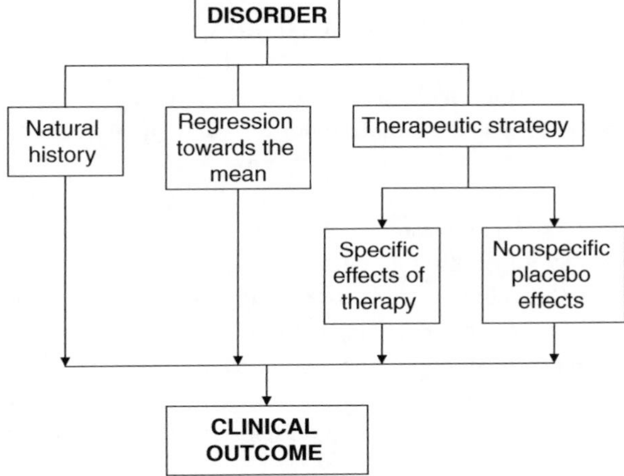

Fig. 12.1 Factors that may affect clinical outcome of a disorder

P.O. Bonetti
Division of Cardiology, Kantonsspital Graubuenden, Chur, Switzerland
e-mail: piero.bonetti@ksgr.ch

G.W. Barsness and D.R. Holmes Jr. (eds.), *Coronary Artery Disease*,
DOI 10.1007/978-1-84628-712-1_12, © Springer-Verlag London Limited 2012

outcomes, especially pain, could not be ruled out. Based on current knowledge it may be concluded that placebo effects may, indeed, play a beneficial role in patients with pain syndromes. However, the often quoted "one third-rule" (i.e., one third of all patients respond to placebo) probably overestimates the significance of placebo effects in clinical practice. Unfortunately, however, the proportional contribution of a placebo effect to an observed benefit in connection with treatment is highly variable and can neither be predicted nor measured in a given individual. In addition, the placebo response may vary considerably in the same individual [8].

The mechanisms responsible for placebo effects are poorly understood. Currently, classical conditioning and cognitive factors such as response expectancy are considered likely mechanisms for the placebo response [9]. Conditioning involves repeated pairing of an active (unconditioned) stimulus with a neutral (conditioned) stimulus until the conditioned stimulus alone elicits the same response as the unconditioned stimulus. In fact, after exposure to a biologically active drug, the efficacy of a subsequently administered placebo that physically resembles the initial active drug will be enhanced. Importantly, the shape and color of pills are not the only conditioned stimuli. Other conditioned stimuli that may produce a placebo response if repeatedly associated with an effective therapy include syringes, stethoscopes, white coats, hospitals, doctors, nurses, and many more [10]. On the other hand, expectation of a beneficial effect appears to be an important factor in the placebo response. Indeed, it was claimed that a placebo responder can be identified by simply asking what he or she would expect after a placebo procedure [10]. Indeed, expectation of pain relief may be particularly pronounced in severely symptomatic patients, which could explain why these patients are more susceptible to experience a positive placebo response than less symptomatic individuals.

Interestingly, growing evidence coming from studies investigating the effect of placebo on pain suggests that placebo stimuli may activate endogenous opioid systems, thereby producing analgesia [10, 11]. On the other hand, there is also evidence for the involvement of nonopioid mechanisms in placebo analgesia [12]. Indeed, it was demonstrated that the involvement of opioid or nonopioid systems depends on the underlying mechanism of activation. Whereas, expectation triggers endogenous opioids, conditioning may affect either the endogenous opioid system or nonopioid systems depending on the nature of the unconditioned stimulus that was used for conditioning [13]. Thus, although the underlying mechanisms have yet to be further elucidated, current evidence supports the notion that placebos may directly modulate pain perception.

Placebo Effect in Patients with Chronic, Stable Angina Pectoris

Placebo effects have been reported to improve outcomes in patients with a wide range of clinical disorders, including cardiovascular diseases [2]. Given the evidence that placebo effects might contribute to pain relief it may be speculated that patients with chronic, stable angina may be a population particularly susceptible to placebo effects. Indeed, Amsterdam et al. found that placebo therapy led to a reduction in the frequency of symptoms in up to 80% of patients with chronic, stable angina [14]. Boissel et al. studied the long-term effects of placebo therapy in a small cohort of patients with stable angina [15]. In this study, 77% of the participants reported subjective, clinical improvement, whereas 27% of patients also experienced objective, clinical improvement as demonstrated by an increase in exercise performance in response to placebo therapy. A positive effect of placebo on exercise tolerance was also demonstrated in the Transdermal Nitroglycerin Cooperative Study [16]. In this study, the therapeutic effect of various doses of transdermal-patch nitroglycerin was tested in comparison with placebo-patch treatment. Tolerance to therapy was demonstrated in all groups including the placebo group. Moreover, an impressive improvement in exercise tolerance, as demonstrated by an increase in walking time on a treadmill by up to 90 s, was observed in both the active treatment and the placebo groups.

Two potential mechanisms have been postulated to contribute to the improvement in exercise performance that is often observed in placebo-treated patients with angina: (1) a "learning phenomenon" (i.e. the unfamiliarity and anxiety that is associated with the first treadmill test is reduced during the second test, which leads to better performance); and (2) a "training effect" (i.e., true improvement in exercise tolerance due to repetitive treadmill testing during the study period) [17].

It is generally accepted that the strength of a drug`s placebo response is related to its route of administration. In 1955, Louis Lasagna, one of the early investigators of the placebo effect, stated that "an injection is thought to be more effective than something taken by mouth" [18].

In this regard, it has been suggested that medical devices and procedures may have particularly potent placebo effects or "enhanced" placebo effects [19]. Surgical procedures are thought to exert such enhanced placebo effects. An excellent example for a placebo effect of surgery in patients with angina pectoris is the ligation of the internal mammary artery, which was performed in the United States in the 1950s in hundreds of patients and was associated with a rate of subjective improvement of up to 90%. This procedure, which was based on the presumption that it would increase coronary blood flow, was finally abandoned after studies by Cobb et al. and Dimond et al., comparing ligation of the internal mammary artery with a sham procedure (skin incision) in a double-blind fashion, had convincingly demonstrated that patients undergoing the sham procedure experienced the same benefit with regard to symptom relief as those who underwent "real ligation" [20, 21].

Placebo Effects in Patients with Refractory Angina Pectoris

Currently, various therapeutic modalities are available for patients with refractory angina pectoris, including optimized medical treatment, enhanced external counterpulsation (EECP) as well as myocardial laser revascularization, neurostimulation techniques, and therapeutic angiogenesis [22]. All of these therapies are associated with a relatively extensive procedure and involve a more or less invasive approach. Thus, given that the use of medical devices and procedures may be associated with enhanced placebo effects, it has been argued that the beneficial effects observed with these techniques are, at least in part, mediated by nonspecific placebo effects, rather than direct physiologic effects of treatment. This suspicion is further fueled by the fact that the primary mechanisms of action of all these techniques are still not fully understood.

Enhanced External Counterpulsation (EECP) and Placebo Effect

Results from various clinical trials including a randomized, double-blinded, sham-controlled trial (Multicenter Study of Enhanced External Counterpulsation: MUST-EECP) as well as data from large patients registries have consistently demonstrated that EECP may lead to a reduction of symptoms in up to 80% of patients with refractory angina [23, 24]. However, although the concept of external counterpulsation was introduced nearly four decades ago, the mechanisms by which EECP exerts its clinical benefit are still not fully understood. EECP leads to an increase in diastolic pressure (diastolic augmentation) and a decrease in systolic pressure (systolic unloading) as well as to an enhancement of venous return by sequential early diastolic inflation and rapid systolic deflation of three pairs of pneumatic cuffs that are wrapped around the calves, the lower thighs, and the upper thighs. Suggested mechanisms responsible for the clinical benefit of EECP include improvement in endothelial function, promotion of coronary collateralization, enhancement of ventricular function, peripheral effects similar to those observed with regular physical exercise but also nonspecific placebo effects [25]. Aside from the impressive device-based procedure *per se*, the likelihood that nonspecific factors may affect the outcome of EECP-treated patients is increased by the prolonged duration of a standard EECP treatment course (7 weeks) and the fact that this therapy is limited to centers where close medical attention is provided. Indeed, as mentioned above, a specific environment, such as a hospital, can serve as a conditioned stimulus that may elicit a placebo response in susceptible individuals. The observation that many patients experience significant symptomatic improvement despite a suboptimal hemodynamic effect of EECP (i.e. inadequate diastolic augmentation during treatment) further supports the presumption that a placebo effect may indeed contribute to the symptomatic benefit associated with this therapy. However, given that various clinical trials found objective evidence for a reduction of myocardial ischemia by demonstrating resolution of myocardial perfusion defects in response to treatment and given the favorable results of the randomized, sham-controlled MUST-EECP trial (Fig. 12.2) it may be concluded that, although nonspecific placebo effects may possibly exist, other EECP-specific mechanisms seem to be more important for the observed clinical benefit of this technique [24, 25].

Myocardial Laser Revascularization and Placebo Effect

Myocardial laser revascularization techniques were introduced with the intention to improve myocardial perfusion by delivering oxygen-rich blood from the

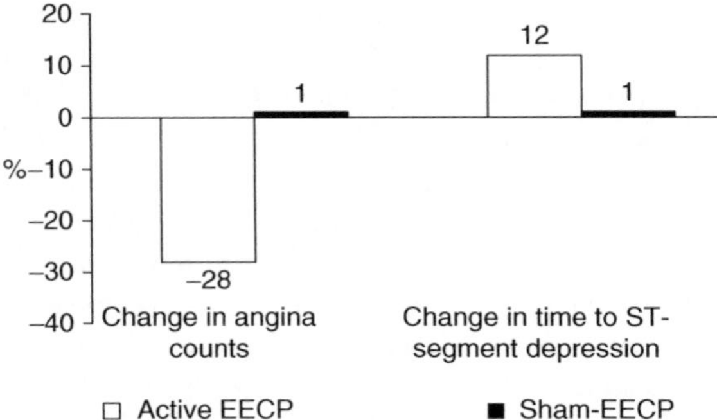

Fig. 12.2 Change in angina counts and change in time to ≥1 mm ST-segment depression during exercise in patients undergoing active EECP or inactive (sham) EECP in the randomized MUST-EECP trial [24]

left ventricle directly into the myocardium via laser-generated channels that can be created either surgically via an epicardial approach (transmyocardial laser revascularization; TMR) or percutaneously via an endocardial approach (percutaneous myocardial laser revascularization; PMR). Similar to EECP, the mechanism of action of myocardial laser revascularization is incompletely understood. In the meantime, the original "open channel" hypothesis has been largely abandoned after various studies have failed to demonstrated long-term patency of the laser-induced channels. Currently, laser-induced denervation of the myocardium and laser-induced angiogenesis are thought to be likely mechanisms responsible for the clinical benefit associated with myocardial laser revascularization. In observational studies, both TMR and PMR have been associated with a reduction of symptoms, improved exercise tolerance, and quality of life in patients with end-stage coronary artery disease, whereas no beneficial effect on survival has been demonstrated for any of the myocardial laser revascularization techniques so far [26, 27]. Although several randomized clinical trial suggested a beneficial effect of TMR in patients with angina, the positive results of TMR therapy have recently been questioned because of methodological limitations of the currently available studies, including the lack of blinding and high crossover rates to TMR, as well as because of the lack of a TMR trial involving a sham control group [26].

In contrast to TMR, the results of three randomized, sham-controlled PMR trials have been published so far (Table 12.1). In the Blinded Evaluation of Laser Intervention Electively For angina pectoris (BELIEF) trial, 82 patients with refractory Class III or IV angina pectoris and a left ventricular ejection fraction of ≥25% were randomly assigned to either PMR with optimized medical therapy ($n=40$) or to a sham PMR procedure with optimized medical therapy ($n=42$) [28]. All patients and investigators were blinded to treatment. Blinding was assured by placing the laser console behind an opaque curtain, such that there was no visual or audible feedback from the laser system to the patient and the investigator. Only a laser technician, who opened the treatment assignment envelope and connected the PMR catheter to either the laser console or a lead box (sham), was aware of the therapy performed. Compared with baseline, significantly more patients of the PMR group than of the sham group improved by ≥2 CCS classes at 6 months (40% vs. 12%, $p<0.01$) and at 12 months (35% vs. 14%, $p=0.04$). Moreover, angina-specific quality-of-life measures, as determined by the Seattle angina questionnaire were significantly higher in PMR-treated patients at 6 and 12 months, whereas exercise capacity was similar among the groups at baseline and during follow-up. Unlike the positive results of the BELIEF trial, the negative results of two other randomized, sham-controlled PMR trials have further strengthened the important role of the placebo effect as a major mechanism responsible for the positive effect of myocardial laser revascularization. In the Direct myocardial revascularization In Regeneration of Endomyocardial Channels Trial (DIRECT) 298 patients with refractory angina were randomized to undergo a low-dose (10–15 channels per zone, $n=98$) PMR, a high-dose (20–25 channels per zone, $n=98$) PMR, or a sham PMR-procedure ($n=102$) [29]. Importantly, there were no differences among the groups with regard to reduction of angina and improvement of exercise time after 6 months (Fig. 12.3). Also, there was no significant difference in MACE-free 1-year survival between patients undergoing high-dose PMR (78.6%), low-dose PMR (85.7%), or sham PMR (88.7%; $P=\mathrm{NS}$). Similar negative results were found in the Prospective, Multicenter, Randomized trial of PMR in Patients with Nonrecanalizable Chronic Total Occlusions [30]. In this trial a total of 141 patients with class III or IV angina due to chronically occluded native coronary arteries were randomized into a PMR + maximal medical therapy (MMT) group ($n=71$) or a MMT only group ($n=70$) after unsuccessful recanalization of the occluded coronary artery by PCI. Blinding was achieved through heavy sedation, dark

Table 12.1 Published, randomized, sham-controlled trials of PMR in patients with refractory angina

Reference	Number of peatients	Persons blinded to treatment	Duration of follow-up	Percentage of patients with symptomatic improvement of ≥2 CCS classes: PMR vs. sham	Improvement in exercise time (s): PMR vs. sham
Salem et al. [28]	82	Patient, investigators	12 months	35% vs. 14%; $p=0.04$	Not assessed
Leon et al. [29]	298	Patients	6 months	65% vs. 56%; $p=$NS	+27 vs. +31; $p=$NS
Stone et al. [30]	141	Patients	6 months	49% vs. 37%; $p=$NS	+64 vs. +52; $p=$NS

Adapted from Saririan and Eisenberg [26], with permission from the American College of Cardiology Foundation
CCS Canadian Cardiovascular Society, *PMR* percutaneous myocardial laser revascularization

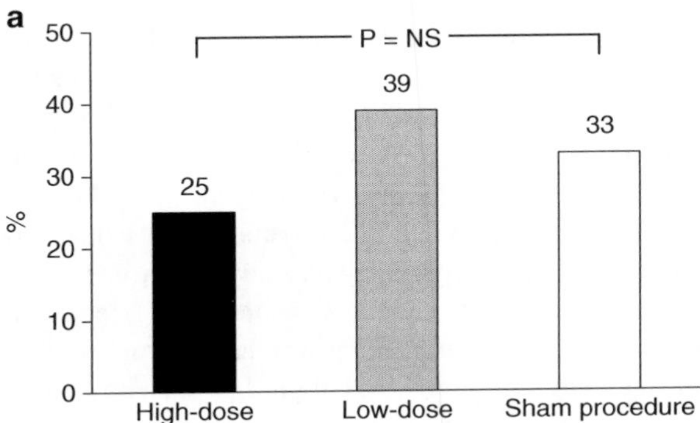

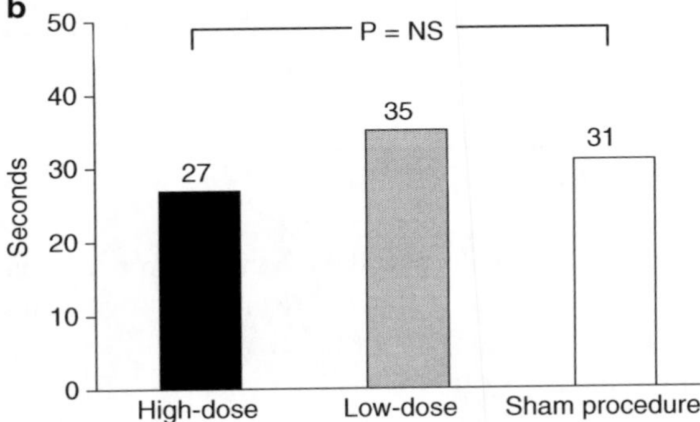

Fig. 12.3 Change in angina (improvement ≥2 CCS classes) (**a**) and change in exercise time (**b**) from baseline to 6-month follow-up in patients undergoing high-dose PMR, low-dose PMR, or sham-PMR in the DIRECT trial [29]

goggles, and the concurrent performance of PCI in all patients. At 6 months, reduction in angina (≥2 classes: 49% vs. 37%), increase in exercise duration from baseline (64 s vs. 52 s), death rates (8.6% vs. 8.8%), myocardial infarction (4.3% vs. 2.9%), or revascularization rates (4.3% vs. 5.9%) were similar in patients of the PMR + MMT group and in MMT only patients ($P=$NS for all). Taken together, the results of these well-performed, randomized and blinded trials suggest a significant placebo response associated with PMR. Moreover, given the current controversy about TMR and the morbidity associated with TMR on the one hand and the scientifically proven placebo effect of thoracotomy in patients with symptomatic coronary artery disease on the other [20, 21], additional randomized and sham-controlled TMR trials would be desperately needed to definitely rule out a significant placebo effect of TMR. However, such trials are considered unethical and are, therefore, unlikely to be performed in the future.

Neurostimulation and Placebo Effect

In the last two decades numerous short- and long-term studies have demonstrated a beneficial effect of transcutaneous electrical nerve stimulation (TENS) and spinal cord stimulation (SCS) on symptoms in patients with refractory angina pectoris. Indeed, clinical long-term follow-up shows that up to 80% of properly selected patients treated with TENS or SCS enjoy a reduction of anginal attacks and use of nitroglycerin as well as an improvement of exercise tolerance and quality of life [31]. The mechanisms by which neurostimulation reduces angina are unclear. The original "gate-control theory" stated that high-frequency stimulation of large non-nociceptive myelinated type A fibers inhibits conduction through smaller, unmyelinated type C fibers, thereby blocking afferent transmission of painful stimuli [32]. Based on this theory, concerns were raised because neurostimulation was considered to deprive patients from the important warning signal of anginal pain. However, to date, various experimental studies suggested that the reduction of symptoms associated with neurostimulation techniques is secondary to a decrease in myocardial ischemia and that treatment does not alter the pain response to myocardial ischemia.

The antiischemic effect of neurostimulation seems to be complex and is thought to involve a decrease in myocardial oxygen consumption, a redistribution of myocardial blood flow as well as neurohormonal mechanisms [31–33]. However, similar to other therapies used in patients with refractory angina the question as to whether a major placebo effect might contribute to the clinical benefit of neurostimulation has been raised. Given the need for surgical implantation of a neurostimulator this holds particularly true for SCS. Unfortunately, however, there is no satisfactory method for using as a placebo control because both TENS and SCS produce a characteristic paresthesia in the area of stimulation. To evaluate the possibility of a placebo effect of the SCS device implantation itself, Hautvast et al. performed a prospective trial in which 25 patients were randomly assigned to either an active treatment ($n=13$) or a control group ($n=12$) [34]. SCS devices were implanted in all patients of both groups. However, in the control group SCS was not activated until 6 weeks after implantation. Compared with the control group, patients of the active treatment demonstrated a significantly longer exercise duration as well as a significant increase in the time to angina. Moreover, actively treated patients had significantly less anginal attacks and lower nitrate consumption. Finally, patients with active stimulators had significantly less ischemic episodes as demonstrated during a 48-h electrocardiogram and reduced ST segment depression during exercise at comparable workload compared with their counterparts with inactivated stimulators. Thus, these results argue against a major placebo effect of SCS implantation. Moreover, although placebo response may affect subjective measures such as number of anginal attacks and nitrate consumption, it is unlikely that a placebo effect could influence objective measures of myocardial ischemia, such as ST segment changes [35]. Taken together, although the exact mechanism of action of neurostimulation in patients with refractory angina is still unknown, placebo effects seem to play only a minor role for the clinical benefit observed with TENS and SCS.

Therapeutic Angiogenesis and Placebo Effect

Therapeutic angiogenesis represents an emerging therapeutic strategy based on the generation of new blood vessels in the ischemic myocardium through administration of exogenous angiogenic growth factors either as recombinant protein or via gene transfer [36]. Strategies to deliver the angiogenic agent to the targets cell include intravenous, intracoronary, and intraatrial injection as well as direct intramyocardial injection through a surgical or percutaneous catheter-based approach. Finally, intrapericardial administration of angiogenic factors has been described [36]. However, despite encouraging results of experimental and smaller clinical trials, therapeutic angiogenesis is still in its infancy and further larger-scale, placebo-controlled and double-blind trials with long-term follow-up will have to demonstrate the true potential of these therapeutic modalities. In addition, such trials will help to estimate the role of a placebo effect for the possible benefit of this therapy. Most angiogenesis trials have been performed in symptomatic patients with exhausted standard therapy. Such patients are known to have a particularly prominent placebo response [37]. Indeed, a surprisingly pronounced improvement in exercise time and anginal symptoms was found in placebo-treated patients in two recently published randomized, double-blind trials of intracoronary infusion of either recombinant fibroblast growth factor-2 (FGF2) or recombinant vascular endothelial growth factor (VEGF) [38, 39].

Conclusion

Placebo effects may contribute to symptom reduction and improvement in quality of life in patients with pain syndromes including those with refractory angina. Thus, although to give a specific therapy just because of its anticipated placebo properties would be considered unethical, a therapeutic modality that, aside from improving myocardial perfusion, evokes an additional beneficial placebo response with subsequent pain reduction may be desirable in individual patients by augmenting the desired effect of this specific treatment and, thereby, adding to the patient`s overall wellbeing. A placebo response may be observed with drug therapy alone but may be particularly prominent in patients undergoing device-based and/or invasive therapeutic strategies (Table 12.2). To further evaluate the efficacy of recently introduced therapies for patients with refractory angina, including novel antianginal drugs such as ranolazine [40, 41] and ivabradine [42], and to assess the magnitude of a placebo response associated with such therapeutic strategies, continued development

Table 12.2 Estimated magnitude of a placebo effect contributing to the clinical benefit of various therapies for patients with refractory angina

Therapeutic modality	Estimated placebo effect
Enhanced external counterpulsation (EECP)	+
Transmyocardial/percutaneous myocardial laser revascularization (TMR/PMR)	+ + (+)
Spinal cord stimulation (SCS)	+ (+)
Therapeutic angiogenesis	?

of large-scale, randomized, sham-controlled and double-blind trials is badly needed. Finally, further understanding of the placebo effect might be used to enhance the therapeutic response of standard and novel therapies in this challenging population.

References

1. Morton V, Torgerson DJ. Effect of regression to the mean on decision making in health care. BMJ. 2003;326:1083–4.
2. Bienenfeld L, Frishman W, Glasser SP. The placebo effect in cardiovascular disease. Am Heart J. 1996;132:1207–21.
3. Gøtzsche PC. Is there logic in the placebo? Lancet. 1994;344: 925–6.
4. Bailar JC. The powerful placebo and the wizard of Oz. N Engl J Med. 2001;344:1630–2.
5. Beecher HK. The powerful placebo. JAMA. 1955;159: 1602–6.
6. Hróbjartsson A, Gøtzsche PC. Is the placebo powerless? An analysis of clinical trials comparing placebo with no treatment. N Engl J Med. 2001;344:1594–602.
7. Hróbjartsson A, Gøtzsche PC. Is the placebo powerless? Update of a systematic review with 52 new randomized trials comparing placebo with no treatment. J Intern Med. 2004;256:91–100.
8. Turner JA, Deyo RA, Loeser JD, Von Korff M, Fordyce WE. The importance of placebo effects in pain treatment and research. JAMA. 1994;271:1609–14.
9. Heeg MJ, Deutsch KF, Deutsch E. The placebo effect. Eur J Nucl Med. 1997;24:1433–40.
10. Benedetti F, Amanzio M. The neurobiology of placebo analgesia: from endogenous opioids to cholezystokinin. Prog Neurobiol. 1997;51:109–25.
11. Levine JD, Gordon NC, Bornstein JC, Fields HL. Role of pain in placebo analgesia. Proc Natl Acad Sci USA. 1979; 76:3528–31.
12. Gracely RH, Dubner R, Wolskee PJ, Deeter WR. Placebo and naloxone can alter postsurgical pain by separate mechanisms. Nature. 1983;306:264–5.
13. Amanzio M, Benedetti F. Neuropharmacological dissection of placebo analgesia: expectation-activated opioid systems versus conditioning-activated specific subsystems. J Neurosci. 1999;19:484–94.
14. Amsterdam EA, Wolfson S, Gorlin R. New aspects of the placebo response in angina pectoris. Am J Cardiol. 1969;24:305–6.
15. Boissel JP, Philippon AM, Gauthier E, Schbath J, Destors JM, and the BIS Research Group. Time course of long-term placebo therapy effects in angina pectoris. Eur Heart J. 1986;7:1030–6.
16. Transdermal Nitroglycerin Cooperative Study Group. Acute and chronic antianginal efficacy and continuous 24 hours application of transdermal nitroglycerin. Am J Cardiol. 1991;68:1263–73.
17. McGraw BF, Hemberger JA, Smith AL, Schroeder JS. Variability of exercise performance during long-term placebo treatment. Clin Pharmacol Ther. 1981;30:321–7.
18. Lasagna L. Placebos. Sci Am. 1955;193:68–71.
19. Kaptchuk TJ, Goldman P, Stone DA, Stason WB. Do medical devices have enhanced placebo effects? J Clin Epidemiol. 2000;53:786–92.
20. Cobb LA, Thomas GI, Dillard DH, Merendino KA, Bruce RA. An evaluation of internal-mammary-artery ligation by a double-blind technic. N Engl J Med. 1959;260:1115–8.
21. Dimond EG, Kittel CF, Crockett JE. Comparison of internal mammary ligation and sham operation for angina pectoris. Am J Cardiol. 1960;5:483–6.
22. Kim MC, Kini A, Sharma SK. Refractory angina pectoris: mechanism and therapeutic options. J Am Coll Cardiol. 2002;39:923–34.
23. Barsness GW. Enhanced external counterpulsation in unrevascularizable patients. Curr Interv Cardiol Rep. 2001;3:37–43.
24. Arora RR, Chou TM, Jain D, Fleishman B, Crawford L, McKiernan T, et al. The Multicenter Study of Enhanced External Counterpulsation (MUST-EECP): effect of EECP on exercise-induced myocardial ischemia and anginal episodes. J Am Coll Cardiol. 1999;33:1833–40.
25. Bonetti PO, Holmes Jr DR, Lerman A, Barsness GW. Enhanced external counterpulsation for ischemic heart disease: what`s behind the curtain? J Am Coll Cardiol. 2003;41:1918–25.
26. Saririan M, Eisenberg MJ. Myocardial laser revascularization for the treatment of end-stage coronary artery disease. J Am Coll Cardiol. 2003;41:173–83.
27. Szatkowski A, Ndubuka-Irobunda C, Oesterle SN, Burkhoff D. Transmyocardial laser revascularization: a review of basic and clinical aspects. Am J Cardiovasc Drugs. 2002;2:255–66.
28. Salem M, Rotevatn S, Stavnes S, Brekke M, Vollset SE, Nordrehaug JE. Usefulness and safety of percutaneous myocardial laser revascularization for refractory angina pectoris. Am J Cardiol. 2004;93:1086–91.
29. Leon MB. DIRECT (DMR in Regeneration of Endomyocardial Channels Trial). Presented at Lake-Breaking Trials, Transcatheter Cardiovascular Therapeutics, Washington D.C., 19 Oct 2000.
30. Stone GW, Teirstein PS, Rubenstein R, Schmidt D, Whitlow PL, Kosinski EJ, et al. A prospective, multicenter randomized trial of percutaneous transmyocardial laser revascularization in patients with nonrecanalizable chronic total occlusions. J Am Coll Cardiol. 2002;39:1581–7.
31. Mannheimer C, Camici P, Chester MR, Collins A, DeJongste M, Eliasson T, et al. The problem of chronic refractory angina: report from the ESC Joint Study Group on the treatment of refractory angina. Eur Heart J. 2002;23:355–70.

32. Murray S, Collins PD, James MA. Neurostimulation treatment for angina pectoris. Heart. 2000;83:217–20.
33. Latif OA, Nedeljkovic SS, Stevenson LW. Spinal cord stimulation for chronic intractable angina pectoris: a unified theory on its mechanism. Clin Cardiol. 2001;24:533–41.
34. Hautvast RW, DeJongste MJ, Staal MJ, van Gilst WH, Lie KI. Spinal cord stimulation in chronic intractable angina pectoris: a randomizedm, controlled efficacy study. Am Heart J. 1998;136:1114–20.
35. Khurmi N, Bowles M, Kohli R, Raftery EB. Does placebo improve indexes of effort-induced myocardial ischemia? An objective study in 150 patients with chronic stable angina pectoris. Am J Cardiol. 1986;57:907–11.
36. Freedman SB, Isner JM. Therapeutic angiogenesis for coronary artery disease. Ann Intern Med. 2002;136:54–71.
37. Simons M. Angiogenesis: where do we stand now? Circulation. 2005;111:1556–66.
38. Simons M, Annex BH, Laham RJ, Kleiman N, Henry T, Dauerman H, et al. Pharmacological treatment of coronary artery disease with recombinant fibroblast growth factor-2: double-blind, randomized, controlled clinical trial. Circulation. 2002;105:788–93.
39. Henry TD, Annex BH, McKendall GR, Azrin MA, Lopez JJ, Giordano FJ, et al. The VIVA trial: vascular endothelial growth factor in ischemia for vascular angiogenesis. Circulation. 2003;107:1359–65.
40. Chaitman BR, Pepine CJ, Parker JO, Skopal J, Chumakova G, Kuch J, et al. Effects of ranolazine with atenolol, amlodipine, or diltiazem on exercise tolerance and angina frequency in patients with severe chronic angina. JAMA. 2004;291:309–16.
41. Chaitman BR, Skettino SL, Parker JO, Hanley P, Meluzin J, Kuch J, et al. Anti-ischemic effects and long-term survival during ranolazine monotherapy in patients with chronic severe angina. J Am Coll Cardiol. 2004;43:1375–82.
42. Borer JS, Fox K, Jaillon P, Lerebours G, for the Ivabradine Investigators Group. Antianginal and antiischemic effects of ivabradine, an I_f inhibitor, in stable angina. A randomized, double-blind, multicentered, placebo-controlled trial. Circulation. 2003;107:817–23.

Prognostic Implications of Depression in Ischemic Syndromes

13

Karen E. Joynt and Christopher M. O'Connor

Introduction

In a nation of almost 300 million people, ischemic heart disease (IHD) and depression remain two of the nation's most pressing public health issues. Cardiovascular disease remains the leading cause of death and hospitalization in the USA, and according to the American Heart Association, IHD alone demonstrated a total prevalence of 13 million individuals (6.9% of the US population) and was responsible for 2,125,000 hospital discharges, 656,000 deaths, and $142 billion in health care spending in 2002 [1]. As a growing proportion of patients survive myocardial infarction (MI), the number of patients with chronic, often nonrevascularizable IHD continues to increase. According to the National Institute of Mental Health (NIMH), 5% of the American population suffers from major depressive disorder (MDD) in any given 1-year period [2], and depression has been identified by the World Health Organization (WHO) as the leading cause of disability worldwide [3].

In recent years, an increasing amount of time and resources has been spent in investigating the relationship between these two conditions. Evidence suggests that depression may actually predispose individuals to the development of IHD, and that depression is present at a higher rate in IHD patients than in the general population. Further, patients with both IHD and depression may suffer increased morbidity and mortality in comparison with patients with IHD alone. These findings are particularly important given the fact that "traditional" IHD risk factors only explain about two-thirds of incident IHD cases; [4] identification and quantification of the impact of "nontraditional" risk factors such as depression could therefore have major public health implications in this country. In the subset of IHD patients with refractory angina, patients that despite optimal medical therapy continue to have angina as well as objective evidence of ischemia, and for whom revascularization is no longer an option, feelings of hopelessness and helplessness may be particularly common and particularly salient. These patients, more than others, may feel that their treatment options are so limited that they have no choice but to resign themselves to a life of limited activity. Patients may fear recurrent cardiac events or have a hard time coming to terms with the understanding that their lifespan is going to be reduced by their heart disease. For these reasons, individuals with refractory angina may be at particularly high risk for depression, and may benefit most from the recognition and modification of this negative prognostic factor.

The purpose of this chapter is to review the available literature regarding the prognostic impact of depression in ischemic syndromes, and to suggest ways in which the relationship between depression and IHD might impact clinical practice as well as future research efforts.

K.E. Joynt (✉)
Cardiovascular Division, Brigham and Women's Hospital, Boston, MA, USA
e-mail: kjoynt@partners.org

C.M. O'Connor
Division of Clinical Pharmacology, Departments of Medicine and Psychiatry and Behavioral Sciences, Duke University Medical Center, Durham, NC, USA
e-mail: oconn002@mc.duke.edu

G.W. Barsness and D.R. Holmes Jr. (eds.), *Coronary Artery Disease*,
DOI 10.1007/978-1-84628-712-1_13, © Springer-Verlag London Limited 2012

Impact of Depression on the Development of Ischemic Syndromes

Recent studies have shown that incident depression may be a significant risk factor for the future development of ischemic heart disease in patients without known heart disease at baseline. (Table 13.1) In fact, two recent meta-analyses have concluded that depression predicts the development of IHD in initially healthy individuals. Rugulies included 11 studies and found a relative risk for the development of IHD of 2.69 (1.63–4.43) for clinical depression and of 1.49 (1.16–1.92) for depressed mood [5]. Similarly, Wulsin and Singal included ten studies (there was significant overlap between the two meta-analyses) and reported a relative risk for IHD of 1.64 (1.41–1.90) [6]. These findings could have enormous public health implications in terms of attempting to further delineate cardiovascular risk factors, in hopes of providing primary prevention or early interventions that might decrease the morbidity and mortality associated with the nation's epidemic of IHD. In fact, emerging technology has allowed us to detect precursors of clinically evident heart disease, and these too, such as coronary artery calcification [7], have recently been associated with depression.

One of the earliest investigations looking at depression as a primary risk factor for the development of heart disease, and, not coincidentally, the study with the longest follow-up to date, is an investigation by Ford et al. that assessed self-reported depression in a sample of 1,190 male medical students who were enrolled in the study at an average age of 26. The students were followed for 37 years; baseline depression was associated with a relative risk (RR) of 2.12 for MI over the follow-up period [8]. In a study by Pratt et al. of patients in Baltimore (roughly 38% male) without known heart disease in which two-thirds of patients were under the age of 45 at the initiation of the study, baseline depression as determined by interview was associated with a RR of incident MI of 4.54 [9].

A majority of the remaining studies looking at the prognostic implication of depression on otherwise healthy people, however, have focused on a slightly older demographic. For example, Ariyo et al. followed 4,493 patients aged 65 and older and found that depression was associated with a relative risk of 1.11 for cardiovascular disease over 6 years of follow-up [10]; and Schwartz et al. enrolled 2,960 patients aged 65 and older and reported that patients with depression had a RR for MI of 2.23 over 3 years of follow-up [11].

The issue of gender differences in the effect of depression on heart disease has also been raised. For example, in a study by Ferketich et al., enrolling nearly 8,000 patients with a mean age of 55, depression conferred a RR of about 1.7 for IHD incidence for both men and women, but an increased risk for IHD mortality was found only in men ($RR=2.34$) [12]. Penninx et al. found no association between depression and 4-year risk of cardiovascular events or mortality in women, while new depression was associated with increased risk in men ($RR=2.07$ for cardiovascular events; $RR=1.74$ for cardiovascular mortality) [13]. Similarly, Marzari et al. reported that depressive symptoms were associated with an increase in death over 4 years of follow-up from "circulatory" disease for men ($RR=2.49$) but not for women, although depression predicted all-cause mortality in both genders [14]. On the other hand, Wasserthiel-Smoller et al. demonstrated that increases in depression scores were associated with a 5-year relative risk of MI or stroke of 1.2 per 5-unit increase in CES-D score for women, while no significant association was noted for men [15]. The Women's Health Initiative (WHI) trial, which enrolled more than 93,000 women, found that among 73,098 women without known cardiovascular disease at baseline, depression predicted a relative risk of 1.5 for cardiovascular death over 4 years of follow-up; the association remained significant when events occurring in the first 6 months were censored [16]. Similarly, a study by Whooley and Browner with a sample limited exclusively to older women enrolled 7,518 subjects over the age of 67, and discovered a RR of 1.8 over 6 years for cardiovascular mortality among those who were depressed based on scores on the Geriatric Depression Scale [17]. The discrepancy in findings may be in part due to the fact that women tend to develop heart disease at a later age than men; therefore, a sample looking at men and women of the same age may underestimate the impact of this risk factor in women if the follow-up period is not long enough or late enough in life to pick up morbid cardiovascular events.

The duration of time over which a patient has had depression may also confound results. For example, Penninx et al. found significant results for new but not chronic depression, with new depression demonstrating a RR of 2.07 for cardiovascular events in men only [13]. As mentioned earlier, Wasserthiel-Smoller et al.

Table 13.1 Prognostic value of depression on the development of ischemic heart disease without known IHD at baseline

Author (year)	*N*	Mean age or range of ages	% female	Diagnostic instrument/ prevalence of depression	Length of follow-up (mean or median)	Primary outcome	Relative risk (95% CI), adjusted when available, for primary outcome, vs. no depression, *p*-values ≤0.05 unless otherwise indicated
Anda et al. (1993) [189]	2,832	45–77		GWS/11.1%	12.4 years	Fatal and nonfatal CAD	1.50 (1.0–2.3)
Aromaa et al. (1994) [190]	5,355	40–64		PSE	6.6 years	Fatal and nonfatal MI	2.62 in men, 1.90 in women
Barefoot and Schroll (1996) [191]	730	Born in 1914	44	MMPI/16.7%	Max 27 years	Fatal and nonfatal MI	1.7 (1.23–2.34) for 2-SD difference in depression score
Pratt et al. (1996) [9]	1,551	18 and older	62.4	DIS/4.7% h/o depression, 23.9% h/o dysphoria	Max 12 years	MI	*OR*=4.54 (1.65–12.44) for h/o depression, *OR*=2.07 (1.16–3.71) for h/o dysphoria
Wassertheil-Smoller et al. (1996) [15]	4,367, HTN at baseline	72	53	CES-D/4.8% at baseline, 12.4% incidence over follow-up	Max 5 years	CV mortality, MI or stroke	Baseline CES-D NS, CV mortality 1.26 (1.12–1.42) and MI/ stroke 1.18 (1.08–1.30) for 5-unit increase in CES-D in women, NS in men
Ford et al. (1998) [8]	1,190	Enrolled at 26	0	Self-reported depression/12% incidence over follow-up	37 years	CAD incidence, MI	2.12 (1.24–3.63) for CAD incidence, 2.12 (1.11–4.06) for MI
Mendes de Leon et al. (1998) [192]	2,391	72	60.5	CES-D/8.4%	Max 9 years	CAD incidence, CAD mortality	1.03 (1.01–1.05) per unit increase in CES-D score in women for both incidence and mortality, NS in men
Penninx et al. (1998) [13]	3,701	78.3	66	CES-D/12.9% (53.6% new, 46.3% chronic)	4 years	CVD events, CVD mortality	New depression: 2.07 (1.44–2.96) for CVD events and 1.75 (1.0–3.05) for CVD mortality in men, NS in women; chronic depression: NS for men or women
Schwartz et al. (1998) [11]	2,960	73	66.5	CES-D/10%	3 years	MI	*OR*=2.23
Sesso et al. (1998) [193]	1,305	40–90	0	MMPI-2 DEP, MMPI-2D, SCL-90	7 years	Total CAD, total CAD and angina	NS for total CAD, 2.07 (1.13–3.81) for MMPI-2 DEP only for total CAD and angina
Whooley and Browner (1998) [17]	7,518	72	100	GDS/6.3%	6 years	All-cause mortality, CVD mortality	2.14 (1.75–2.61) for all-cause mortality, 1.8 (1.2–2.5) for CVD mortality
Ariyo et al. (2000) [10]	4,493	72	61	CES-D	6 years	Development of CVD, all-cause mortality	1.11 (1.01, 1.22) for CVD, 1.13 (1.03, 1.23) for mortality for every 5-unit increase in score

(continued)

Table 13.1 (continued)

Author (year)	*N*	Mean age or range of ages	% female	Diagnostic instrument/ prevalence of depression	Length of follow-up (mean or median)	Primary outcome	Relative risk (95% CI), adjusted when available, for primary outcome, vs. no depression, *p*-values ≤0.05 unless otherwise indicated
Ferketich et al. (2000) [12]	7,893	55	63.4	CES-D/17.5% in women, 9.7% in men	8.3 years	CAD incidence and mortality	1.73 (1.11–2.68) in women and 1.71 (1.14–2.56) in men for CAD incidence, NS in women and 2.34 (1.54–3.56) in men for CAD mortality
Penninx et al. (2001) [24]	2,397	70.2	52	CES-D, DIS	4.2 years	Cardiac mortality	NS for minor depression, 5.2 (1.5–17.7) for major depression
Wasserthiel-Smoller et al. (2004) [16]	73,098	50–79	100	CES-D/15.8%	4.1 years	CVD mortality	1.5 (1.10–2.03)
Marzari et al. (2005) [14]	2,766	74	50	GDS/3.9% severe in men, 11.9% severe in women	4 years	All-cause mortality, circulatory mortality	1.43 (1.04–1.95) in women and 2.02 (1.58–2.58) in men for all-cause mortality, NS in women and 2.49 (1.60–3.87) in men for circulatory mortality

Note: when a study included both patients with and without IHD at baseline, only the data for the patients without IHD at baseline was included here

BDI Beck Depression Inventory, *CABG* coronary artery bypass grafting, *CAD* coronary artery disease, *CES-D* Center for Epidemiological Studies Depression Scale, *CVD* cardiovascular disease, *DIS* Diagnostic Interview Schedule, *GDS* Geriatric Depression Scale, *GWS* General Well-being Scale, *MI* myocardial infarction, *MMPI* Minnesota Multiphasic Personality Inventory, *NS* nonsignificant, *PSE* Present State Examination

found a significant association between an increase in CES-D scores and incident MI or stroke in women but not in men; baseline depression was not associated with an increased risk of cardiovascular or cerebrovascular events [15].

Again, significant methodologic variability complicates attempts to compare and contrast studies. Many of these analyses, the majority of which were epidemiologic rather than clinical in nature, used patient self-report instruments to assess depression; these instruments are unlikely to be as highly specific as the diagnostic interview used in a minority of the studies. Additionally, a wide range of instruments were used, which can lead to heterogeneity of disease-finding. It should also be noted that the primary outcomes differed among these studies; some studies used cardiovascular disease mortality in general, while others looked at incident coronary artery disease or MI, and others included stroke in their analysis.

The major advantage of these studies is size; the large number of patients included in these investigations should theoretically improve the precision of the observed effect size. It should also be noted, however, that studies of this type may suffer from publication bias, that is, the preferential reporting of analyses in which associations are found to be significant over those analyses showing no linkage.

Prevalence of Depression in Established Ischemic Syndromes

As mentioned previously, NIMH figures suggest that the point prevalence of depression in the general population is roughly 5% [2]. Studies have consistently shown that the prevalence of depression in patients with IHD is significantly higher, with estimates ranging from 16% to 30% (Table 13.2). The largest studies

Table 13.2 Prevalence of depression in known ischemic heart disease

Author (year)	*N*	Mean age	% female	Patient selection	Diagnostic instrument	Prevalence of depression
Frasure-Smith et al. (1995) [25]	222	60	22	Admitted for acute MI	BDI	16%
Barefoot et al. (1996) [18]	1,250	52	17.2	Admitted for angiography, CAD present	Zung SDS	25.7% mild, 11.2% mod/sev
Kaufmann et al. (1999) [26]	391			Admitted for acute MI	DIS	27.2%
Lesperance et al. (2000) [194]	430	62	28.6	Admitted for unstable angina	BDI	41.4%
Mayou et al. (2000) [30]	344	63	27	Admitted for acute MI	HAD	7.6% probable, 9.9% borderline
Bush et al. (2001) [22]	271	64.8	42	Admitted for acute MI	BDI, interview	19.9% by BDI, 9.5% major by interview
Connerney et al. (2001) [23]	309	63.1	33	Post-CABG	BDI, DIS	20% major by DIS
Lane et al. (2001) [28]	288	62.7	25	Admitted for acute MI	BDI	30.9%
Penninx et al. (2001) [24]	2,847	70.5	52	Community sample	CES-D, interview	17.8% minor, 2.4% major among those with cardiac disease c/w 12.0%/1.8% among those without ($p<0.001$)
Lesperance et al. (2002) [19]	896	59.4	31.8	Admitted for acute MI	BDI	23.5% mild, 8.8% mod/sev
Burg et al. (2003) [31]	89	66.3	0	Admitted for nonemergent CABG	BDI	28.1%
Strik et al. (2003) [27]	318	58	0	1 month after first MI	SCL-90	47.1%
Bankier et al. (2004) [20]	100	67.1	31	Outpatients with CAD	SCID/DSM-IV	Single past MDE in full remission 29%, current dysthymic disorder 15%, recurrent MDD with current MDE 31%
Moore et al. (2005) [21]	69	62.3	81	Outpatients with chronic refractory angina	HAD	32.3%

BDI Beck Depression Inventory, *CABG* coronary artery bypass grafting, *CAD* coronary artery disease, *CES-D* Center for Epidemiological Studies Depression Scale, *DIS* Diagnostic Interview Schedule, *HAD* Hospital Anxiety and Depression Scale, *MDD* major depressive disorder, *MDE* major depressive episode, *MI* myocardial infarction, *NS* nonsignificant, *SCID/DSM-IV* Structured Clinical Interview for the Diagnostic and Statistical Manual of Mental Disorders, 4th Edition, *SCL-90* 90-item Symptom Check List, *SDS* Self-Rating Depression Scale

were performed by Barefoot et al. [18] and Lesperance et al. [19] in a sample of 1,250 patients with CAD who were admitted for angiography, Barefoot et al. reported that minor depression was present in 25.7% and major depression in 11.2% [18]. Lesperance et al., collecting data on 896 patients admitted for acute MI, noted similar prevalence figures of 23.5% for minor depression and 8.8% for moderate to severe depression [19]. Perhaps the most comprehensive appraisal was undertaken by Bankier et al., who performed complete psychiatric evaluations on 100 consecutive outpatients with known IHD [20]. The results were striking; single past major depressive episode was detected in 29% of patients, current dysthymic disorder in 15%, and recurrent major depressive disorder with current major depressive episode in 31%. Post-traumatic stress disorder (29%) and generalized anxiety disorder (24%) were also common [20].

It should be noted that there is significant methodologic variance between and among the many studies that have assessed depression in cardiovascular disease, including the inclusion and exclusion criteria used to define study populations, the application of numerous diagnostic instruments to detect depression, and a fairly wide range of sample sizes and male-to-female ratios. In addition, a lack of information regarding the severity of patients' IHD makes it nearly impossible to determine if disease severity may impact or even confound the findings. One study that focused on patients with chronic refractory angina found the prevalence of depression in the outpatient setting to be 32.3%, suggesting that disease severity – or perhaps perceived disease severity – may play a role [21]. Additionally, there is little longitudinal data for an unselected population, that is, a group chosen on the basis of the presence of IHD and then followed to determine whether worsening IHD correlates with the development of or worsening of depressive symptoms.

One interesting discrepancy deserves particular mention; studies that have drawn on data exclusively from an inpatient cardiac population and that have reported rates for both major and minor depression have reported major depression rates between 8% and 20% [18, 19, 22, 23], while studies of stable outpatients have shown rates of roughly 30% [20, 21], and the single large community study of patients with heart disease reported a major depression rate of only 2.4% [24].

Impact of Depression on Prognosis in Established Ischemic Syndromes

Depression may be associated with increased morbidity and mortality in patients with established IHD (Table 13.3). Although many of the studies are limited by a small number of events, authors have reported that depression is associated with a 1.5 to 4-fold increased risk of mortality.

The predominance of investigations in this field have been undertaken in the post-MI population, with mean enrollee ages usually in the 60s and a study population that is generally a third or less female. Frasure-Smith et al. followed 222 patients who were admitted for acute MI, and found that depressed patients' odds of 18-month mortality was 6.64 times higher than nondepressed patients (95% CI 1.76–25.09) [25]. In analysis of data from 271 patients, Bush et al. reported that the presence of any depression carried a RR for all-cause mortality of 3.5 in the 4 months following admission for acute MI [22]. Kaufmann et al. showed that 12-month mortality was predicted by baseline depression (RR 4.29), although the 6-month data was not statistically significant [26]. Lesperance et al. reported on 896 patients admitted for acute MI, and demonstrated over 5 years of follow-up that mild depression ($RR = 2.35$) and moderate to severe depression ($RR = 3.57$) were both associated with an increased risk for cardiac mortality [19]. Strik et al. found that depression was associated with a RR of 2.32 for fatal or nonfatal MI 1 month after first MI in a group of 318 male patients, but that this relationship became nonsignificant when anxiety was concurrently added to the model [27].

Here, too, however, there have been negative results. Lane et al. reported that depression had no impact on all-cause mortality at 12 months [28] or 3 years [29] in a group of 288 post-MI patients, while Mayou et al. demonstrated that a combined depression and anxiety score was not associated with outcomes over 6 months of follow-up for 344 post-MI patients [30].

Although, as outlined above, the bulk of the research in this field has been conducted in the post-MI population, other populations have been studied as well. The largest inpatient study was done by Barefoot et al., who enrolled a group of 1,250 patients admitted for angiography; this analysis showed that mild depression was associated with a RR of 1.38 for cardiac mortality over more than 10 years of follow-up, and that major depression was associated with a RR of 1.69 [18]. In a post-CABG population, Burg et al. reported the odds of cardiac mortality in 2 years of follow-up to be 23 times higher in the subset of patients found to be depressed prior to their surgery ($OR = 23.16$, 95% CI 1.38–398.08) [31].

Fewer studies have examined this issue in the outpatient setting, and the ones that have report conflicting results. Penninx et al. enrolled nearly 3,000 individuals in a community sample, and of the 450 with known baseline cardiac disease, a 4-year relative risk of cardiac mortality of 3.9 (1.3–11.8) was noted when major depression was present [24]. Wassertheil-Smoller, utilizing data from the Women's Health Initiative (WHI), found that depression did not confer an elevated risk of cardiovascular mortality in the

Table 13.3 Prognostic value of depression on patients with known ischemic heart disease

Author (year)	*N*	Mean age	% Female	Patient selection	Diagnostic instrument	Follow-up	Primary outcome	Rate of outcome in group without depression	Rate of outcome in group with depression	Relative risk (95% CI), adjusted when available, for primary outcome, vs. no depression, *p*-values ≤0.05 unless otherwise indicated
Frasure-Smith et al. (1995) [25]	222	60	22	Admitted for acute MI	BDI/DIS	18 months	Cardiac mortality	2.7%	17.6%	*OR*=6.64 (1.76–25.09)
Barefoot et al. (1996) [18]	1,250	52	17.3	Admitted for angiography, CAD present	Zung SDS	Median 15.2 years	Cardiac mortality	35.5%	42.2% mild, 51.4% mod/sev	1.38 mild, 1.69 mod/sev
Kaufmann et al. (1999) [26]	391			Admitted for acute MI	DIS	12 months	All-cause mortality			NS at 6 months, 4.29 at 12 months
Lesperance et al. (2000) [194]	430	62	28.6	Admitted for unstable angina	BDI	12 months	Cardiac death or nonfatal MI	2.8%	11.8%	*OR*=6.73 (2.43–18.64)
Mayou et al. (2000) [30]	344	63	27	Admitted for acute MI	HAD	18 months	All-cause mortality	7.5%	11.8%	NS for "distress," combined measure of depression or anxiety
Bush et al. (2001) [22]	271	64.8	27	Admitted for acute MI	BDI, interview	4 months	All-cause mortality	3.6%	13.6%	3.5 for any depression
Connerney et al. (2001) [23]	309	63.1	33	Post-CABG	BDI, DIS	12 months	Cardiac events	10%	27%	2.31 (1.17–4.56)
Penninx et al. (2001) [24]	450	70.2	52	Community sample	CES-D, interview	4 years	IHD mortality	11.9%	20.5% minor, 36.4% major	2.1 (1.1–3.8) minor, 3.9 (1.13–11.8) major
Lane et al. (2002) [29]	288	62.7	25	Admitted for acute MI	BDI	3 years	Cardiac mortality, all-cause mortality	NR	NR	NS
Lesperance et al. (2002) [19]	896	59.4	31.8	Admitted for acute MI	BDI	5 years	Cardiac mortality	7.2%	18.5% mild, 26.6% mod/sev	2.8 mild (1.68–4.66), 4.32 (2.4–7.75) mod/sev
Burg et al. (2003) [31]	89	66.3	0	Nonemergent CABG	BDI	2 years	Cardiac mortality	1.6%	16%	*OR*=23.16 (1.38–389.08)
Strik et al. (2003) [27]	318	58	0	1 month after first MI	SCL-90	3.4 years	Fatal or nonfatal MI	NR	NR	2.32 (1.04–5.18), NS when anxiety added to model
Wassertheil-Smoller et al. (2004) [16]	18,572	50–79	100	Community sample	CES-D	4.1 years	Cardiac mortality	NR	NR	NS

Note: absolute event rates may not always correspond precisely to relative risk figures in the table above due to the impact of adjusting for other risk factors on the reported relative risk

BDI Beck Depression Inventory, *CABG* coronary artery bypass grafting, *CAD* coronary artery disease, *CES-D* Center for Epidemiological Studies Depression Scale, *DIS* Diagnostic Interview Schedule, *HAD* Hospital Anxiety and Depression Scale, *MI* myocardial infarction. *NR* not reported, *NS* nonsignificant, *SCL-90* 90-item Symptom Check List, *SDS* Self-Rating Depression Scale

18,572 women in the WHI with heart disease at baseline (RR 1.22, 95% CI 0.92–1.61) [16].

Again, the bulk of the data seems to suggest that depression is a poor prognostic factor in established coronary disease, although a quantitative summary of the somewhat variable data reviewed above has not yet been published. The generalizability of results is limited by the variability between studies in terms of diagnostic instrument (and the cutoff values for depression used on any one instrument), patient population, and study inclusion criteria. Additional investigations have looked at such factors as anxiety, personality traits, social isolation, social support, and stress, and these may contribute as well, be it via modulation of depression or via independent causatory relationships [32].

Possible Mechanisms Connecting Depression and IHD

The available evidence presented above suggests that depression may increase the risk of developing IHD, is highly prevalent in patients with IHD, and is an independent risk factor for poor outcomes in the presence of known IHD. The exact mechanisms underlying this relationship have not been determined, and a complete review of the postulated pathways is beyond the scope of this chapter. However, clinicians caring for patients with nonrevascularizable coronary disease should be aware of the proposed mechanisms and how these may impact both current and future therapeutic intervention.

A good deal of both clinical and basic science research has begun to suggest that such factors as inflammation, platelet aggregation, sympathetic nervous system activation, cardiac rhythm abnormalities, endothelial dysfunction, mental or emotional stress, adherence to medical regimens, social support, and clustering of typical IHD risk factors may play a role in the connection between cardiovascular disease and depression (Table 13.4) (for review, see [33, 34]).

Inflammation

Patients with depression have been shown to demonstrate elevated plasma levels of proinflammatory cytokines such as interleukin (IL)-1, IL-6, and tissue necrosis factor alpha (TNFα) [35–39]. Additionally, patients with depression tend to have elevated levels of acute-phase reactants such as C-reactive protein (CRP) and alpha-1-acid glycoprotein (AGP) when compared to controls [38, 40, 41]. These findings may be the result of a response to acute or chronic psychological distress, as cytokine production is increased in the setting of stressors, be they local or generalized, acute or chronic; the release of cytokines may be regulated in part by beta-adrenergic receptor signaling [37, 42, 43]. In turn, inflammatory cytokines signal the liver to increase production of acute-phase reactants, including CRP and AGP as well as fibrinogen and haptoglobin. On the other hand, research suggests that inflammatory cytokines could actually be causative of depression rather than simply reflecting the presence of depression. For example, studies following patient groups receiving infusions of IL-1, IL-2, TNF, or interferon alpha for cancer or chronic viral infection have shown that these patients have a very high risk for development of depressed mood and anxiety after the initiation of therapy [37, 44].

There is also a growing body of evidence suggesting that inflammation, as demonstrated by plasma levels of inflammatory cytokines and acute-phase reactants, might play an important role in the initiation and progression of cardiovascular disease (for review see [45–47]). Pathophysiologically, it has been shown that endothelial damage signals the release of inflammatory cytokines, which in turn induce leukocyte chemoattraction. As leukocytes enter and degrade the plaque matrix, it can become unstable and eventually rupture; this predisposes to acute thrombosis and vascular occlusion [45, 46]. Many clinical investigations have shown that elevated plasma levels of CRP, which as mentioned above is an acute-phase reactant that reflects the overall level of systemic inflammation in the body, are predictive of poor cardiovascular outcomes. Elevated plasma CRP has been reported in patients with acute coronary syndromes, and predicts recurrent cardiovascular events among patients with unstable angina; [48–50] additionally, elevated CRP independently predicts poor outcomes in patients with chronic heart failure [51]. Therefore, whether depression leads to release of inflammatory cytokines and consequent negative cardiac impact, or whether a proinflammatory state predisposes to both depression and ischemic heart disease, inflammation is one possible mechanism linking the two conditions.

Table 13.4 Parameters that may link depression and cardiovascular disease

Parameter associated with depression	Nature of change	Impact on cardiovascular system or outcomes
Inflammation	• Elevated plasma concentration of inflammatory molecules (IL-1, IL-6, TNF)	• Acceleration of atherosclerosis
	• Elevated plasma concentration of acute-phase reactants (CRP)	• Instability of atherosclerotic plaques • Increased risk of MI and stroke
Platelet activation	• Increased platelet activation and aggregability	• Microvascular and/or macrovascular clotting • Increased risk of MI and stroke
HPA and SNS activation	• Hypercortisolemia	• Acceleration of atherosclerosis
	• Nonsuppression with dexamethasone challenge	• Hypertension
	• Elevated plasma norepinephrine	• Elevated heart rate
Cardiac rhythm disturbances	• Decreased HRV	• Susceptibility to arrhythmias
	• Increased frequency of ventricular tachycardia	• Increased risk of sudden cardiac death
	• Increased frequency of arrhythmia after ICD implantation	
Endothelial dysfunction	• Impaired flow-mediated vasodilation as measured in the brachial artery	• Predictive of poor cardiovascular outcomes
Stress	• Mental stress-induced myocardial ischemia	• Increased ambulatory myocardial ischemia
	• HPA/SNS hyperactivity	• Increased risk of recurrent cardiovascular events
	• Inflammation	
Compliance	• Decreased compliance with medications, diet, appointments, and rehabilitation programs	• Less use of evidence-based therapies • Poor outcomes independently associated with noncompliance
Social support	• Decreased social support	• Increased cardiovascular mortality
Smoking	• Increased risk of depression if a smoker	• Risk of cardiovascular mortality 1.39 per pack smoked per day
	• Increased risk of smoking if depressed	
	• Less likely to quit successfully if depressed	
Hypertension	• Possible higher risk of developing hypertension over many years if depressed	• Dose-related increased risk of cardiovascular disease with elevated blood pressure
Diabetes	• Increased risk of depression	• Increased cardiovascular mortality
	• Poor glycemic control	• Increased risk of complications such as retinopathy, neuropathy, nephropathy
Hypercholesterolemia	• Depression is associated with low cholesterol	• Potentially beneficial

CRP C-reactive protein, *HRV* heart rate variability, *ICD* implantable cardioverter defibrillator, *IL-1* interleukin-1, *IL-6* interleukin-6, *MI* myocardial infarction, *TNF* tumor necrosis factor

Platelet Aggregation

Depression is associated with a number of abnormalities in platelet function that are associated with increased platelet aggregation (for review see [52–54]), and thus may predispose depressed patients to poor cardiovascular outcomes. For example, depressed patients' platelets have been shown to have increased numbers of functional GPIIb/IIIa receptors, the proteins which act as fibrinogen receptors to initiate or propagate thrombosis. By measuring receptor levels, as well as plasma factors such as beta-thromboglobulin (β-TG), platelet factor 4, and antiligand-induced binding site antibody levels, researchers have demonstrated platelet reactivity and activation in depressed patients that is as much as 40% greater than nondepressed controls [55–57].

Platelet activation is also an important factor in the development and progression of IHD. In both initially healthy individuals [58] as well as patients with known IHD, elevated platelet aggregability has been shown to predict cardiovascular events [59]. The armamentarium of physicians and providers treating patients with ischemic heart disease is full of agents that target this very pathway; for example, aspirin and the glycoprotein IIb/IIIa inhibitors are a mainstay of therapy for patients with both acute and chronic ischemic syndromes. The proven ability of these medications to improve both short-term and long-term outcomes in patients presenting with acute coronary syndromes as well as patients with stable coronary disease supports the centrality of platelets in cardiovascular outcomes [60], and represents one possible link between depression and ischemic heart disease.

Sympathetic Nervous System Activation

Depression is associated with significant hyperactivity of the hypothalamic-pituitary-adrenal (HPA) axis in depressed patients, demonstrated by hypercortisolemia, elevated corticotropin-releasing factor (CRF) in cerebrospinal fluid, decreased adrenocorticotropic hormone (ACTH) response to CRF challenge, and pituitary and adrenal gland enlargement (for review see [32, 61–63]). In turn, the upregulation of the HPA axis leads to upregulation of the sympathetic nervous system (SNS); in patients with depression, SNS hyperactivity can be independently demonstrated by elevated plasma norepinephrine and urinary catecholamine metabolites as well as a hypersecretory catecholamine response to orthostatic challenge (for review see [64, 65]).

HPA and SNS activation may cause physiologic changes that have been shown to influence the development and progression of IHD. For example, elevated plasma cortisol levels can lead to vascular injury by promoting damage to endothelial cells, and via a cascade of effects on the peripheral vasculature as well as renal handling of electrolyte and fluid balance, may accelerate the development of atherosclerosis and hypertension [66, 67]. High plasma levels of catecholamines such as epinephrine and norepinephrine cause vasoconstriction, platelet activation, and an increase in resting heart rate, all of which may be damaging to the cardiovascular system both in the acute and chronic setting [68]. As with other potential links between depression and IHD, it is not entirely clear whether depression is causative of, reflective of, or a result of HPA and SNS activation, but regardless of the directionality of the relationship, may be an important contributor to poor outcomes in IHD.

Cardiac Rhythm Abnormalities

Another type of physiologic derangement commonly seen in depressed patients is cardiac rhythm abnormalities, including a reduction in heart rate variability (HRV). Measures of HRV can quantify the balance between sympathetic and parasympathetic influence on the heart, which as noted in the preceding section can be altered in the setting of depression. A reduction in HRV suggests a decrease in vagal modulation of the heart and therefore less parasympathetic protection from arrhythmias [68, 69]. Depressed patients have been found to have lower HRV on both linear and nonlinear measures; [70, 71] further, a dose-response effect has been described, that is, more severe depression is associated with a more severe reduction in HRV [72]. Other rhythm abnormalities have been demonstrated in patients with depression; depressed patients with IHD may have a higher likelihood of episodic ventricular tachycardia during ambulatory monitoring than those who are not depressed [73], and mood disturbance has been shown to be an independent predictor of arrhythmias after internal cardioverter defibrillator (ICD) implantation, even after controlling for LVEF, arrhythmia history, and medication use [74].

The presence of cardiac rhythm abnormalities in patients with IHD is associated with a poor prognosis. Roughly half of the deaths in patients with cardiovascular disease are ascribed to sudden cardiac death [75–77], and a majority of these events result from ventricular arrhythmias [78, 79]. Decreased HRV is a known risk factor for sudden death and ventricular arrhythmias in patients with IHD (for review see [69, 80]). Interestingly, abnormalities in cardiac rhythm might be particularly salient in patients with both IHD and depression; one study that enrolled over 200 patients after MI found that, while depressed patients had an odds ratio for mortality of 6.64 compared with nondepressed patients, depressed patients with a high frequency of premature ventricular contractions had an odds ratio for mortality of 29.1, and the excess death was primarily attributable to arrhythmic causes [25]. Therefore, rhythm disturbances may play a significant role in mediating the relationship between depression and IHD.

Endothelial Dysfunction

Depression has also been found to be associated with endothelial dysfunction; studies have demonstrated that even young, otherwise healthy individuals who suffer from depression show markedly abnormal flow-mediated vasodilation when compared with controls [81, 82]. Abnormalities in nitric oxide production by the vascular wall have been seen in patients with depression and may underlie this finding [83]. Depressed patients with IHD have also been shown to have impairment of endothelial reactivity, in comparison with nondepressed patients with IHD, and use of antidepressant medication was found to attenuate this relationship [84]. This is particularly important since endothelial dysfunction has been shown to have poor prognostic impact in patients with known IHD, an area of research which is rapidly growing and carries great therapeutic potential for the future [85, 86].

Stress

The relationship between depression and stress has historically been somewhat difficult to quantify; this may be due in part to difficulty in defining the concept of stress. The biological definition of stress is "a state of threatened homeostasis provoked by a psychological, environmental, or physiologic stressor" [87]. The definition of stress for practical purposes, however, becomes less strict when moving from controlled laboratory experiments to real-life observations, and many studies use an imprecise measure of self-reported stress when attempting to clarify the relationship. These studies have shown that stress in daily life might be related to both the development and the subsequent outcomes of depression (for review see [88–90]). For example, in both clinic and broader community samples, stressful life experiences have been shown to correlate with the onset and course of depressive disorders [91–97].

Stress may predispose to the development and progression of IHD, as has been demonstrated in a number of studies [98–100], although there have been negative studies in this field as well [101, 102]. The pathophysiology of the impact of stress on cardiac health is also imprecisely understood, largely because of the interaction between stress, autonomic function, and inflammation; the body's "stress response" is carried out by the HPA and SNS, raising the possibility that stress might underlie both depression and HPA/SNS hyperactivity [87, 103]. Several studies have proposed that inflammation is the mediating factor; stress may induce cytokine production [104, 105], and as mentioned previously, cytokine production may have a negative impact on cardiovascular health. Additionally, mentally stressful tasks can directly induce myocardial ischemia in susceptible individuals with IHD, potentially contributing to worsening cardiac status (for review, see [87, 106–108]); patients who test "positive" for mental stress-induced ischemia may have a higher long-term risk of poor cardiovascular outcomes [109, 110]. Stress may reflect or mediate the connection between depression and IHD, possibly via physiologic pathways outlined in the preceding sections.

Compliance

Depressed patients with a range of medical illnesses, including IHD and heart failure but also patients with end-stage renal disease, cancer, and rheumatoid arthritis, are less likely to comply with medical recommendations [111–115]. It is easy to understand how a person who suffers from symptoms of depression, including fatigue, poor concentration, anhedonia, insomnia, and hopelessness, could have difficulty with maintaining compliance, which may include taking medication as prescribed, following a specific diet, initiating and sticking with an exercise program, attending appointments, and making healthy lifestyle choices such as smoking cessation [111].

Compliance with recommended treatments for IHD can include each of the above components, and may involve complex medication regimens with dosing at intervals throughout the day. For example, a large number of randomized, placebo-controlled trials in the post-MI population suggest that therapy with aspirin, beta-blockers, ACE inhibitors, and HMG-CoA reductase inhibitors (statins) may cumulatively confer a 70–75%

reduction in recurrent cardiac events [116]. However, for these medications to be effective they must be taken – patients who do not comply with pharmaceutical or lifestyle recommendations will not reap these benefits. There is, in fact, evidence to suggest that many proven therapies are not being taken by roughly half of the patients to whom they are prescribed; studies have reported a 40–60% medication compliance rate over the 1–2 years following cardiovascular events [117, 118].

Evidence also suggests that noncompliance itself may be associated with poor outcomes. The Coronary Drug Project Research Group found a relative mortality risk for subjects nonadherent with clofibrate and placebo of 1.7 and 1.9, respectively, when compared to patients adherent with each ($p<0.001$ for each) [119], while the Beta-Blocker Heart Attack Trial showed that nonadherers to either propanolol or placebo had an odds ratio for mortality of 2.6 ($p=0.03$) [120]. There have been negative studies in this field of research, but a recent meta-analysis concluded that noncompliance to either placebo or active medication was associated with worse outcomes in terms of both rehospitalization and mortality [121]. Therefore, attention to compliance is essential when looking for connections between depression and IHD.

Social Support

The presence of social support, defined generally as the friends, family, or community that patients turn to for emotional, spiritual, or functional needs, has been shown to correlate with a lower risk for prevalent depression [122] as well as better outcomes in known depression, as evidenced by a higher chance of remission [123]. Further, depression in elderly patients, which is often associated with significant functional decline, may be buffered by high levels of social support [124].

Although the reasons why this might be the case are not entirely clear, low levels of social support are associated with poor outcomes in cardiovascular disease. Studies including patients with IHD [125–129] as well as stroke [130, 131] have demonstrated that patients with good support systems do better than those who have poor support systems. Compliance with medical recommendations can also be improved by the presence of social support [115], which may help to explain this relationship.

Traditional Risk Factors

There are a number of well-recognized risk factors for the development of IHD, among which smoking, hypertension, diabetes, and hypercholesterolemia are some of the most important [132, 133]. In addition to the association that has been noted between IHD and depression, links between risk factors and depression have been recognized as well.

Cigarette smoking significantly increases the risk of poor cardiovascular outcomes; the relative risk of cardiovascular mortality associated with each additional pack of cigarettes smoked per day is approximately 1.39 [134]. Depression is strongly associated with a higher prevalence of cigarette smoking; in the USA, 49% of individuals with depression are habitual smokers, significantly higher than the 20–30% prevalence in the overall US population [135], and a history of major depression is associated with a three-fold increased risk of becoming a smoker [136]. Not only is smoking more common in individuals with depression, but depression is more common in individuals who are smokers. Depression occurs at a lifetime frequency of 30–45% in smokers, compared with 5–10% in the general population [137, 138]. Depressed smokers are less likely to successfully quit, and more likely to experience problematic symptoms of withdrawal during efforts at abstinence [135, 137, 138].

Hypertension is also recognized as an important IHD risk factor; a prolonged increase of 10 mm Hg above normal in diastolic pressure is associated with a 37% increased risk for development of IHD [133]. Although there have been a number of both prospective and retrospective studies attempting to determine whether there might be a connection between depression and hypertension, these studies have thus far produced conflicting results [139–141].

Cardiovascular mortality in general and IHD mortality in particular are increased three to four-fold in the presence of diabetes. Additionally, outcomes are related to the degree of glycemic control, with worse control associated with higher rates of IHD, stroke, and peripheral vascular disease [142]. There is a documented relationship between depression and diabetes, although the directionality is unclear; depression is roughly twice as common in individuals with diabetes as in the general population [143]. Further, the presence of depression is associated with worse glycemic control in known diabetics [144], and a higher risk of long-term complications such as nephropathy, neuropathy, and retinopathy [145].

Hypercholesterolemia is also a well-documented risk factor for IHD. Cardiovascular mortality increases 9% for each 10 mg/dL increase in plasma cholesterol [146], and individuals in the highest quartile of plasma cholesterol levels are three times more likely to die of cardiovascular disease than those in the lowest quartile [134]. Depression, however, has been associated with low cholesterol levels rather than high cholesterol levels [147–150], and cholesterol-lowering agents have actually been reported to cause depressive symptoms in a small subset of individuals [151]. Tryptophan, which is a precursor of serotonin, competes with serum fatty acids for binding to albumin; therefore, when higher levels of fatty acids are present in the blood, there are fewer albumin molecules available to bind up tryptophan. This leads to an increase in the amount of free tryptophan in the body, increasing the availability of this protein for conversion to serotonin in the brain. In theory, high serotonin availability should be indicative of a lower propensity for depression. As of yet, this has not been utilized clinically, but may have consequences at some point for treatment of elevated cholesterol in patients who have a history of depression or are actively suffering from a major depressive episode.

Implications for the Clinician

The connection between depression and IHD has significant implications for the clinician in the detection and treatment of depression in individuals referred for evaluation of risk factors for the development of IHD as well as in patients with established IHD who present for management. Particularly in patients for whom further revascularization is not an option, optimal medical management of known cardiac disease requires careful evaluation of all potential therapeutic targets for intervention. Evidence from the observational studies cited earlier in this chapter would suggest that routine screening for depression is warranted as part of a cardiac evaluation.

Unfortunately, evidence also suggests that routine screening is rarely performed, and suggests that depression is likely overwhelmingly underdiagnosed in patients with heart disease. In the general population, recent data suggests that 30–50% of cases of depression are never detected by a medical professional [152–154]. Nonpsychiatrist physicians and other clinicians may be limited by high-volume clinical setting and consequent time constraints, may not have been trained to assess for depression, and may not feel comfortable treating depression when it is suspected [155]. Further, patients may be hesitant to share feelings of depression with their medical providers due to a misconception that their emotional distress is part of their physical illness, or because they fear the ramifications of being labeled with a mental illness [155, 156].

Additionally, assessing depressive symptoms in the setting of chronic heart disease, a condition that frequently causes symptoms that mimic depression, can be complex [157, 158]. Depression is characterized by low mood, loss of interest in usual activities, weight loss or gain, difficulty sleeping, low energy, feelings of worthlessness, and decreased ability to concentrate [154, 159], while chronic IHD, particularly when complicated by heart failure, can be associated with fatigue, malaise, and insomnia [160]. Pharmacotherapy for IHD, often consisting of complex regimens, may worsen or mimic symptoms traditionally associated with depression. As a result, patients or physicians may attribute fatigue or malaise to components of the medical regimen such as beta-blockers, which have been reported to carry an increased risk of depression [161, 162]. A recent meta-analysis found no increase in depression attributable to beta-blockade [163], but this is a common misconception that could negatively impact appropriate diagnosis and treatment for a depressive disorder.

Clinicians attempting to utilize a case-finding instrument for depression in patients with chronic IHD may also notice that most depression inventories do not take medical illness into account [164]. Consequently, diagnosis can be inconsistent; for example, Koenig et al. showed that the prevalence of major depression in a population of 460 medically ill older inpatients varied from 10% to 21% depending on which diagnostic scheme was utilized [165]. In response to this problem, the Depression Interview and Structured Hamilton (DISH) was specifically developed to diagnose and assess the severity of depression via interview in the setting of medical illness; it was utilized in the Enhancing Recovery in Coronary Heart Disease (ENRICHD) trial and was found to be valid as well as efficient to administer [164].

A practical, efficient alternative is also needed for use in a busy clinical setting with significant time constraints. Although currently recommended by the US Preventive Services Task Force as part of routine medical care, screening for depression is perceived as prohibitively time-consuming [166]. Fortunately, a two-question screening tool tested in a population of 590 patients at an urgent care clinic was shown to have 96% sensitivity and 57% specificity for depression, similar to the six lengthier instruments tested [159]. The two questions were "During the past month, have you often been bothered by feeling down, depressed, or hopeless?" and "During the past month, have you often been bothered by little interest or pleasure in doing things?" [159] Although it has not yet been validated in a population of patients with chronic IHD, utilization of this simple instrument would improve the identification of depression that is currently going undiagnosed.

As a result of these difficulties with diagnosis, depression, both in the general population and in patients with known IHD, is vastly undertreated. A recent study that assessed 100 patients with known heart disease demonstrated that only one-third of patients diagnosed with recurrent major depressive disorder with current major depressive episode were being treated with antidepressant medication [20]. On a wider scale, the figures might be somewhat better; data from the National Comorbidity Survey Replication interviewed 9,090 individuals, and found that 57.3% of those with current depression had received treatment for depression in the 12 months preceding their interview. Interestingly, only 64.3% of those who were treated received treatment that was considered to meet criteria for minimal adequacy [167]. Major public information campaigns have helped to increase awareness of depression, and the number of patients seeking treatment for depression is increasing yearly [168], but underdiagnosis and consequent undertreatment remain major public health concerns [169].

Further complicating matters, it was unclear until recently whether treatment of depression in patients with heart disease was safe or efficacious. Patients with IHD have traditionally been excluded from trials of antidepressants, or present in such small numbers that little was known regarding the use of these medications in a cardiac population. Recently, the Sertraline Anti-Depressant Heart Attack Trial (SADHART) enrolled 369 patients with major depressive disorder and either acute MI or unstable angina in a randomized, double-blind, placebo-controlled trial of 24 weeks' duration [170]. Results of the trial were encouraging; sertraline was shown to be safe in this population, with no detected changes in mean left ventricular ejection fraction, QTc interval, or other cardiac measures [170]. This is particularly important when compared with the available evidence for tricyclic antidepressants, which are known to have potentially harmful cardiac effects and are generally contraindicated in patients with known IHD [171]. Efficacy data was mixed, with sertraline showing superiority to placebo on the Clinical Global Impression Improvement (CGI-I) scale (2.57 vs. 2.75, $p=0.049$) but not on the Hamilton Depression (HAM-D) change score (−8.4 vs. −7.6, $p=0.14$). No statistically significant difference was seen in severe cardiac events (death, myocardial infarction, congestive heart failure, stroke, and recurrent angina), although the event rate was numerically lower among patients receiving sertraline than those receiving placebo (14.5% vs. 22.4%, RR 0.77, 95% CI 0.51–1.16) [170]. Ongoing trials, powered to detect survival differences, will undoubtedly clarify this relationship in the coming years.

Nonpharmacologic treatment of depression in patients with IHD has been investigated as well, but results are difficult to interpret. Most of these trials have consisted of multidisciplinary programs for patients, incorporating support from nurses, counselors, pharmacists, etc., and few have specifically targeted depression, instead focusing on stress management. Frasure-Smith and Prince conducted a stress-reducing program with 229 post-MI patients and showed a 50% decrease in cardiac mortality (4.5% vs. 9%), although no change was found in readmission rates [172]. Blumenthal et al. enrolled 40 post-MI patients in a stress management program and noted a relative risk for cardiac events of 0.26 compared to 33 controls [173]. Conversely, the Montreal Heart Attack Readjustment Trial (M-HART) offered an anxiety-reduction program to 684 female post-MI patients and found that those women in the intervention group were actually more likely to die ($RR=1.39$) when compared with 692 controls, with the increased mortality primarily related to sudden cardiac death [174].

The ENRICHD (ENhancing Recovery In Coronary Heart Disease) trial enrolled 2,481 patients with myocardial infarction as well as depression and/or low perceived social support to receive a cognitive-behavioral therapy intervention of 6 months' duration [175]. Mean BDI scores at the 6-month evaluation were 9.1 in the intervention group vs. 12.2 in the control group ($p<0.001$), but these effects did not persist to the 30-month evaluation. There was no difference in event-free survival between the two groups (75.9% vs. 75.8%, p=NS) [175]. A 1996 meta-analysis evaluated the addition of psychosocial interventions to standard care for patients with CAD and found a decrease in disease recurrence and mortality rates; however, many of the studies included in the analysis were limited by sample size and length of follow-up [176].

The utility of exercise training, with or without formal cardiac rehabilitation programs, to improve both physical and emotional symptoms is also worth noting. Many patients cannot tolerate or choose not to pursue pharmacotherapy for the treatment of depression; further, exercise is cost-effective compared with pharmacotherapy and psychotherapy, and less time-intensive, it generally has fewer side effects, and it is independently sustainable as a long-term measure. Studies have shown that depressed post-MI patients have lower peak oxygen consumption and lower total work capacity than nondepressed post-MI patients [177], particularly important because exercise capacity is a predictor of survival in IHD [178]. Trials of exercise therapy in otherwise-healthy depressed patients have consistently shown that exercise is more effective than no treatment in reducing depressive symptoms, and is similarly effective to psychotherapy [179]. Cardiac rehabilitation has been shown to decrease depression scores [180, 181], and a recent trial of exercise and stress management in patients with IHD showed that both interventions produced improvements in BDI scores as well as potentially mediating factors such as heart rate variability, endothelial dysfunction, and left ventricular wall motion abnormalities, although no survival data was collected [182].

Depression itself is a condition that causes great detriment to quality of life, and in fact is the leading cause of disability worldwide [3]. Even if it were not associated with poor prognosis in IHD, it would still be important to increase the recognition and treatment of this commonly underdiagnosed disease [156]. Successful treatment of depression has been shown to significantly improvement patient-rated quality of life in both cardiac and noncardiac patients [183, 184].

New Approaches

As ongoing research in genetics and genomics continues to progress in sophistication and applicability, the molecular mechanisms underlying the relationship between IHD and depression may be further elucidated. Ischemic heart disease is a complex syndrome that does not follow straightforward Mendelian inheritance, but nonetheless genomic studies suggest possible susceptibility regions on chromosomes 1, 2, 14, and 16 [185]. Research regarding the genetic basis of depression has identified candidate regions on chromosomes 4, 5, 11, 12, 18, 21, and X, although no single region has been shown to consistently predict depression [186]. Even more subtle relationships are being explored; for example, depressed patients with the serotonin-transporter-linked promoter region *l/l* genotype (associated with a greater number of serotonin transporters) had increased platelet activation relative to both nondepressed controls and depressed patients without the *l/l* genotype, suggesting that genetic differences may influence the effect of depression-related serotonin dysregulation on platelet activation [187], and the *l/l* genotype has also been shown in healthy volunteers to predict increased cardiovascular reactivity to stress [188]. Genetic studies such as these as well as genomic studies seeking candidate genes may one day allow us to target therapy at the particular abnormality underlying an individual's susceptibility to depression, IHD, or both.

Conclusions

In conclusion, research suggests that depression is a risk factor for the development of IHD, is common in IHD, and is associated with a poor prognosis in IHD. Research is ongoing, and much needed, to clarify the pathophysiologic nature of this relationship. Depression may represent a therapeutic target via which to improve outcomes in patients with IHD, particularly as a component of aggressive medical management for patients who lack options for further revascularization. As such, patients with known IHD should be screened for depression during routine clinic visits. When present, depression should be treated with pharmacologic and/or nonpharmacologic modalities. Although existing data has shown that utilizing sertraline in patients with IHD is safe and efficacious, further research is needed to clarify the precise impact of pharmacologic and nonpharmacologic treatment of depression on well-defined parameters of morbidity and mortality, as well as the generalizability of these results.

References

1. American Heart Association. Heart disease and stroke statistics – 2004 update. Dallas: American Heart Association; 2003.
2. National Institute of Mental Health. The numbers count: mental disorders in America. NIH publication 01–4584. Bethesda: National Institutes of Health; 2001.
3. Murray CJL, Lopez AD, editors. The global burden of disease and injury series, volume 1: a comprehensive assessment of mortality and disability from diseases, injuries, and risk factors in 1990 and projected to 2020. Cambridge: Harvard School of Public Health on behalf of the World Health Organization and the World Bank, Harvard University Press; 1996.
4. Beaglehole R, Magnus P. The search for new risk factors for coronary heart disease: occupational therapy for epidemiologists? Int J Epidemiol. 2002;31:1117–22.
5. Rugulies R. Depression as a predictor for coronary heart disease. A review and meta-analysis. Am J Prev Med. 2002;23: 51–61.
6. Wulsin LR, Singal BM. Do depressive symptoms increase the risk for the onset of coronary disease? A systematic quantitative review. Psychosom Med. 2003;65:201–10.
7. Agatisa PK, Matthews KA, Bromberger JT, Edmundowicz D, Chang YF, Sutton-Tyrrell K. Coronary and aortic calcification in women with a history of major depression. Arch Intern Med. 2005;165:1229–36.
8. Ford DE, Mead LA, Chang PP, Cooper-Patrick L, Wang NY, Klag MJ. Depression is a risk factor for coronary artery disease in men: the precursors study. Arch Intern Med. 1998;158:1422–6.
9. Pratt LA, Ford DE, Crum RM, Armenian HK, Gallo JJ, Eaton WW. Depression, psychotropic medication, and risk of myocardial infarction. Prospective data from the Baltimore ECA follow-up. Circulation. 1996;94:3123–9.
10. Ariyo AA, Haan M, Tangen CM, Rutledge JC, Cushman M, Dobs A, et al. Depressive symptoms and risks of coronary heart disease and mortality in elderly. Americans Cardiovascular Health Study Collaborative Research Group. Circulation. 2000;102:1773–9.
11. Schwartz SW, Cornoni-Huntley J, Cole SR, Hays JC, Blazer DG, Schocken DD. Are sleep complaints an independent risk factor for myocardial infarction? Ann Epidemiol. 1998;8:384–92.
12. Ferketich AK, Schwartzbaum JA, Frid DJ, Moeschberger ML. Depression as an antecedent to heart disease among women and men in the NHANES I study. National Health and Nutrition Examination Survey. Arch Intern Med. 2000;160:1261–8.
13. Penninx BW, Guralnik JM, de Mendes LCF, Pahor M, Visser M, Corti MC, et al. Cardiovascular events and mortality in newly and chronically depressed persons>70 years of age. Am J Cardiol. 1998;81:988–94.
14. Marzari C, Maggi S, Manzato E, Destro C, Noale M, Bianchi D, et al. Depressive symptoms and development of coronary heart disease events: the Italian longitudinal study on aging. J Gerontol A Biol Sci Med Sci. 2005;60:85–92.
15. Wassertheil-Smoller S, Applegate WB, Berge K, Chang CJ, Davis BR, Grimm Jr R, et al. Change in depression as a precursor of cardiovascular events. SHEP Cooperative Research Group (Systoloc Hypertension in the elderly). Arch Intern Med. 1996;156:553–61.
16. Wassertheil-Smoller S, Shumaker S, Ockene J, Talavera GA, Greenland P, Cochrane B, et al. Depression and cardiovascular sequelae in postmenopausal women. The Women's Health Initiative (WHI). Arch Intern Med. 2004;164: 289–98.
17. Whooley MA, Browner WS. Association between depressive symptoms and mortality in older women. Study of Osteoporotic Fractures Research Group. Arch Intern Med. 1998;158:2129–35.
18. Barefoot JC, Helms MJ, Mark DB, Blumenthal JA, Califf RM, Haney TL, et al. Depression and long-term mortality risk in patients with coronary artery disease. Am J Cardiol. 1996;78:613–7.
19. Lesperance F, Frasure-Smith N, Talajic M, Bourassa MG. Five-year risk of cardiac mortality in relation to initial severity and one-year changes in depression symptoms after myocardial infarction. Circulation. 2002;105:1049–53.
20. Bankier B, Januzzi JL, Littman AB. The high prevalence of multiple psychiatric disorders in stable outpatients with coronary heart disease. Psychosom Med. 2004;66:645–50.
21. Moore RK, Groves D, Bateson S, Barlow P, Hammond C, Leach AA, et al. Health related quality of life of patients with refractory angina before and one year after enrolment onto a refractory angina program. Eur J Pain. 2005;9: 305–10.
22. Bush DE, Ziegelstein RC, Tayback M, Richter D, Stevens S, Zahalsky H, et al. Even minimal symptoms of depression increase mortality risk after acute myocardial infarction. Am J Cardiol. 2001;88:337–41.
23. Connerney I, Shapiro PA, McLaughlin JS, Bagiella E, Sloan RP. Relation between depression after coronary artery bypass surgery and 12-month outcome: a prospective study. Lancet. 2001;358:1766–71.
24. Penninx BW, Beekman AT, Honig A, Deeg DJ, Schoevers RA, van Eijk JT, et al. Depression and cardiac mortality: results from a community-based longitudinal study. Arch Gen Psychiatry. 2001;58:221–7.
25. Frasure-Smith N, Lesperance F, Talajic M. Depression and 18-month prognosis after myocardial infarction. Circulation. 1995;91:999–1005.
26. Kaufmann MW, Fitzgibbons JP, Sussman EJ, Reed III JF, Einfalt JM, Rodgers JK, et al. Relation between myocardial infarction, depression, hostility, and death. Am Heart J. 1999;138:549–54.
27. Strik JJ, Denollet J, Lousberg R, Honig A. Comparing symptoms of depression and anxiety as predictors of cardiac events and increased health care consumption after myocardial infarction. J Am Coll Cardiol. 2003;42:1801–7.
28. Lane D, Carroll D, Ring C, Beevers DG, Lip GY. Mortality and quality of life 12 months after myocardial infarction: effects of depression and anxiety. Psychosom Med. 2001;63:221–30.

29. Lane D, Carroll D, Ring C, Beevers DG, Lip GY. In-hospital symptoms of depression do not predict mortality 3 years after myocardial infarction. Int J Epidemiol. 2002;31: 1179–82.
30. Mayou RA, Gill D, Thompson DR, Day A, Hicks N, Volmink J, et al. Depression and anxiety as predictors of outcome after myocardial infarction. Psychosom Med. 2000;62:212–9.
31. Burg MM, Benedetto MC, Soufer R. Depressive symptoms and mortality two years after coronary artery bypass graft surgery (CABG) in men. Psychosom Med. 2003;65: 508–10.
32. Rozanski A, Blumenthal JA, Kaplan J. Impact of psychological factors on the pathogenesis of cardiovascular disease and implications for therapy. Circulation. 1999;99: 2192–217.
33. Musselman DL, Evans DL, Nemeroff CB. The relationship of depression to cardiovascular disease: epidemiology, biology, and treatment. Arch Gen Psychiatry. 1998;55:580–92.
34. Joynt KE, Whellan DJ, O'Connor CM. Depression and cardiovascular disease: mechanisms of interaction. Biol Psychiatry. 2003;54:248–61.
35. Sluzewska A, Rybakowski J, Bosmans E, Sobieska M, Berghmans R, Maes M, et al. Indicators of immune activation in major depression. Psychiatry Res. 1996;64:161–7.
36. Anisman H, Merali Z. Cytokines, stress, and depressive illness. Brain Behav Immun. 2002;16:513–24.
37. Maes M, Bosmans E, Meltzer HY, Scharpe S, Suy E. Interleukin-1 beta: a putative mediator of HPA axis hyperactivity in major depression? Am J Psychiatry. 1993;150:1189–93.
38. Kop WJ, Gottdiener JS, Tangen CM, Fried LP, McBurnie MA, Walston J, et al. Inflammation and coagulation factors in persons>65 years of age with symptoms of depression but without evidence of myocardial ischemia. Am J Cardiol. 2002;89:419–24.
39. Appels A, Bar FW, Bar J, Bruggeman C, de Baets M. Inflammation, depressive symptomtology, and coronary artery disease. Psychosom Med. 2000;62:601–5.
40. Seidel A, Arolt V, Hunstiger M, Rink L, Behnisch A, Kirchner H. Cytokine production and serum proteins in depression. Scand J Immunol. 1995;41:534–8.
41. Lanquillon S, Krieg JC, Bening-Abu-Shach U, Vedder H. Cytokine production and treatment response in major depressive disorder. Neuropsychopharmacology. 2000;22:370–9.
42. Papanicolaou DA, Wilder RL, Manolagas SC, Chrousos GP. The pathophysiologic roles of interleukin-6 in human disease. Ann Intern Med. 1998;128:127–37.
43. Leonard BE. The immune system, depression and the action of antidepressants. Prog Neuropsychopharmacol Biol Psychiatry. 2001;25:767–80.
44. Capuron L, Gumnick JF, Musselman DL, Lawson DH, Reemsnyder A, Nemeroff CB, et al. Neurobehavioral effects of interferon-alpha in cancer patients: phenomenology and paroxetine responsiveness of symptom dimensions. Neuropsychopharmacology. 2002;26:643–52.
45. Koenig W. Inflammation and coronary heart disease: an overview. Cardiol Rev. 2001;9:31–5.
46. Mulvihill NT, Foley JB. Inflammation in acute coronary syndromes. Heart. 2002;87:201–4.
47. Robbins M, Topol EJ. Inflammation in acute coronary syndromes. Cleve Clin J Med. 2002;69 Suppl 2:SII130–42.
48. Liuzzo G, Biasucci LM, Gallimore JR, Grillo RL, Rebuzzi AG, Pepys MB, et al. The prognostic value of C-reactive protein and serum amyloid a protein in severe unstable angina [comment]. N Engl J Med. 1994;331:417–24.
49. Thompson SG, Kienast J, Pyke SD, Haverkate F, van de Loo JC. Hemostatic factors and the risk of myocardial infarction or sudden death in patients with angina pectoris. European Concerted Action on Thrombosis and Disabilities Angina Pectoris Study Group. N Engl J Med. 1995;332:635–41.
50. Ridker PM, Cushman M, Stampfer MJ, Tracy RP, Hennekens CH. Inflammation, aspirin, and the risk of cardiovascular disease in apparently healthy men. N Engl J Med. 1997;336:973–9.
51. Yin WH, Chen JW, Jen HL, Chiang MC, Huang WP, Feng AN, et al. Independent prognostic value of elevated high-sensitivity C-reactive protein in chronic heart failure. Am Heart J. 2004;147:931–8.
52. Markovitz JH, Matthews KA. Platelets and coronary heart disease: potential psychophysiologic mechanisms. Psychosom Med. 1991;53:643–68.
53. Nair GV, Gurbel PA, O'Connor CM, Gattis WA, Murugesan SR, Serebruany VL. Depression, coronary events, platelet inhibition, and serotonin reuptake inhibitors. Am J Cardiol. 1999;84:321–3.
54. Nemeroff CB, Musselman DL. Are platelets the link between depression and ischemic heart disease? Am Heart J. 2000;140:S57–62.
55. Kuijpers PM, Hamulyak K, Strik JJ, Wellens HJ, Honig A. Beta-thromboglobulin and platelet factor 4 levels in post-myocardial infarction patients with major depression. Psychiatry Res. 2002;109:207–10.
56. Laghrissi-Thode F, Wagner WR, Pollock BG, Johnson PC, Finkel MS. Elevated platelet factor 4 and beta-thromboglobulin plasma levels in depressed patients with ischemic heart disease. Biol Psychiatry. 1997;42:290–5.
57. Musselman DL, Tomer A, Manatunga AK, Knight BT, Porter MR, Kasey S, et al. Exaggerated platelet reactivity in major depression. Am J Psychiatry. 1996;153: 1313–7.
58. Thaulow E, Erikssen J, Sandvik L, Stormorken H, Cohn PF. Blood platelet count and function are related to total and cardiovascular death in apparently healthy men. Circulation. 1991;84:613–7.
59. Heeschen C, Dimmeler S, Hamm CW, van den Brand MJ, Boersma E, Zeiher AM, et al. Soluble CD40 ligand in acute coronary syndromes. N Engl J Med. 2003;348:1104–11.
60. Antithrombotic Trialists' Collaboration. Collaborative meta-analysis of randomised trials of antiplatelet therapy for prevention of death, myocardial infarction, and stroke in high risk patients. BMJ. 2002;324:71–86.
61. Arborelius L, Owens MJ, Plotsky PM, Nemeroff CB. The role of corticotropin-releasing factor in depression and anxiety disorders. J Endocrinol. 1999;160:1–12.
62. Ehlert U, Gaab J, Heinrichs M. Psychoneuroendocrinological contributions to the etiology of depression, posttraumatic stress disorder, and stress-related bodily disorders: the role of the hypothalamus-pituitary-adrenal axis. Biol Psychol. 2001;57:141–52.
63. Plotsky PM, Owens MJ, Nemeroff CB. Psychoneuroendocrinology of depression. Hypothalamic-pituitary-adrenal axis. Psychiatr Clin North Am. 1998;21:293–307.

64. Gold PW, Gabry KE, Yasuda MR, Chrousos GP. Divergent endocrine abnormalities in melancholic and atypical depression: clinical and pathophysiologic implications. Endocrinol Metab Clin North Am. 2000;31:37–62.
65. Maas JW, Katz MM, Koslow SH, Swann A, Davis JM, Berman N, et al. Adrenomedullary function in depressed patients. J Psychiatr Res. 1994;28:357–67.
66. Colao A, Pivonello R, Spiezia S, Faggiano A, Ferone D, Filippella M, et al. Persistence of increased cardiovascular risk in patients with Cushing's disease after five years of successful cure. J Clin Endocrinol Metab. 1999;84: 2664–72.
67. Troxler RG, Sprague EA, Albanese RA, Fuchs R, Thompson AJ. The association of elevated plasma cortisol and early atherosclerosis as demonstrated by coronary angiography. Atherosclerosis. 1977;26:151–62.
68. Remme WJ. The sympathetic nervous system and ischaemic heart disease. Eur Heart J. 1998;19(Suppl):F62–71.
69. Huikuri HV, Makikallio TH. Heart rate variability in ischemic heart disease. Auton Neurosci. 2001;90:95–101.
70. Gorman JM, Sloan RP. Heart rate variability in depressive and anxiety disorders. Am Heart J. 2000;140:77–83.
71. Yeragani VK, Rao KA, Smitha MR, Pohl RB, Balon R, Srinivasan K. Diminished chaos of heart rate time series in patients with major depression. Biol Psychiatry. 2002;51: 733–44.
72. Agelink MW, Boz C, Ullrich H, Andrich J. Relationship between major depression and heart rate variability. Clinical consequences and implications for antidepressive treatment. Psychiatry Res. 2002;113:139–49.
73. Carney RM, Freedland KE, Rich MW, Smith LJ, Jaffe AS. Ventricular tachycardia and psychiatric depression in patients with coronary artery disease. Am J Med. 1993; 95:23–8.
74. Dunbar SB, Kimble LP, Jenkins LS, Hawthorne M, Dudley W, Slemmons M, et al. Association of mood disturbance and arrhythmia events in patients after cardioverter defibrillator implantation. Depress Anxiety. 1999;9:163–8.
75. Buxton AE, Lee KL, Hafley GE, Wyse DG, Fisher JD, Lehmann MH, et al. MUSTT I: relation of ejection fraction and inducible ventricular tachycardia to mode of death in patients with coronary artery disease: an analysis of patients enrolled in the multicenter unsustained tachycardia trial. Circulation. 2002;106:2466–72.
76. Goldstein S, Friedman L, Hutchinson R, Canner P, Romhilt D, Schlant R, et al. Timing, mechanism and clinical setting of witnessed deaths in postmyocardial infarction patients. J Am Coll Cardiol. 1984;3:1111–7.
77. Rouleau JL, Talajic M, Sussex B, Potvin L, Warnica W, Davies RF, et al. Myocardial infarction patients in the 1990s–their risk factors, stratification and survival in Canada: the Canadian Assessment of Myocardial Infarction (CAMI) Study. J Am Coll Cardiol. 1996;27:1119–27.
78. de Bayes LA, Coumel P, Leclercq JF. Ambulatory sudden cardiac death: mechanisms of production of fatal arrhythmia on the basis of data from 157 cases. Am Heart J. 1989; 117:151–9.
79. Pires LA, Lehmann MH, Steinman RT, Baga JJ, Schuger CD. Sudden death in implantable cardioverter-defibrillator recipients: clinical context, arrhythmic events and device responses. J Am Coll Cardiol. 1999;33:24–32.
80. Curtis BM, O'Keefe Jr JH. Autonomic tone as a cardiovascular risk factor: the dangers of chronic fight or flight. Mayo Clin Proc. 2002;77:45–54.
81. Rajagopalan S, Brook R, Rubenfire M, Pitt E, Young E, Pitt B. Abnormal brachial artery flow-mediated vasodilation in young adults with major depression. Am J Cardiol. 2001;88: 196–8, A7.
82. Broadley AJ, Korszun A, Jones CJ, Frenneaux MP. Arterial endothelial function is impaired in treated depression. Heart. 2002;88:521–3.
83. Chrapko WE, Jurasz P, Radomski MW, Lara N, Archer SL, Le Melledo JM. Decreased platelet nitric oxide synthase activity and plasma nitric oxide metabolites in major depressive disorder. Biol Psychiatry. 2004;56:129–34.
84. Sherwood A, Hinderliter A, Watkins L, Waugh R, Blumenthal JA. Impaired endothelial function in coronary heart disease patients with depressive symptomatology. J Am Coll Cardiol. 2005;46(4):656–9.
85. Heitzer T, Schlinzig T, Krohn K, Meinertz T, Munzel T. Endothelial dysfunction, oxidative stress, and risk of cardiovascular events in patients with coronary artery disease. Circulation. 2001;104:2673–8.
86. Halcox JP, Schenke WH, Zalos G, Mincemoyer R, Prasad A, Waclawiw MA, et al. Prognostic value of coronary vascular endothelial dysfunction. Circulation. 2002;106:653–8.
87. Black PH, Garbutt LD. Stress, inflammation and cardiovascular disease. J Psychosom Res. 2002;52:1–23.
88. Brown GW, Harris TO. Social origins of depression: a study of psychiatric disorder in women. New York: Free Press; 1978.
89. Harris T. Recent developments in understanding the psychosocial aspects of depression. Br Med Bull. 2001;57:17–32.
90. Kessler RC. The effects of stressful life events on depression. Annu Rev Psychol. 1997;48:191–214.
91. Lora A, Fava E. Provoking agents, vulnerability factors and depression in an Italian setting: a replication of Brown and Harris's model. J Affect Disord. 1992;24:227–35.
92. Monroe SM, Bellack AS, Hersen M, Himmelhoch JM. Life events, symptom course, and treatment outcome in unipolar depressed women. J Consult Clin Psychol. 1983;51:604–15.
93. Monroe SM, Harkness K, Simons AD, Thase ME. Life stress and the symptoms of major depression. J Nerv Ment Dis. 2001;189:168–75.
94. Ravindran AV, Griffiths J, Waddell C, Anisman H. Stressful life events and coping styles in relation to dysthymia and major depressive disorder: variations associated with alleviation of symptoms following pharmacotherapy. Prog Neuropsychopharmacol Biol Psychiatry. 1995;19:637–53.
95. Kendler KS, Kessler RC, Neale MC, Heath AC, Eaves LJ. The prediction of major depression in women: toward an integrated etiologic model. Am J Psychiatry. 1993;150: 1139–48.
96. Chevalier A, Bonenfant S, Picot MC, Chastang JF, Luce D. Occupational factors of anxiety and depressive disorders in the French National Electricity and Gas Company. The Anxiety-Depression Group. J Occup Environ Med. 1996;38: 1098–107.
97. Bosworth HB, Steffens DC, Kuchibhatla M, Jiang W, Arias R, O'Connor C. The relationship of social support, social networks and negative events with depression in patients with coronary artery disease. Aging Ment Health. 2000;4: 253–8.

98. Iso H, Date C, Yamamoto A, Toyoshima H, Tanabe N, Kikuchi S, et al. Perceived mental stress and mortality from cardiovascular disease among Japanese men and women: the Japan Collaborative Cohort Study for Evaluation of Cancer Risk Sponsored by Monbusho (JACC Study). Circulation. 2002;106:1229–36.
99. Rosengren A, Tibblin G, Wilhelmsen L. Self-perceived psychological stress and incidence of coronary artery disease in middle-aged men. Am J Cardiol. 1991;68:1171–5.
100. Tennant CC, Palmer KJ, Langeluddecke PM, Jones MP, Nelson G. Life event stress and myocardial reinfarction: a prospective study. Eur Heart J. 1994;15:472–8.
101. Jenkinson CM, Madeley RJ, Mitchell JR, Turner ID. The influence of psychosocial factors on survival after myocardial infarction. Public Health. 1993;107:305–17.
102. Welin C, Lappas G, Wilhelmsen L. Independent importance of psychosocial factors for prognosis after myocardial infarction. J Intern Med. 2000;247:629–39.
103. McEwen BS. The neurobiology of stress: from serendipity to clinical relevance. Brain Res. 2000;886:172–89.
104. Song C, Kenis G, van Gastel A, Bosmans E, Lin A, de Jong R, et al. Influence of psychological stress on immune-inflammatory variables in normal humans. Part II. Altered serum concentrations of natural anti- inflammatory agents and soluble membrane antigens of monocytes and T lymphocytes. Psychiatry Res. 1999;85:293–303.
105. Uchakin PN, Tobin B, Cubbage M, Marshall Jr G, Sams C. Immune responsiveness following academic stress in first-year medical students. J Interferon Cytokine Res. 2001;21:687–94.
106. Bairey Merz CN, Dwyer J, Nordstrom CK, Walton KG, Salerno JW, Schneider RH. Psychosocial stress and cardiovascular disease: pathophysiological links. Behav Med. 2002;27:141–7.
107. Chrousos GP, Gold PW. The concepts of stress and stress system disorders. Overview of physical and behavioral homeostasis. JAMA. 1992;267:1244–52.
108. Esch T, Stefano GB, Fricchione GL, Benson H. Stress in cardiovascular diseases. Med Sci Monit. 2002;8: RA93–101.
109. Jiang W, Babyak M, Krantz DS, Waugh RA, Coleman RE, Hanson MM, et al. Mental stress–induced myocardial ischemia and cardiac events. JAMA. 1996;275:1651–6.
110. Sheps DS, McMahon RP, Becker L, Carney RM, Freedland KE, Cohen JD, et al. Mental stress-induced ischemia and all-cause mortality in patients with coronary artery disease: results from the Psychophysiological Investigations of Myocardial Ischemia study. Circulation. 2002;105:1780–4.
111. DiMatteo MR, Lepper HS, Croghan TW. Depression is a risk factor for noncompliance with medical treatment: meta-analysis of the effects of anxiety and depression on patient adherence. Arch Intern Med. 2000;160:2101–7.
112. Wang PS, Bohn RL, Knight E, Glynn RJ, Mogun H, Avorn J. Noncompliance with antihypertensive medications: the impact of depressive symptoms and psychosocial factors. J Gen Intern Med. 2002;17:504–11.
113. Blumenthal JA, Williams RS, Wallace AG, Williams Jr RB, Needles TL. Physiological and psychological variables predict compliance to prescribed exercise therapy in patients recovering from myocardial infarction. Psychosom Med. 1982;44:519–27.
114. Glazer KM, Emery CF, Frid DJ, Banyasz RE. Psychological predictors of adherence and outcomes among patients in cardiac rehabilitation. J Cardiopulm Rehabil. 2002;22:40–6.
115. Evangelista LS, Berg J, Dracup K. Relationship between psychosocial variables and compliance in patients with heart failure. Heart Lung. 2001;30:294–301.
116. Yusuf S. Two decades of progress in preventing vascular disease. Lancet. 2002;360:2–3.
117. Butler J, Arbogast PG, BeLue R, Daugherty J, Jain MK, Ray WA, et al. Outpatient adherence to beta-blocker therapy after acute myocardial infarction. J Am Coll Cardiol. 2002;40:1589–95.
118. Jackevicius CA, Mamdani M, Tu JV. Adherence with statin therapy in elderly patients with and without acute coronary syndromes. JAMA. 2002;288:462–7.
119. The Coronary Drug Project Research Group. Influence of Adherence to Treatment and Response of Cholesterol on Mortality in the Coronary Drug Project. N Engl J Med. 1980;303:1038–41.
120. Horwitz RI, Viscoli CM, Berkman L, Donaldson RM, Horwitz SM, Murray CJ, et al. Treatment adherence and risk of death after a myocardial infarction. Lancet. 1990;336:542–5.
121. McDermott MM, Schmitt B, Wallner E. Impact of medication nonadherence on coronary heart disease outcomes. A critical review. Arch Intern Med. 1997;157:1921–9.
122. Penninx BW, van Tilburg T, Boeke AJ, Deeg DJ, Kriegsman DM, van Eijk JT. Effects of social support and personal coping resources on depressive symptoms: different for various chronic diseases? Health Psychol. 1998;17:551–8.
123. Bosworth HB, Hays JC, George LK, Steffens DC. Psychosocial and clinical predictors of unipolar depression outcome in older adults. Int J Geriatr Psychiatry. 2002;17: 238–46.
124. Hays JC, Steffens DC, Flint EP, Bosworth HB, George LK. Does social support buffer functional decline in elderly patients with unipolar depression? Am J Psychiatry. 2001;158:1850–5.
125. Berkman LF, Leo-Summers L, Horwitz RI. Emotional support and survival after myocardial infarction. A prospective, population-based study of the elderly. Ann Intern Med. 1992;117:1003–9.
126. Gorkin L, Schron EB, Brooks MM, Wiklund I, Kellen J, Verter J, et al. Psychosocial predictors of mortality in the Cardiac Arrhythmia Suppression Trial-1 (CAST-1). Am J Cardiol. 1993;71:263–7.
127. Williams RB, Barefoot JC, Califf RM, Haney TL, Saunders WB, Pryor DB, et al. Prognostic importance of social and economic resources among medically treated patients with angiographically documented coronary artery disease. JAMA. 1992;267:520–4.
128. Case RB, Moss AJ, Case N, McDermott M, Eberly S. Living alone after myocardial infarction. Impact on prognosis. JAMA. 1992;267:515–9.
129. Kawachi I, Colditz GA, Ascherio A, Rimm EB, Giovannucci E, Stampfer MJ, et al. A prospective study of social networks in relation to total mortality and cardiovascular disease in men in the USA. J Epidemiol Community Health. 1996;50:245–51.
130. Colantonio A, Kasl SV, Ostfeld AM, Berkman LF. Psychosocial predictors of stroke outcomes in an elderly population. J Gerontol. 1993;48:S261–8.

131. Kwakkel G, Wagenaar RC, Kollen BJ, Lankhorst GJ. Predicting disability in stroke–a critical review of the literature. Age Ageing. 1996;25:479–89.
132. Fuster V, Gotto AM, Libby P, Loscalzo J, McGill HC. 27th Bethesda Conference: matching the intensity of risk factor management with the hazard for coronary disease events. Task Force 1. Pathogenesis of coronary disease: the biologic role of risk factors. [Review] [82 refs]. J Am Coll Cardiol. 1996;27:964–76.
133. Wilson PW, D'Agostino RB, Levy D, Belanger AM, Silbershatz H, Kannel WB. Prediction of coronary heart disease using risk factor categories. Circulation. 1998; 97:1837–47.
134. Multiple Risk Factor Intervention Trial Research Group. Relationship between baseline risk factors and coronary heart disease and total mortality in the Multiple Risk Factor Intervention Trial. Prev Med. 1986;15:254–73.
135. Quattrocki E, Baird A, Yurgelun-Todd D. Biological aspects of the link between smoking and depression. Harv Rev Psychiatry. 2000;8:99–110.
136. Breslau N, Peterson EL, Schultz LR, Chilcoat HD, Andreski P. Major depression and stages of smoking. A longitudinal investigation. Arch Gen Psychiatry. 1998;55:161–6.
137. Anda RF, Williamson DF, Escobedo LG, Mast EE, Giovino GA, Remington PL. Depression and the dynamics of smoking. A national perspective. JAMA. 1990;264:1541–5.
138. Hall SM, Munoz RF, Reus VI, Sees KL. Nicotine, negative affect, and depression. J Consult Clin Psychol. 1993;61: 761–7.
139. Shinn EH, Poston WS, Kimball KT, St Jeor ST, Foreyt JP. Blood pressure and symptoms of depression and anxiety: a prospective study. Am J Hypertens. 2001;14:660–4.
140. Jonas BS, Lando JF. Negative affect as a prospective risk factor for hypertension. Psychosom Med. 2000;62: 188–96.
141. Davidson K, Jonas BS, Dixon KE, Markovitz JH. Do depression symptoms predict early hypertension incidence in young adults in the CARDIA study? Coronary Artery Risk Development in Young Adults. Arch Intern Med. 2000;160:1495–500.
142. Garcia MJ, McNamara PM, Gordon T, Kannel WB. Morbidity and mortality in diabetics in the Framingham population. Sixteen year follow-up study. Diabetes. 1974;23:105–11.
143. Anderson RJ, Freedland KE, Clouse RE, Lustman PJ. The prevalence of comorbid depression in adults with diabetes: a meta- analysis. Diabetes Care. 2001;24:1069–78.
144. Lustman PJ, Anderson RJ, Freedland KE, de Groot M, Carney RM, Clouse RE. Depression and poor glycemic control: a meta-analytic review of the literature. Diabetes Care. 2000;23:934–42.
145. de Groot M, Anderson R, Freedland KE. Association of depression and diabetes complications: a meta-analysis. Psychosom Med. 2001;63:619–30.
146. Anderson KM, Castelli WP, Levy D. Cholesterol and mortality. 30 years of follow-up from the Framingham study. JAMA. 1987;257:2176–80.
147. Horsten M, Wamala SP, Vingerhoets A, Orth-Gomer K. Depressive symptoms, social support, and lipid profile in healthy middle-aged women. Psychosom Med. 1997;59: 521–8.
148. Olusi SO, Fido AA. Serum lipid concentrations in patients with major depressive disorder. Biol Psychiatry. 1996;40: 1128–31.
149. Steegmans PH, Fekkes D, Hoes AW, Bak AA, van der Does E, Grobbee DE. Low serum cholesterol concentration and serotonin metabolism in men. BMJ. 1996; 312:221.
150. Steegmans PH, Hoes AW, Bak AA, van der Does E, Grobbee DE. Higher prevalence of depressive symptoms in middle-aged men with low serum cholesterol levels. Psychosom Med. 2000;62:205–11.
151. Hyyppa MT, Kronholm E, Virtanen A, Leino A, Jula A. Does simvastatin affect mood and steroid hormone levels in hypercholesterolemic men? A randomized double-blind trial. Psychoneuroendocrinology. 2003;28:181–94.
152. Ormel J, Koeter MW, van den Brink W, van de Willige G. Recognition, management, and course of anxiety and depression in general practice. Arch Gen Psychiatry. 1991;48:700–6.
153. Simon GE, VonKorff M. Recognition, management, and outcomes of depression in primary care. Arch Fam Med. 1995;4:99–105.
154. Spitzer RL, Williams JB, Kroenke K, Linzer M, de Gruy III FV, Hahn SR, et al. Utility of a new procedure for diagnosing mental disorders in primary care The PRIME-MD 1000 study. JAMA. 1994;272:1749–56.
155. Davidson JR, Meltzer-Brody SE. The underrecognition and undertreatment of depression: what is the breadth and depth of the problem? J Clin Psychiatry. 1999;60 Suppl 7:4–9.
156. Goldman LS, Nielsen NH, Champion HC. Awareness, diagnosis, and treatment of depression. J Gen Intern Med. 1999;14:569–80.
157. Alexopoulos GS, Borson S, Cuthbert BN, Devanand DP, Mulsant BH, Olin JT, et al. Assessment of late life depression. Biol Psychiatry. 2002;52:164–74.
158. Charlson M, Peterson JC. Medical comorbidity and late life depression: what is known and what are the unmet needs? Biol Psychiatry. 2002;52:226–35.
159. Whooley MA, Avins AL, Miranda J, Browner WS. Case-finding instruments for depression. Two questions are as good as many. J Gen Intern Med. 1997;12:439–45.
160. Juenger J, Schellberg D, Kraemer S, Haunstetter A, Zugck C, Herzog W, et al. Health related quality of life in patients with congestive heart failure: comparison with other chronic diseases and relation to functional variables. Heart. 2002;87:235–41.
161. Avorn J, Everitt DE, Weiss S. Increased antidepressant use in patients prescribed beta-blockers. JAMA. 1986;255: 357–60.
162. Thiessen BQ, Wallace SM, Blackburn JL, Wilson TW, Bergman U. Increased prescribing of antidepressants subsequent to beta-blocker therapy. Arch Intern Med. 1990;150:2286–90.
163. Ko DT, Hebert PR, Coffey CS, Sedrakyan A, Curtis JP, Krumholz HM. Beta-blocker therapy and symptoms of depression, fatigue, and sexual dysfunction. JAMA. 2002;288:351–7.
164. Freedland KE. The Depression Interview and Structured Hamilton (DISH): rationale, development, characteristics, and clinical validity. Psychosom Med. 2002;64:897–905.

165. Koenig HG, George LK, Peterson BL, Pieper CF. Depression in medically ill hospitalized older adults: prevalence, characteristics, and course of symptoms according to six diagnostic schemes. Am J Psychiatry. 1997;154:1376–83.
166. Pignone MP, Gaynes BN, Rushton JL, Burchell CM, Orleans CT, Mulrow CD, et al. Screening for depression in adults: a summary of the evidence for the U.S. Preventive Services Task Force. Ann Intern Med. 2002;136:765–76.
167. Kessler RC, Berglund P, Demler O, Jin R, Koretz D, Merikangas K, et al. The epidemiology of major depressive disorder: results from the National Comorbidity Survey Replication (NCS-R). JAMA. 2003;289:3095–105.
168. Olfson M, Marcus SC, Druss B, Elinson L, Tanielian T, Pincus HA. National trends in the outpatient treatment of depression. JAMA. 2002;287:203–9.
169. Hirschfeld RM, Keller MB, Panico S, Arons BS, Barlow D, Davidoff F, et al. The National Depressive and Manic-Depressive Association consensus statement on the undertreatment of depression. JAMA. 1997;277:333–40.
170. Glassman AH, O'Connor CM, Califf RM, Swedberg K, Schwartz P, Bigger Jr JT, et al. Sertraline treatment of major depression in patients with acute MI or unstable angina. Sertraline Antidepressant Heart Attack Randomized Trial. JAMA. 2002;288:701–9.
171. Glassman AH, Bigger Jr JT. Cardiovascular effects of therapeutic doses of tricyclic antidepressants. A review. Arch Gen Psychiatry. 1981;38:815–20.
172. Frasure-Smith N, Prince R. Long-term follow-up of the Ischemic Heart Disease Life Stress Monitoring Program. Psychosom Med. 1989;51:485–513.
173. Blumenthal JA, Jiang W, Babyak MA, Krantz DS, Frid DJ, Coleman RE, et al. Stress management and exercise training in cardiac patients with myocardial ischemia. Effects on prognosis and evaluation of mechanisms. Arch Intern Med. 1997;157:2213–23.
174. Frasure-Smith N, Lesperance F, Prince RH, Verrier P, Garber RA, Juneau M, et al. Randomised trial of home-based psychosocial nursing intervention for patients recovering from myocardial infarction. Lancet. 1997;350:473–9.
175. Writing Committee for the ENRICHD Investigators. The effects of treating depression and low perceived social support on clinical events after myocardial infarction: the Enhancing Recovery in Coronary Heart Disease Patients (ENRICHD) Randomized Trial. JAMA. 2003;289:3106–16.
176. Linden W, Stossel C, Maurice J. Psychosocial interventions for patients with coronary artery disease: a meta-analysis. Arch Intern Med. 1996;156:745–52.
177. Marchionni N, Fattirolli F, Fumagalli S, Oldridge NB, Del Lungo F, Bonechi F, et al. Determinants of exercise tolerance after acute myocardial infarction in older persons. J Am Geriatr Soc. 2000;48:146–53.
178. Ghayoumi A, Raxwal V, Cho S, Myers J, Chun S, Froelicher VF. Prognostic value of exercise tests in male veterans with chronic coronary artery disease. J Cardiopulm Rehabil. 2002;22:399–407.
179. Moore KA, Blumenthal JA. Exercise training as an alternative treatment for depression among older adults. Altern Ther Health Med. 1998;4:48–56.
180. Maines TY, Lavie CJ, Milani RV, Cassidy MM, Gilliland YE, Murgo JP. Effects of cardiac rehabilitation and exercise programs on exercise capacity, coronary risk factors, behavior, and quality of life in patients with coronary artery disease. South Med J. 1997;90:43–9.
181. Lavie CJ, Milani RV, Cassidy MM, Gilliland YE. Effects of cardiac rehabilitation and exercise training programs in women with depression. Am J Cardiol. 1999;83:1480–3, A7.
182. Blumenthal JA, Sherwood A, Babyak MA, Watkins LL, Waugh R, Georgiades A, et al. Effects of exercise and stress management training on markers of cardiovascular risk in patients with ischemic heart disease: a randomized controlled trial. JAMA. 2005;293:1626–34.
183. Heiligenstein JH, Ware Jr JE, Beusterien KM, Roback PJ, Andrejasich C, Tollefson GD. Acute effects of fluoxetine versus placebo on functional health and well-being in late-life depression. Int Psychogeriatr. 1995;7(Suppl):125–37.
184. Swenson JR, O'Connor CM, Barton D, van Zyl LT, Swedberg K, Forman LM, et al. Influence of depression and effect of treatment with sertraline on quality of life after hospitalization for acute coronary syndrome. Am J Cardiol. 2003;92:1271–6.
185. Lusis AJ, Mar R, Pajukanta P. Genetics of atherosclerosis. Annu Rev Genomics Hum Genet. 2004;5:189–218.
186. Souery D, Rivelli SK, Mendlewicz J. Molecular genetic and family studies in affective disorders: state of the art. J Affect Disord. 2001;62:45–55.
187. Whyte EM, Pollock BG, Wagner WR, Mulsant BH, Ferrell RE, Mazumdar S, et al. Influence of serotonin-transporter-linked promoter region polymorphism on platelet activation in geriatric depression. Am J Psychiatry. 2001;158:2074–6.
188. Williams RB, Marchuk DA, Gadde KM, Barefoot JC, Grichnik K, Helms MJ, et al. Central nervous system serotonin function and cardiovascular responses to stress. Psychosom Med. 2001;63:300–5.
189. Anda R, Williamson D, Jones D, Macera C, Eaker E, Glassman A, et al. Depressed affect, hopelessness, and the risk of ischemic heart disease in a cohort of U.S. adults. Epidemiology. 1993;4:285–94.
190. Aromaa A, Raitasalo R, Reunanen A, Impivaara O, Heliovaara M, Knekt P, et al. Depression and cardiovascular diseases. Acta Psychiatr Scand Suppl. 1994;377:77–82.
191. Barefoot JC, Schroll M. Symptoms of depression, acute myocardial infarction, and total mortality in a community sample. Circulation. 1996;93:1976–80.
192. de Mendes LCF, Krumholz HM, Seeman TS, Vaccarino V, Williams CS, Kasl SV, et al. Depression and risk of coronary heart disease in elderly men and women: New Haven EPESE, 1982–1991. Established Populations for the Epidemiologic Studies of the Elderly. Arch Intern Med. 1998;158:2341–8.
193. Sesso HD, Kawachi I, Vokonas PS, Sparrow D. Depression and the risk of coronary heart disease in the Normative Aging Study. Am J Cardiol. 1998;82:851–6.
194. Lesperance F, Frasure-Smith N, Juneau M, Theroux P. Depression and 1-year prognosis in unstable angina. Arch Intern Med. 2000;160:1354–60.

Secondary Prevention Strategies 14

Romero Corral Abel, Lopez Jimenez Francisco,
Josef Korinek, Virend Somers,
and Thomas E. Kottke

Introduction

Nearly all patients with coronary artery disease have at least one modifiable cardiovascular risk factor and most risk factors remain inadequately controlled after patients are diagnosed with coronary heart disease (CHD). The suboptimal management of cardiovascular risk factors in secondary prevention contributes to high rates of recurrent coronary events in patients with a history of myocardial infarction.

There are solid clinical trial data supporting the use of aspirin, beta blockers, statins, and ACE inhibitors in nearly all patients with CHD who do not have specific contraindications. This is especially true for patients with a history of myocardial infarction.

Up to 85% of recurrent events in patients with coronary disease could be prevented or delayed with the use of these medications [1, 2]. It is likely that this percentage could be increased by adding exercise and dietary changes.

This chapter reviews the most recent evidence that control of cardiovascular disease risk factors in patients with established coronary disease improves outcomes. It also reviews the futility of several widely used interventions that failed to show benefit in clinical trials.

R.C. Abel (✉) • J. Korinek
Cardiovascular Division, Mayo Clinic Rochester,
Rochester, MN, USA

Cardiovascular Department, Albert Einstein Medical Center,
Philadelphia, PA, USA
e-mail: romeroab@einstein.edu

L.J. Francisco • V. Somers
Cardiovascular Division, Mayo Clinic College of Medicine,
Rochester, MN, USA

T.E. Kottke
Cardiovascular Division, HealthPartners Research Foundation,
Minneapolis, MN, USA

Lipid-Lowering Therapy

Dyslipidemia, especially hypercholesterolemia, is a key modifiable CHD risk factor. The level of serum cholesterol is most strongly related to saturated fat in the diet, but in some individuals hypercholesterolemia is caused by mutations or polymorphisms of the genes involved in lipid metabolism [3]. Low-density lipoprotein cholesterol (LDL-C) has been identified as a potent atherogenic component of serum cholesterol and is strongly related to CHD risk. Placebo-controlled randomized clinical trials of 3-hydroxy-3-methylglutaryl (HMG-CoA) reductase inhibitors (statins) provide clear evidence that lowering LDL-C reduces CHD-related morbidity and mortality in patients with documented CHD [4, 5]. The same is true for individuals without a history of CHD [6, 7].

There are data that suggest that there is no threshold LDL-C below which no cardioprotective effect of lipid-lowering is apparent. Results of the Heart Protection Study (HPS) [8] and the Anglo-Scandinavian Cardiac Outcomes Trial (ASCOT) [9] suggest that statin therapy may be beneficial for patients at high risk of cardiovascular disease regardless of their baseline values: patients with baseline LDL-C levels less than 100 mg/dL or greater than 130 mg/dL both benefited from statin therapy. Moreover the dosage of statins affects progression of CHD as was shown in Reversing Atherosclerosis with Aggressive Lipid Lowering therapy trial (REVERSAL) [10]. Using intravascular ultrasonography, intensive therapy with atorvastatin

G.W. Barsness and D.R. Holmes Jr. (eds.), *Coronary Artery Disease*,
DOI 10.1007/978-1-84628-712-1_14,

Table 14.1 Recent randomized clinical trial of cholesterol lowering in secondary prevention of CHD

Study	Study population	Intervention	F/u	CVD event reduction RR 95% CI	Overall mortality RR 95% CI
4S	4,444 men and women; mean age 59 years	Simvastatin , titration	5.4	0.58 (0.46–0.73)	0.70 (0.58–0.85)
CARE [1]	4,159 men and women; mean age 59 years	Pravastatin, 40 mg	5	0.76 (0.64–0.91)	0.91(0.74–1.12)
LIPID	9,014 men and women age 31–75 years	Pravastatin, 40 mg	6.1	0.76 (0.65–0.88)	0.78 (0.69–0.87)
VA-HIT [1]	2,531 men age <74 years	Gemfibrozil, 1,200 mg	5.1	0.78 (0.65–0.93)	0.89 (0.73–1.08)
HPS	20,526 men and women age 40–80 years	Simvastatin, 40 mg	5.5	0.83 (0.75–0.91)	0.87 (0.81–0.94)
PROSPER [1]	5,804 men and women age 70–82 years	Pravastatin, 40 mg	3.2	0.85 (0.74–0.97)	*
GREACE [1]	1,600 men and women; mean age 58 years	Atorvastatin, 10–80 mg	3	0.49 (0.27–0.73)	0.57 (0.39–0.78)
ASCOT	19,342 men and women age 40–79 years	Atorvastatin, 10 mg	3.3	0.64 (0.54–0.83)	0.87 (0.71–1.06)
TNT	10,001 men and women:mean age 61 years	Atorvastatin 10 mg vs. Atorvastatin 80 mg	4.9	0.78 (0.69–0.89)	1.01 (0.85–1.19)
PROVE-IT	4,162 men and women; mean age 58 years	Pravastatin 40 mg vs. Atorvastatin 80 mg	2.0	0.87 (0.70–1.08)	0.72 (0.48–1.02)

ASCOT Anglo-Scandinavian Cardiac Outcomes Trial-Lipid-Lowering Arm, *CARE* Coronary Events After Myocardial Infarction in Patients with Average Cholesterol levels, *4S* Scandinavian Simvastatin Survival Study, *GREACE* Greek Atorvastatin and Coronary-Heart-Disease Evaluation, *HPS* Heart Protection Study, *LIPID* Long-Term Intervention with Pravastatin in Ischemic Disease, *PROSPER* Prospective Study of Pravastatin in the Elderly at Risk, *VA-HIT* Veterans Affairs High-Density Lipoprotein Intervention Trial, *PROVE-IT* Pravastatin or Atorvastatin Evaluation and Infection trial, *TNT* Treating New Target
F/u follow-up. *No data available

(80 mg) was superior to moderate therapy with pravastatin (40 mg) in slowing progression of atherosclerosis, but none of the treatments appears to reverse atherosclerotic process. The reduction of atherosclerotic progression was proportional to the reduction in LDL-C levels. Pravastatin or Atorvastatin Evaluation and Infection Trial (PROVE-IT) [11] using the same medications and doses as REVERSAL included a large number of patients with acute coronary syndromes who were followed by a mean of 24 months in order to assess the cardiovascular events and mortality of all causes. When compared to pravastatin, atorvastatin showed a 16% reduction in the hazard ratio for primary endpoints (composite death of any cause, myocardial infarction, documented unstable angina, revascularization, and stroke). Treating New Target (TNT) [12] using atorvastatin 10 and 80 mg (intensive therapy) showed 22% relative reduction in risk in favor of the 80 mg dose, but there was no difference in the overall mortality between groups. On the other hand, treatment with higher dose of atorvastatin increased overall rate of adverse events (8.1% vs. 5.8%). Interestingly, 3 of the 5 cases of rhabdomyolysis were reported in low-dose treatment group.

Statins have proven to be an effective treatment for secondary prevention in patients with CHD and an aggressive treatment appears to be guaranteed to obtain the most benefit Table 14.1. Adverse events could be a limiting factor of high dose of statins, but the absolute risk of major adverse events appears to be low. Current goals recommended by the National Cholesterol education Program Adult Treatment Panel III [13] for LDL-C are shown on Table 14.2.

Antihypertensive Treatment

Arterial hypertension contributes significantly to the pathogenesis of coronary atherosclerosis and worsens outcome of patients with CHD. The most common manifestation of end-organ target damage in hypertension is heart disease. According to the World Health

Table 14.2 National cholesterol education program adult treatment panel III for lipid-lowering therapy recommendations

Risk category	LDL-C goal	Initiate TLC[⊥]	Consider drug therapy
High risk: CHD or CHD	<100 mg/dL	≥100 mg/dL	≥100 mg/dL[3] (≤100 mg/dL optional)
Risk equivalents* (10-year risk >20%)	Optional goal: <70 mg/dL[+]		
Moderately high risk: 2+	<130 mg/dL	≥130 mg/dL	≥130 mg/dL (100–129 mg/dL optional)
Risk factors^ (10-year risk 10–20%)	Optional goal: <100 mg/dL		
Moderate risk: 2+ risk	<130 mg/dL	≥130 mg/dL	≥160 mg/dL
Factors (10-year risk <10%)			
Lower risk: 0–1 risk Factor	160 mg/dL	≥160 mg/dL	≥190 mg/dL (160–190 mg/dL optional)

[⊥]Therapeutic life style changes
[*]CHD risk equivalents includes history of MI, unstable angina, coronary artery procedures (angioplasty or bypass surgery), or evidence of clinically significant myocardial ischemia
[^]Risk Factors include cigarette smoking, hypertension, low HDL cholesterol (<40 mg/dL), family history of premature CHD (first-degree male relative < 55 years; female < 65 years), and age (men ≥ 45 years; women ≥ years)
[3]If TG 200–499 mg/dL: Consider fibrate or niacin after LDL-lowering therapy, If TG ≥ 500 mg/dL: Consider fibrate or niacin before LDL-lowering therapy Consider omega-3 fatty acids as adjunct for high TG
[+]Patients with recent MI; Smoking and previous MI; Diabetes Mellitus and previous MI

Table 14.3 AHA/ACC recommendation for management of arterial hypertension adapted for secondary prevention

BP control: *Goal*:	Initiate lifestyle modification (weight control, physical activity, alcohol moderation, moderate sodium restriction, and emphasis on fruits, vegetables, and low-fat dairy products) in all patients with blood pressure ≤130 mmHg systolic or 80 mmHg diastolic.
<140/90 mmHg or *<130/85* mmHg if heart failure or renal insufficiency *<130/80* mmHg if diabetes	Add blood pressure medication, individualized to other patient requirements and characteristics (i.e., age, race, need for drugs with specific benefits) *if* blood pressure is not <140 mmHg systolic or 90 mmHg diastolic *or* if blood pressure is not <130 mmHg systolic or 85 mmHg diastolic for individuals with heart failure or renal insufficiency (<80 mmHg diastolic for individuals with diabetes).

Organization, about 50% of CHD burden and 66% of cerebrovascular events can be attributed to poor blood pressure control [14]. Data from the National Health and Nutrition Survey [15] reports that only 34% of the hypertensive population has achieved target blood pressure values less than 140/90 mmHg.

Hypertension treatment trials have demonstrated than even small reductions in blood pressure can reduce hypertension-related morbidity and mortality [16–18]. With one exception, alpha$_1$-blockers, this effect appears to be independent of the medication used [19]. Antihypertensive drugs, such as low-dose diuretics, ACE inhibitors, beta blockers, calcium channel blockers, and angiotensin receptor blockers have all been shown to decrease cardiovascular mortality and morbidity in hypertensive patients.

Two large-scale meta-analyses [20, 21] of hypertension trials have been conducted to assess which antihypertensive medications provide better outcomes. All the major antihypertensive drugs mentioned above were examined in the meta-analyses. None of the medications used as first-line treatments strategies were superior to low-dose diuretics. Blood pressure changes were similar among treatments. Important from a pharmacoeconomic perspective was the observation that, in comparison with calcium channel blockers, beta blockers and ACE inhibitors, low-dose diuretics were associated with a slightly greater reduction in risk of cardiovascular disease events (RR, 0.94, 0.94, and 0.89, respectively). Interestingly, there was no difference in risk of coronary artery disease between angiotensin receptor blockers based and control regimens, despite greater blood pressure reduction. These meta-analyses indicate that alpha$_1$ blockers, another group of antihypertensive therapy previously used as first-line treatment for arterial hypertension, may be harmful in patients with CHD. In fact, the treatment arm in ALLHAT study with alpha$_1$ blockers was discontinued because of a higher incidence of combined CVD events. Therefore, the use of alpha$_1$ blockers is not recommended in patients with CHD. The ACC/AHA recommendation for blood pressure control is listed on Table 14.3.

Table 14.4 Current antihypertensive recommendation for specific conditions in secondary prevention

Comorbidities							
Medication	Post-MI	Heart failure	Diabetes	Renal disease	Recurrent stroke prevention	High coronary disease risk	Angina
Diuretic		*Yes*	*Yes*		*Yes*	*Yes*	
BB	*Yes*	*Yes*	*Yes*			*Yes*	*Yes*
ACEI	*Yes*	*Yes*	*Yes*	*Yes*	*Yes*	*Yes*	
CCBs			*Yes*			*Yes*	*Yes*
ARB		*Yes*	*Yes*	*Yes*			
Aldosterone Antagonist	*Yes*	*Yes*					

BB Beta Blockers, *ACEI* Angiotensin Conversing Enzyme Inhibitors, *CCBs* Calcium Channel BlockerS, (*ARB*) Angiotensin Receptor Blockers

Table 14.5 Benefit from antiplatelet therapy versus adjusted controls in secondary prevention in patients with CHD without previous MI and in patients with prior MI

Patients baseline comorbidities	No of RT with data	No patients enrolled	% risk reduction
Stable angina/CHD	7	2,920	33
Unstable angina	12	5,031	46
Coronary artery bypass[a]	25	6,231	4
Heart Failure[a]	2	134	41
Coronary angioplasty	9	3,212	53
Subtotal	*55*	*17,528*	*37*
Benefit from antiplatelet therapy versus adjusted controls in secondary prevention in patients with prior or acute MI:			
Previous MI	12	20,006	25
Acute MI	15	19,302	30

Based on data from: Antithrombotic Trialists' Collaboration [38]
RT Randomized trials, *MI* myocardial infarction
[a]Did not reach statistical significance

The type of medication for arterial hypertension becomes important in patient with certain conditions, such as CHD, congestive heart failure, angina pectoris, chronic renal disease, recurrent stroke, or previous MI [22]. In these diseases specific antihypertensive medications must be considered. In patients with stable angina, the first drug of choice is usually a beta blocker, but a calcium channel blocker can also be used in patients who have preserved left ventricular systolic function. Nitrates may be particularly useful in treating hypertension in patients with angina pectoris. In acute coronary syndromes, a beta blocker and ACE inhibitor should be the initial treatment. Nitrates and other drugs can be added as needed for blood pressure or angina pectoris control. In patients who have suffered a myocardial infarction, ACE inhibitors, beta blockers, and aldosterone antagonists have all improved outcomes, especially if the left ventricular ejection fraction is reduced [23–25] (Table 14.4).

Aspirin, Other Antiplatelet and Anticoagulant Agents

The effect and mechanism of action of antiplatelet agents are well known. There is strong evidence of benefit in secondary prevention after myocardial infarction. The Antithrombotic Trialists' Collaboration meta-analysis compared randomized controlled trials of antiplatelet therapy [26]. Patients with stable angina/CHD receiving antiplatelet therapy experienced an adjusted 33% risk reduction when compared to control group patients. Patients at high risk for cardiac death due to other causes also benefited from antiplatelet therapy, (Table 14.5). A dose of aspirin ranging from 75 to 150 mg appears to confer the same protection as larger doses.

The three trials comparing dipyridamole with aspirin did not show any difference on any outcome. Other antiplatelet agents, such as clopidogrel, have

Table 14.6 Oral anticoagulants alone and combined versus placebo or aspirin alone.

Therapy used	Benefits (% risk reduction)	Increase in major bleeding
High-intensity oral anticoagulants vs. control (placebo) INR 2.8–4.8	Mortality 22% MI 42% Thromboembolic complications including stroke 63%	6 fold
Moderate -intensity Oral anticoagulants vs. control (placebo) INR 2–3	Mortality 18% MI 52% Stroke 53%	7.7 fold
Moderately high Oral anticoagulants + aspirin vs. aspirin INR ≥ 2	Mortality, MI, and stroke 56%	1.9 fold
Low-intensity Oral anticoagulants + aspirin vs. aspirin INR <2	No significant reduction was observed	1.3 fold

INR International Normalized Ratio
Based on data from: Anand and Yusuf [30]

also been studied for the secondary prevention of CHD. Long-term administration of clopidogrel plus aspirin to patients with atherosclerotic disease is more effective than aspirin alone in reducing the combined endpoint of stroke, MI, and vascular death. Risk of major bleeding appeared to be similar among medications [27, 28]. Clopidogrel in addition to aspirin has also been studied in patients undergoing elective percutaneous coronary intervention. In this scenario clopidogrel plus aspirin, when compared to aspirin alone, showed a 26% relative risk reduction (3% absolute reduction) in the combined risk of death, MI, or stroke. On the other hand, major ischemic bleeding events increased 1.1% [29].

Oral anticoagulants (warfarin/Coumarins) have also been studied for secondary prevention of CHD. Yusuf et al. [30] published a meta-analysis of oral anticoagulants of 16 randomized trials in 10,056 patients with CHD. Patients were divided into three groups based on the International Normalized Radio (INR): high (2.8–4.8), moderately high (≥2), and low intensity (<2) and were compared to a control group (placebo or aspirin). In comparison to placebo, high-intensity and moderate-intensity therapy reduced mortality and thromboembolic complications including stroke, but anticoagulation was associated with a 6–7.7 fold increase in risk of bleeding complications. No benefit in outcomes was noted when moderately high-intensity anticoagulation was compared to aspirin, but a 1.9 fold increase of bleeding complications was observed with coumadin. The results of other comparisons are listed in Table 14.6.

The ACC/AHA Guidelines regarding Antiplatelet and Anticoagulant Use to Prevent MI in Patients with CHD Are:

- Daily dose of 75–325 mg aspirin and, if contraindicated, 75 mg a day of clopidogrel or warfarin (INR 2–3) when clinically indicated or unable to take aspirin or clopidogrel [31].
- Clopidogrel is indicated in the management of unstable angina and non-ST elevation MI.

Smoking Cessation

Smoking is the most important cause of preventable death in the USA. One of every five deaths is related to cigarette smoking. CHD is responsible for 43% of deaths caused by smoking [32, 33]. A recent analysis has found evidence that environmental tobacco smoke and nearly any concentration is highly toxic [34].

Two major meta-analyses assessing the effect of smoking cessation in patients with established CHD attributed a 36% reduction of cardiovascular mortality and a 46% reduction in overall mortality to smoking cessation [35, 36]. In comparison with other risk-lowering tactics (lipid-lowering treatments (25–35% reduction), aspirin (15–25% reduction) beta blockers and ACE inhibitors (20–25% reduction)), smoking cessation reduces risk to a similar extent but is far less expensive than all other interventions [37–40].

The AHA/ACC recommendation for smoking cessation in secondary prevention is to achieve a complete cessation by providing counseling and pharmacological therapy (which may include nicotine replacement and bupropion). Although most patients who smoke will want to quit after a myocardial infarction, relapse rates can be high [41]. Nicotine replacement therapy, the most frequent pharmacological intervention, has shown minimum benefit when compared to placebo [42]. Because nicotine appears to have cardiotoxic effects during acute ischemic events, nicotine replacement therapy should not be used in a patient experiencing an acute coronary syndrome [43]. For many smokers, however, the question is not whether they will get nicotine, but rather how they will get their nicotine. Because nicotine replacement delivers only about half the dose of nicotine and none of the tar and carbon monoxide delivered by cigarettes, the authors feel comfortable prescribing nicotine replacement to smokers with stable coronary artery disease [44, 45]. Although bupropion has not been studied in patients with CHD, a panel of experts has concluded that use of bupropion increases the odds of success [46]. If the patient can be entered into a structured program of support, the odds of cessation increase markedly [47].

Weight Loss

Obesity is a worldwide epidemic and its prevalence is steadily increasing [48, 49]. Excess weight is associated with increased mortality and risk of cardiovascular events [50, 51]. The mechanisms whereby excess body fat affects the cardiovascular system include not only an indirect effect on the vascular system through risk factors like dyslipidemia, hypertension, obstructive sleep apnea, or insulin resistance, but also by an enhanced inflammatory state, a high turnover of free fatty acids with a lipotoxic effect on myocardial cells [52], and the potential effects of high levels of leptin [53, 54]. The American Heart Association has declared that obesity is an independent cardiovascular risk factor [55]. Recent data from myocardial infarction surveillance studies suggest that excess weight is the most common cardiovascular risk factor in patients with MI and that its prevalence has increased over time [56]. Nevertheless, obesity is underrecognized, underdiagnosed, and undertreated in persons with acute MI [57].

Data from weight loss programs in patients with CHD are limited. Data from small trials have shown that a combination of exercise and diet can effectively induce weigh loss in patients with CHD, but attrition is high. When this approach fails, patients can be offered bariatric surgery which is an effective option for treatment of high-risk obese patients (BMI ≥ 40). Bariatric surgery, especially gastric bypass, has shown great improvements in many of the major cardiovascular risk factors, such as hypertension, dyslipidemia, diabetes, and obstructive sleep apnea. Mortality for gastric bypass is estimated to be less than 1%, although postoperative complications may occur in up to 20% of patients [58, 59].

The evidence for long-term efficacy of pharmacologic intervention in weight loss is limited to two medications: sibutramine and orlistat. Treatment with sibutramine produces significantly more maintained weight loss at 2 years than placebo, but the drug is contraindicated in patients with CHD. Orlistat, a medication that blocks the absorption of fat, causes weight loss of about 2.2 kg greater than placebo at 4 years, with significantly more patients achieving ≥10% loss of initial body weight (26.2% and 15.6%, respectively) [60].

New drugs like the cannabinoid-1 receptor blocker rimonabant (previously discussed) are being studied both for weight loss and smoking cessation. The drug appears to act by decreasing appetite in the brain and stimulating satiety in the gastrointestinal tract. A recent randomized control trial has shown a 6.6 kg greater weight loss with rimonabant (20 mg) when compared to placebo after 1 year of treatment. Moreover, triglycerides and insulin levels were reduced and HDL-C was increased [61]. Side effects, mild and well tolerated, were mainly limited to dizziness, nausea, and diarrhea.

Other medications, for example, thyroid hormone, amphetamines, phentermine, amfepramone (diethylpropion), phenylpropanolamine, mazindol, and fenfluramines increase risk of angina pectoris, myocardial infarction, and death because they increase oxygen demand and vasospasm. Therefore, these medications are contraindicated for weight loss in the secondary prevention of CHD.

The AHA/ACC recommendations for weight control in patients with CHD include: calculating BMI and measuring waist circumference during the clinical evaluation, and using these measures to monitor response to therapy. The goal of weight management is to achieve a BMI between 18.5 and 24.9 kg/m^2. When the BMI *is* 25 kg/m^2 or greater, *the* waist circumference goal is <40 in. in men and <35 in. in women.

Exercise and Physical Activity

Physical activity can be defined as movements produced by skeletal muscles that result in energy expenditure beyond basal normal energy expenditure. The three major components of exercise and physical fitness are:

Dose, intensity, and type. Dose refers to the amount of energy expended in physical activity (kilocalories) and intensity reflects the rate of energy expended during activity [62]. Absolute intensity is usually measured in metabolic equivalents or METs (1 MET = resting metabolic rate ≅ 3.5 mL O2/kg/min), and relative intensity is the percent of aerobic power utilized during exercise and is expressed as the percent of the maximal heart rate or percent of maximum oxygen consumption (VO2 max): moderate-intensity activities are those performed at a relative intensity of 40–60% of VO2max (absolute of 4–6 METs), and vigorous intensity >60% of VO2max (>6 METs) [63]. Type of exercise refers to the type of stress on the muscles: isometric (load without movement), isotonic (movement without load), or resistance (movement against a load).

Exercise as a treatment for patients with CHD in cardiac rehabilitations programs should be increased gradually. Vigorous physical activity increases the risk of MI [64, 65] and sudden death, especially in sedentary patients or those with preexisting CHD [66]. Indeed, approximately 5–10% of myocardial infarctions are preceded by vigorous physical activity. These facts emphasize the need for a well-established physical activity programs that must be gradually in time and intensity and with proper supervision.

However, a properly implemented exercise program can decrease mortality rates by up to 27% after MI, and a comprehensive rehabilitation program that includes psychosocial and/or educational interventions can decrease mortality rates by up to 31% [67–69].

Health professionals should prescribe a well-supervised physical activity program to patients with CHD regardless of age, as elderly patients have similar trainability when compared to younger patients [70]. Therefore, older patients should be encouraged to follow a guided exercise cardiac rehabilitation to prevent musculoskeletal injuries [71]. About one-quarter of adults who participate in an exercise program will suffer injuries within a year and, as a result, one third will stop exercising [72]. An exercise stress test should be used to assess risk and guide prescription.

A typical exercise prescription would recommend a minimum of 30–60 min of activity, preferably daily, or at least 3 or 4 times weekly (walking, jogging, cycling, or other aerobic activity) supplemented by an increase in daily lifestyle activities (e.g., walking breaks at work, gardening, household work). Patients should be asked to monitor their heart rate and not exceed 85% of their maximum predicted heart rate (220 bpm – age or 85% of the maximal heart rate on a graded exercise test). Medically supervised programs are recommended for moderate- to high-risk patients, including patients who have suffered an MI and or undergone revascularization.

Diet and Supplements in Secondary Prevention

Many different diets have been advocated for patients with CHD. In recent years, the Mediterranean diet has emerged as the diet of choice [73–75]. The Mediterranean diet consists mainly of legumes, cereals, fruits, and vegetables with moderate amounts of fish, olive oil, and wine. Consumption of dairy products and meats is limited. The Mediterranean diet is low in saturated fat and high in omega-3 fatty acids. Randomized controlled secondary prevention trials have demonstrated that the diet reduces both cardiovascular and overall mortality. The Lyon Diet Heart Study [76] included patients with known MI and compared a Mediterranean diet to the AHA step 1 diet. Although, there was no improvement in the lipid profile, lipoproteins or body mass index, a 76% risk reduction in mortality was observed in the Mediterranean diet group.

Another trial, The Indo-Mediterranean Diet Heart study randomized patients with angina pectoris, MI, or risk factors for CHD to either a diet rich in whole grains, fruits, vegetables, walnuts, and almonds or to the step I National Cholesterol Education Program prudent diet. Compared to control group subjects, subjects in the intervention group experienced a 51% risk reduction in nonfatal MI, a 64% reduction in sudden cardiac death, and a 50% risk reduction in total cardiac endpoints [77].

Omega-3 Polyunsaturated Fatty Acids

Omega-3 (or n-3) polyunsaturated fatty acids are comprised of α-linolenic acid, eicosapentaenoic acid (EPA), and docosahexaenoic acid (DHEA). Common sources of α-linolenic acid are flaxseed oil, canola oil, soybean oil, walnuts, and flaxseed. The most common sources of EPA and DHEA are oily fish such as salmon, tuna, and mackerel.

Omega-3 fatty acids from fish and oil fish are associated with lower rates of coronary events, particularly sudden death [78]. Several mechanisms of action had been proposed by which omega-3 fatty acids can be cardioprotective, including: electrical stabilization of myocytes; increased heart rate variability; reduction in blood pressure; reduction in platelet aggregation; anti-atherogenic mechanisms; anti-inflammatory effect, and lowering triglycerides [79].

Cohort studies [80] have shown lower rates of all-cause mortality and a reduced risk of sudden death in individuals with high levels of omega-3 fatty acids in their diet. Recent trial data have confirmed those observations. The Diet and Re-infarction Trial (DART) showed a 29% all-cause mortality reduction over 2 years in men with previous MI who had a diet rich omega-3 fatty acids. Interestingly nonfatal events and lipid levels were not affected [81]. The GISSI-Prevenzione trial [82] studied the effect of omega-3 fatty acid supplementation in addition to proven secondary prevention measures in patients with a recent MI. Omega-3 fatty acid supplementation reduced sudden death by 45% and reduced overall mortality by 20%.

The American Heart Association recommends that patients with documented CHD consume about 1 g of EPA + DHEA per day, preferably from oily fish [83]. American College of Cardiology guidelines suggest that physicians encourage their patients with coronary heart disease to increase omega-3 fatty acid consumption, that omega-3 fatty acids be considered as adjunct therapy for lowering triglycerides, and that high-risk women be advised to consider omega-3 fatty acid supplements [84, 85].

One recent trial of omega-3 fatty acid supplementation in patients with defibrillators found an increased propensity toward ventricular tachycardia events in the active treatment group [86]. However, the increase in ventricular tachycardia was not associated with increased mortality.

Vitamin E

Vitamin E is the major antioxidant substance in lipid metabolism [87]. In animal models, several mechanisms have been proposed for the reduction in atherosclerotic lesions that have been produced by the administration of vitamin E [88, 89]. It has been postulated that vitamin E improves endothelial function in humans [90]. Trial data, however, demonstrate a dose response relationship between vitamin E supplementation and risk of all-cause mortality. Several trials have shown no benefit from vitamin E intake [91]. Recently, the HOPE and HOPE-TOO trial evaluated long-term supplementation of vitamin E. An increase in heart failure was observed in patients with CHD who took vitamin E [92]. Given the lack of benefit and potential harm, vitamin E supplements should not be recommended to patients with CHD.

Beta-Carotene

Like vitamin E, beta-carotene is a lipophilic vitamin carried in lipoproteins. It has been suggested that beta-carotene acts as a singlet oxygen quencher [93] and assists in the metabolism of vitamin A, C, and E [94]. Some observational studies suggest that beta-carotene reduces CVD and certain types of cancer [95, 96]. However, randomized trials have not confirmed any benefit in CVD prevention. The CARET [97] and the Physician Health Study [98] tested beta-carotene for primary prevention of CVD. CARET combined beta-carotene with vitamin A and showed an increase in all-cause mortality, lung cancer, and a trend toward increased CV mortality. Beta-carotene administration in the Physician Health Study showed no benefit in overall death and CV mortality. The effect of beta-carotene supplementation on primary prevention for CHD was also addressed in the Alpha-Tocopherol and Beta-Carotene supplementation on coronary heart disease study (ATBC) [99]. Beta-carotene was associated with an increased risk of first-ever nonfatal MI. Because of the lack of effectiveness in primary prevention and lack of information in secondary prevention, beta carotene supplementation should not be prescribed to any patient.

Folic Acid

Folic acid is a B-complex vitamin that metabolizes homocysteine. High homocysteine levels are associated with a high risk of CHD [100, 101]. It has been suggested that folic acid plays an important role in the vasopressin–nitric oxide pathway and maintains endothelial function [102, 103]. Despite encouraging mechanistic studies suggesting beneficial effects of folic acid on cardiovascular health, clinical trials have

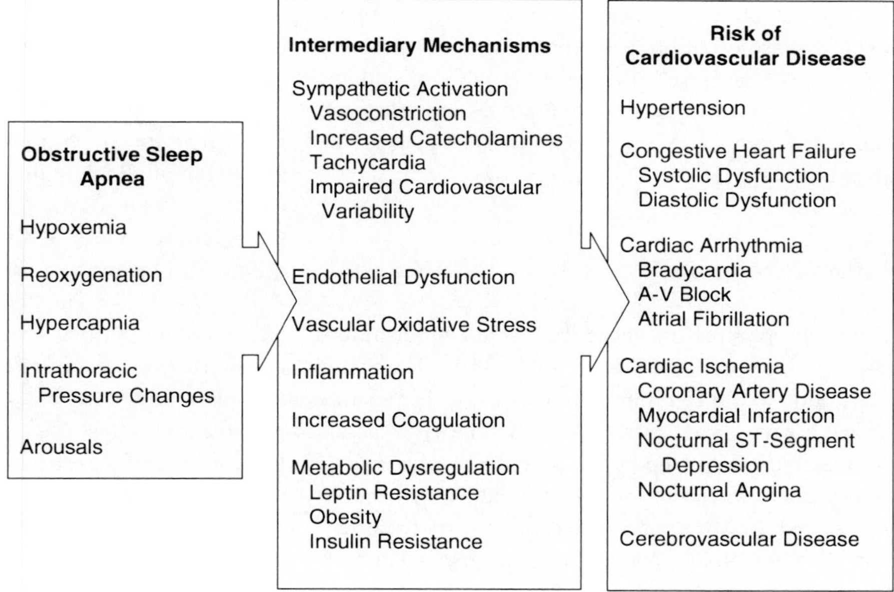

Fig. 14.1 Risk of cardiovascular disease related to OSA [1]. (Caples et al. [122])

failed to show any benefit. The FOLARDA pilot study was designed to assess the benefit of folic acid when added to statin treatment for CVD prevention. Neither cardiovascular morbidity nor mortality was reduced in post-MI in patients with hypercholesterolemia when folic acid was added to statin treatment [104]. The available evidence does not support prescribing folic acid for secondary prevention.

Obstructive Sleep Apnea

Obstructive sleep apnea has been recently identified as an independent and highly prevalent cardiovascular risk factor. Obstructive sleep apnea is both common and commonly unrecognized in clinical practice. This disease can be found in one of every five adults with a BMI of 25–28 kg/m^2, and the prevalence increases in patients who are overweight or obese [105]. The diagnosis of sleep apnea should be suspected in patients with daytime sleepiness and nocturnal snoring, but it must be confirmed with an overnight polysomnography study to determine the total number of apneas and hypopneas during sleep [106].

Several pathophysiological principles relate obstructive sleep apnea to CHD and CHD risk factors. Patients with OSA have a high prevalence of hypertension, metabolic syndrome, type 2 diabetes mellitus, and obesity [107–109]. There are multiple mechanisms though which sleep apnea can cause CHD [110] Fig. 14.1. Sympathetic tone is increased in OSA [111, 112] and can be manifested by faster resting heart rates, blunted heart rate variability, and increased blood pressure [113]. Patients with sleep apnea also have dysfunctional peripheral chemoreceptors and an impaired vagal activity that predisposes them to severe bradyarrhythmias during apneic events. These events can be fatal [114–116]. Endothelial dysfunction and inflammatory markers such as C-reactive protein and serum amyloid A appear to be increased in patients with sleep apnea [117, 118]. Sleep apnea patients also have periodic nocturnal myocardial ischemia and have a nocturnal increase in the incidence of sudden cardiac death [119]. These associations and pathophysiologic findings strongly suggest an important role of obstructive sleep apnea in patients with CHD.

The treatment of sleep apnea includes weight loss (10% weight loss results in significant clinical improvement and improvement of the apnea–hypopnea index) and the use of continuous positive airway pressure. Continuous positive airway pressure eliminates upper-airway flow limitation in almost every patient and it is associated with improvement of most of the pathophysiological mechanisms mentioned previously and significantly improves daytime symptoms. Other treatments include uvulopalatopharyngoplasty or bariatric surgery, which have proven significant improvement and even resolution of sleep apnea [120]. Mandibular devices are successful in a limited number of patients [121, 122]. Whether treatment improves mortality and morbidity from CHD is not yet known and needs to be elucidated.

Future Directions

Three observations in particular should guide future efforts in the secondary prevention of CHD: The first is the finding in a recent international case-control study of acute myocardial infarction that nine risk factors account for 90% of the population attributable risk of myocardial infarction for both men and women: smoking, raised ApoB/ApoA1 ratio, history of hypertension, diabetes, abdominal obesity, psychosocial factors, daily consumption of fruits and vegetables, regular alcohol consumption, and regular physical activity [123]. The second is the finding that subjects in the 4S intervention group who were also on aspirin and a beta-blocker had event rates that were 70% lower than rates for subjects in the control group who were on neither a beta blocker nor aspirin [124]. The third is the finding that English patients who were on a statin, a beta-blocker and aspirin after their first myocardial infarction had event rates that were 85% lower than event rates for patients who were on none of these drugs [125]. These observations imply that, while future etiologic research will increase our understanding of the pathways between the root causes of CHD and clinical events, the root causes of CHD have been identified and the tools are in hand to markedly reduce secondary attack rates of CHD.

The major breakthroughs in the future will come from effective measures to prevent the emergence of risk factors– "primordial prevention" – and the development of secondary prevention tools to help patients optimize risk factor levels through pharmacologic intervention and lifestyles that lead to optimal nutrition and adequate levels of physical activity.

The products of information science, particularly the electronic medical record, remote measuring and recording devices, remote coaching programs that utilize techniques of mass customization, and the internet, are likely to be the major new contributors to the control of CHD in the next decade. The electronic medical record will enable physicians to track both individual patients and groups of patients to assure that individuals are not lost to follow-up, that their risk factors remain in optimal control, and that they are on optimal doses of medication. Remote measuring devices like sphygmomanometers or scales that communicate with a doctor's office or other resource, will allow longitudinal, unbiased collection of data that reflect the status of the patient as she or he goes about their daily business of living. Remote coaching programs, similar to those used to assist athletes in their training, will help patients remain motivated to achieve and maintain optimal levels of risk. The internet will allow patients to communicate with their health care providers more efficiently and with less expense than with the traditional office visit. With the advent of public reporting of performance, the health care organizations that learn how to use these technologies to improve patient outcomes will attract patients to their programs and improve profitability.

Conclusion

Just nine risk factors account for nearly all of the population attributable risk for myocardial infarction: smoking, raised ApoB/ApoA1 ratio, hypertension, diabetes, abdominal obesity, psychosocial factors, daily consumption of fruits and vegetables, regular alcohol consumption, and regular physical activity. While it can be expected that research will produce even more effective pharmaceutical agents for secondary prevention of CHD, clinicians now have the ability to reduce recurrent events by up to 85% with the prescription of just three agents: an aspirin, a beta blocker, and a statin. In addition to reducing the risk of a recurrent CHD event, behavioral interventions that help patients improve their diets and increase physical activity have the potential to synergistically reduce the risk of many other conditions. In contrast to focusing on the most recent novel intervention of hypothesized but undocumented efficacy, clinicians can produce the best outcomes for their patients by controlling established causal risk factors with therapies that are clearly documented as highly efficacious. The communication tools of the electronic age allow them to follow their patients and help them adhere to the lifestyles and medication programs that minimize risk of recurrent CHD events.

Total Word Count:

- With tables and figures: 6,012
- Without tables and figures: 5,004

References

1. Hippisley-Cox J, Coupland C. Effect of combinations of drugs on all cause mortality in patients with ischaemic heart disease: nested case-control analysis. BMJ. 2005;330(7499):1059–63.
2. Kjekshus J, Pedersen TR. Reducing the risk of coronary events: evidence from the Scandinavian Simvastatin Survival Study (4S). Am J Cardiol. 1995;76(9):64C–8.
3. Masson LF, McNeill G. The effect of genetic variation on the lipid response to dietary change: recent findings. Curr Opin Lipidol. 2005;16(1):61–7.
4. The Scandinavian Simvastatin Survival Study (4S). Randomised trial of cholesterol lowering in 4444 patients with coronary heart disease. Lancet. 1994;344(8934):1383–9.
5. (LIPID) Study Group. Prevention of cardiovascular events and death with pravastatin in patients with coronary heart disease and a broad range of initial cholesterol levels. The long-term intervention with pravastatin in ischaemic disease. N Engl J Med. 1998;339(19):1349–57.
6. Shepherd J, Cobbe SM, Ford I, Isles CG, Lorimer AR, MacFarlane PW, et al. Prevention of coronary heart disease with pravastatin in men with hypercholesterolemia. West of Scotland Coronary Prevention Study Group. N Engl J Med. 1995;333(20):1301–7.
7. Downs JR, Clearfield M, Weis S, Whitney E, Shapiro DR, Beere PA, et al. Primary prevention of acute coronary events with lovastatin in men and women with average cholesterol levels: results of AFCAPS/TexCAPS. Air Force/Texas Coronary Atherosclerosis Prevention Study. JAMA. 1998;279(20):1615–22.
8. Heart Protection Study Collaborative Group. MRC/BHF Heart Protection Study of cholesterol lowering with simvastatin in 20536 high-risk individuals: a randomized placebo-controlled trial. Lancet. 2002;360:7–22.
9. Sever PS, Dahlof B, Poulter NR, Wedel H, Beevers G, Caulfield M, et al. Prevention of coronary and stroke events with atorvastatin in hypertensive patients who have average or lower-than-average cholesterol concentrations, in the Anglo-Scandinavian Cardiac Outcomes Trial–Lipid Lowering Arm (ASCOT-LLA): a multicentre randomised controlled trial. Lancet. 2003;361(9364):1149–58.
10. Nissen SE, Tuzcu EM, Schoenhagen P, Brown BG, Ganz P, Vogel RA, et al. Effect of intensive compared with moderate lipid-lowering therapy on progression of coronary atherosclerosis: a randomized controlled trial. JAMA. 2004;291(9):1071–80.
11. Cannon CP, Braunwald E, McCabe CH, Rader DJ, Rouleau JL, Belder R, et al. Intensive versus moderate lipid lowering with statins after acute coronary syndromes. N Engl J Med. 2004;350(15):1495–504. Epub 2004 Mar 08.
12. LaRosa JC, Grundy SM, Waters DD, Shear C, Barter P, Fruchart JC, et al. Intensive lipid lowering with atorvastatin in patients with stable coronary disease. N Engl J Med. 2005;352(14):1425–35. Epub 2005 Mar 8.
13. Grundy SM, Cleeman JI, Merz CN, Brewer Jr HB, Clark LT, Hunninghake DB, et al. Implications of recent clinical trials for the National Cholesterol Education Program Adult Treatment Panel III guidelines. Circulation. 2004;110(2):227–39.
14. WHO. World health report 2002; reducing risk, promoting healthy life. Geneva: World Health Organization, 2002.
15. National Center for Health Statistics. Plan and operation of the third National Health and Nutrition Examination survey, 1988–1994. US Department of Health and Human Services. Publication No. 94–1308. 1994
16. The sixth report of the Joint National Committee on prevention, detection, evaluation, and treatment of high blood pressure. Arch Intern Med. 1997; 157:2413–46.
17. Chalmers J, Todd A, Chapman N, Beilin L, Davis S, Donnan G, et al. International Society of Hypertension (ISH): statement on blood pressure lowering and stroke prevention. J Hypertens. 2003;21(4):651–63.
18. Collins R, Peto R, Godwin J, MacMahon S. Blood pressure and coronary heart disease. Lancet. 1990;336(8711):370–1.
19. Cutler JA, MacMahon SW, Furberg CD. Controlled clinical trials of drug treatment for hypertension. A review. Hypertension. 1989;13(5 Suppl):I36–44.
20. Psaty BM, Lumley T, Furberg CD, Schellenbaum G, Pahor M, Alderman MH, et al. Health outcomes associated with various antihypertensive therapies used as first-line agents: a network meta-analysis. JAMA. 2003;289(19):2534–44.
21. Blood pressure Lowering Treatment Trialists Collaboration. Effects of different blood-pressure-lowering regimens on major cardiovascular events: results of prospectively-designed overviews of randomized trials. Lancet. 2003;362:1527–35.
22. Chobanian AV, Bakris GL, Black HR, Cushman WC, Green LA, Izzo Jr JL, et al. The Seventh Report of the Joint National Committee on Prevention, Detection, Evaluation, and Treatment of High Blood Pressure: the JNC 7 report. JAMA. 2003;289(19):2560–72. Epub 2003 May 14.
23. Dargie HJ. Effect of carvedilol on outcome after myocardial infarction in patients with left-ventricular dysfunction: the CAPRICORN randomised trial. Lancet. 2001;357(9266):1385–90.
24. Pitt B, Remme W, Zannad F, Neaton J, Martinez F, Roniker B, et al. Eplerenone, a selective aldosterone blocker, in patients with left ventricular dysfunction after myocardial infarction. N Engl J Med. 2003;348(14):1309–21. Epub 2003 Mar 31.
25. Solomon SD, Skali H, Anavekar NS, Bourgoun M, Barvik S, Ghali JK, et al. Changes in ventricular size and function in patients treated with valsartan, captopril, or both after myocardial infarction. Circulation. 2005;111(25):3411–9. Epub 2005 Jun 20.
26. Antithrombotic Trialists' Collaboration. Collaborative meta-analysis of randomized trials of antiplatelet therapy for prevention of death, myocardial infarction, and stroke in high risk patients. BMJ. 2002;324:71–86.
27. CAPRIE Steering Committee. A randomised, blinded, trial of clopidogrel versus aspirin in patients at risk of ischaemic events (CAPRIE). Lancet. 1996;348(9038):1329–39.
28. Cure I. Effects of clopidogrel in addition to aspirin in patients with acute coronary syndromes without ST-segment elevation. N Engl J Med. 2001;345:494–502.
29. Steinhubl SR, Berger PB, Mann 3rd JT, et al. Early and sustained dual oral antiplatelet therapy following percutaneous coronary intervention: a randomized controlled trial. JAMA. 2002;288:2411–20 (Erratum JAMA 2003;289:987).
30. Anand SS, Yusuf S. Oral anticoagulant therapy in patients with coronary artery disease: a meta-analysis. JAMA. 2000;284(1):45.

31. Smith Jr SC, Blair SN, Bonow RO, Brass LM, Cerqueira MD, Dracup K, et al. AHA/ACC Guidelines for Preventing Heart Attack and Death in Patients with Atherosclerotic Cardiovascular disease: 2001 update. J Am Coll Cardiol. 2001;38(5):1581–3.
32. McGinnis JM, Foege WH. Actual causes of death in the United States. JAMA. 1993;270(18):2207–12.
33. Rigotti NA, Pasternak RC. Cigarette smoking and coronary heart disease: risks and management. Cardiol Clin. 1996;14(1):51–68.
34. Barnoya J, Glantz SA. Cardiovascular effects of secondhand smoke: nearly as large as smoking. Circulation. 2005;111(20): 2684–98.
35. Wilson K, Gibson N, Willan A, Cook D. Effect of smoking cessation on mortality after myocardial infarction: meta-analysis of cohort studies. Arch Intern Med. 2000;160(7): 939–44.
36. Critchley JA, Capewell S. Mortality risk reduction associated with smoking cessation in patients with coronary heart disease: a systematic review. JAMA. 2003;290(1):86–97.
37. Pignone M, Phillips C, Mulrow C. Use of lipid lowering drugs for primary prevention of coronary heart disease: meta-analysis of randomised trials. BMJ. 2000;321(7267):983–6.
38. Antithrombotic Trialists' Collaboration. Collaborative meta-analysis of randomised trials of antiplatelet therapy for prevention of death, myocardial infarction, and stroke in high risk patients. BMJ. 2002;324(7329):71–86.
39. Freemantle N, Cleland J, Young P, Mason J, Harrison J. beta Blockade after myocardial infarction: systematic review and meta regression analysis. BMJ. 1999;318(7200):1730–7.
40. Flather MD, Yusuf S, Kober L, Pfeffer M, Hall A, Murray G, et al. Long-term ACE-inhibitor therapy in patients with heart failure or left-ventricular dysfunction: a systematic overview of data from individual patients. ACE-Inhibitor Myocardial Infarction Collaborative Group. Lancet. 2000; 355(9215):1575–81.
41. Wiggers LC, Smets EM, de Haes JC, Peters RJ, Legemate DA. Smoking cessation interventions in cardiovascular patients. Eur J Vasc Endovasc Surg. 2003;26(5):467–75.
42. Joseph AM, Norman SM, Ferry LH, Prochazka AV, Westman EC, Steele BG, et al. The safety of transdermal nicotine as an aid to smoking cessation in patients with cardiac disease. N Engl J Med. 1996;335(24):1792–8.
43. Benowitz NL, Gourlay SG. Cardiovascular toxicity of nicotine: implications for nicotine replacement therapy. J Am Coll Cardiol. 1997;29(7):1422–31.
44. Kottke TE. Smoking cessation therapy for the patient with heart disease. J Am Coll Cardiol. 1993;22(4):1168–9.
45. Kottke TE. Managing nicotine dependence. J Am Coll Cardiol. 1997;30(1):131–2.
46. The Tobacco Use and Dependence Clinical Practice Guideline Panel, Staff, and Consortium Representatives. A clinical practice guideline for treating tobacco use and dependence: A US Public Health Service report. JAMA. 2000;283(24):3244–54.
47. Taylor CB, Houston-Miller N, Killen JD, DeBusk RF. Smoking cessation after acute myocardial infarction: effects of a nurse-managed intervention. Ann Intern Med. 1990; 113(2):118–23.
48. Bray GA. Obesity: a time bomb to be defused. Lancet. 1998;352:160–1.
49. Flegal KM, Carroll MD, Ogden CL, Johnson CL. Prevalence and trends in obesity among US adults, 1999–2000. JAMA. 2002;288:1723–7.
50. Melanson KJ, McInnis KJ, Rippe JM, Blackburn G, Wilson PF. Obesity and cardiovascular disease risk: research update. Cardiol Rev. 2002;9:202–7.
51. Ezzati M, Lopez AD, Rodgers A, Hoorn SV, Murray CJL. Selected major risk factors and global and regional burden of disease. Lancet. 2002;360:1347–60.
52. Eckel RH, Barouch WW, Ershow AG. Report of the National Heart, Lung, and Blood Institute—National Institute of Diabetes and Digestive and Kidney Diseases Working Group on the Pathophysiology of Obesity-Associated Cardiovascular Disease. Circulation. 2002;105:2923–8.
53. Mark AL, Correia ML, Rahmouni K, Haynes WG. Selective leptin resistance: a new concept in leptin physiology with cardiovascular implications. J Hypertens. 2002;20: 1245–50.
54. Haynes WG, Morgan DA, Walsh SA, Sivitz WI, Mark AL. Cardiovascular consequences of obesity: role of leptin. Clin Exp Pharmacol Physiol. 1998;25:65–9.
55. Eckel RH. Obesity and heart disease: a statement for healthcare professionals from the Nutrition Committee, American Heart Association. Circulation. 1997;96:3248–50.
56. Lopez-Jimenez F, Jacobsen SJ, Reeder GS, Weston SA, Killian JM, Meverden R, et al. Prevalence of risk factors for coronary disease in myocardial infarction in the community. J Am Coll Cardiol. 2003;41:291-A.
57. Lopez-Jimenez F, Malinski M, Gutt M, Sierra-Johnson J, Wady Aude Y, Rimawi AA, et al. Recognition, diagnosis and management of obesity after myocardial infarction. Int J Obes Relat Metab Disord. 2005;29(1):137–41.
58. Buchwald H, Avidor Y, Braunwald E, Jensen MD, Pories W, Fahrbach K, et al. Bariatric surgery: a systematic review and meta-analysis. JAMA. 2004;292(14):1724–37.
59. Maggard MA, Shugarman LR, Suttorp M, Maglione M, Sugarman HJ, Livingston EH, et al. Meta-analysis: surgical treatment of obesity. Ann Intern Med. 2005;142(7):547–59.
60. Ioannides-Demos LL, Proietto J, McNeil JJ. Pharmacotherapy for obesity. Drugs. 2005;65(10):1391–418.
61. Van Gaal LF, Rissanen AM, Scheen AJ, Ziegler O, Rossner S, RIO-Europe Study Group. Effects of the cannabinoid-1 receptor blocker rimonabant on weight reduction and cardiovascular risk factors in overweight patients: 1-year experience from the RIO-Europe study. Lancet. 2005;365(9468): 1389–97.
62. Pate RR, Pratt M, Blair SN, Haskell WL, Macera CA, Bouchard C, et al. Physical activity and public health. A recommendation from the Centers for Disease Control and Prevention and the American College of Sports Medicine. JAMA. 1995;273(5):402–7.
63. Fletcher GF, Balady GJ, Amsterdam EA, Chaitman B, Eckel R, Fleg J, et al. Exercise standards for testing and training: a statement for healthcare professionals from the American Heart Association. Circulation. 2001;104(14):1694–740.
64. Mittleman MA, Maclure M, Tofler GH, Sherwood JB, Goldberg RJ, Muller JE. Triggering of acute myocardial infarction by heavy physical exertion. Protection against triggering by regular exertion. Determinants of Myocardial Infarction Onset Study Investigators. N Engl J Med. 1993;329(23):1677–83.

65. Giri S, Thompson PD, Kiernan FJ, Clive J, Fram DB, Mitchel JF, et al. Clinical and angiographic characteristics of exertion-related acute myocardial infarction. JAMA. 1999;282(18):1731–6.
66. Thompson PD, Funk EJ, Carleton RA, Sturner WQ. Incidence of death during jogging in Rhode Island from 1975 through 1980. JAMA. 1982;247(18):2535–8.
67. O'Connor GT, Buring JE, Yusuf S, Goldhaber SZ, Olmstead EM, Paffenbarger Jr RS, et al. An overview of randomized trials of rehabilitation with exercise after myocardial infarction. Circulation. 1989;80(2):234–44.
68. Oldridge NB, Guyatt GH, Fischer ME, Rimm AA. Cardiac rehabilitation after myocardial infarction. Combined experience of randomized clinical trials. JAMA. 1988; 260(7):945–50.
69. Jolliffe JA, Rees K, Taylor RS, Thompson D, Oldridge N, Ebrahim S. Exercise-based rehabilitation for coronary heart disease. Cochrane Database Syst Rev. 2001;1:CD001800.
70. Lavie CJ, Milani RV. Benefits of cardiac rehabilitation and exercise training programs in elderly coronary patients. Am J Geriatr Cardiol. 2001;10(6):323–7.
71. Wannamethee SG, Shaper AG, Walker M. Physical activity and mortality in older men with diagnosed coronary heart disease. Circulation. 2000;102(12):1358–63.
72. Hootman JM, Macera CA, Ainsworth BE, Addy CL, Martin M, Blair SN. Epidemiology of musculoskeletal injuries among sedentary and physically active adults. Med Sci Sports Exerc. 2002;34(5):838–44.
73. Panagiotakos DB, Pitsavos Ch, Chrysohoou Ch, Stefanadis Ch, Toutouzas P. The role of traditional mediterranean type of diet and lifestyle, in the development of acute coronary syndromes: preliminary results from CARDIO 2000 study. Cent Eur J Public Health. 2002;10(1–2):11–5.
74. Pitsavos C, Panagiotakos DB, Chrysohoou C, Papaioannou I, Papadimitriou L, Tousoulis D, et al. The adoption of mediterranean diet attenuates the development of acute coronary syndromes in people with the metabolic syndrome. Nutr J. 2003;2(1):1.
75. Trichopoulou A, Bamia C, Trichopoulos D. Mediterranean diet and survival among patients with coronary heart disease in Greece. Arch Intern Med. 2005;165(8):929–35.
76. De Lorgeril M, Salen P, Martin JL, Monjaud I, Delaye J, Mamelle N. Mediterranean diet, traditional risk factors, and the rate of cardiovascular complications after myocardial infarction: final report of the Lyon Diet Heart Study. Circulation. 1999;99(6):779–85.
77. Singh RB, Dubnov G, Niaz MA, Ghosh S, Singh R, Rastogi SS, et al. Effect of an Indo-Mediterranean diet on progression of coronary artery disease in high risk patients (Indo-Mediterranean Diet Heart Study): a randomised single-blind trial. Lancet. 2002;360(9344):1455–61.
78. Bang HO, Dyerberg J, Hjoorne N. The composition of food consumed by Greenland Eskimos. Acta Med Scand. 1976; 200(1–2):69–73.
79. Harrison N, Abhyankar B. The mechanism of action of omega-3 fatty acids in secondary prevention post-myocardial infarction. Curr Med Res Opin. 2005;21(1):95–100.
80. He K, Song Y, Daviglus ML, Liu K, Van Horn L, Dyer AR, et al. Accumulated evidence on fish consumption and coronary heart disease mortality: a meta-analysis of cohort studies. Circulation. 2004;109(22):2705–11.
81. Ness AR, Gunnell D, Hughes J, Elwood PC, Davey Smith G, Burr ML. Height, body mass index, and survival in men with coronary disease: follow up of the diet and reinfarction trial (DART). J Epidemiol Community Health. 2002;56(3): 218–9.
82. Marchioli R, Barzi F, Bomba E, Chieffo C, Di Gregorio D, Di Mascio R, et al. Early protection against sudden death by n-3 polyunsaturated fatty acids after myocardial infarction: time-course analysis of the results of the Gruppo Italiano per lo Studio della Sopravvivenza nell'Infarto Miocardico (GISSI)-Prevenzione. Circulation. 2002;105(16): 1897–903.
83. Kris-Etherton PM, Harris WS, Appel LJ. Fish consumption, fish oil, omega-3 fatty acids, and cardiovascular disease. Circulation. 2002;106(21):2747–57.
84. Smith Jr SC, Blair SN, Bonow RO, Brass LM, Cerqueira MD, Dracup K, et al. AHA/ACC Guidelines for Preventing Heart Attack and Death in Patients with Atherosclerotic Cardiovascular Disease: 2001 update. A statement for healthcare professionals from the American Heart Association and the American College of Cardiology. J Am Coll Cardiol. 2001;38(5):1581–3.
85. Mosca L, Appel LJ, Benjamin EJ, et al. Evidence-based guidelines for cardiovascular disease prevention in women. J Am Coll Cardiol. 2004;43(5):900–21.
86. Raitt MH, Connor WE, Morris C, et al. Fish oil supplementation and risk of ventricular tachycardia and ventricular fibrillation in patients with implantable defibrillators: a randomized controlled trial. JAMA. 2005;293(23):2884–91.
87. Traber MG, Sies H. Vitamin E in humans: demand and delivery. Annu Rev Nutr. 1996;16:321–47.
88. Meydani M. Vitamin E. Lancet. 1995;345(8943):170–5.
89. Bursell SE, King GL. Can protein kinase C inhibition and vitamin E prevent the development of diabetic vascular complications? Diabetes Res Clin Pract. 1999;45(2–3): 169–82.
90. Skyrme-Jones RA, O'Brien RC, Berry KL, Meredith IT. Vitamin E supplementation improves endothelial function in type I diabetes mellitus: a randomized, placebo-controlled study. J Am Coll Cardiol. 2000;36(1):94–102.
91. Miller 3rd ER, Pastor-Barriuso R, Dalal D, Riemersma RA, Appel LJ, Guallar E. Meta-analysis: high-dosage vitamin E supplementation may increase all-cause mortality. Ann Intern Med. 2005;142(1):37–46. Epub 2004 Nov 10.
92. Lonn E, Bosch J, Yusuf S, Sheridan P, Pogue J, Arnold JM, et al. Effects of long-term vitamin E supplementation on cardiovascular events and cancer: a randomized controlled trial. JAMA. 2005;293(11):1338–47.
93. Cantrell A, McGarvey DJ, Truscott TG, Rancan F, Bohm F. Singlet oxygen quenching by dietary carotenoids in a model membrane environment. Arch Biochem Biophys. 2003;412(1):47–54.
94. Bohm F, Edge R, McGarvey DJ, Truscott TG. Beta-carotene with vitamins E and C offers synergistic cell protection against NOx. FEBS Lett. 1998;436(3):387–9.
95. Peto R, Doll R, Buckley JD, Sporn MB. Can dietary beta-carotene materially reduce human cancer rates? Nature. 1981;290(5803):201–8.
96. Gaziano JM, Manson JE, Buring JE, Hennekens CH. Dietary antioxidants and cardiovascular disease. Ann N Y Acad Sci. 1992;669:249–58; discussion 258–9.

97. Omenn GS, Goodman GE, Thornquist MD, Balmes J, Cullen MR, Glass A, et al. Effects of a combination of beta carotene and vitamin A on lung cancer and cardiovascular disease. N Engl J Med. 1996;334(18):1150–5.
98. Hennekens CH, Buring JE, Manson JE, Stampfer M, Rosner B, Cook NR, et al. Lack of effect of long-term supplementation with beta carotene on the incidence of malignant neoplasms and cardiovascular disease. N Engl J Med. 1996;334(18):1145–9.
99. Tornwall ME, Virtamo J, Korhonen PA, Virtanen MJ, Taylor PR, Albanes D, et al. Effect of alpha-tocopherol and beta-carotene supplementation on coronary heart disease during the 6-year post-trial follow-up in the ATBC study. Eur Heart J. 2004;25(13):1171–8.
100. Nygard O, Nordrehaug JE, Refsum H, Ueland PM, Farstad M, Vollset SE. Plasma homocysteine levels and mortality in patients with coronary artery disease. N Engl J Med. 1997;337(4):230–6.
101. Ozkan Y, Ozkan E, Simsek B. Plasma total homocysteine and cysteine levels as cardiovascular risk factors in coronary heart disease. Int J Cardiol. 2002;82(3):269–77.
102. Verhaar MC, Wever RM, Kastelein JJ, van Loon D, Milstien S, Koomans HA, et al. Effects of oral folic acid supplementation on endothelial function in familial hypercholesterolemia. A randomized placebo-controlled trial. Circulation. 1999;100(4):335–8.
103. Doshi SN, McDowell IF, Moat SJ, Payne N, Durrant HJ, Lewis MJ, et al. Folic acid improves endothelial function in coronary artery disease via mechanisms largely independent of homocysteine lowering. Circulation. 2002; 105(1):22–6.
104. Liem AH, van Boven AJ, Veeger NJ, Withagen AJ, Robles de Medina RM, Tijssen JG, van Veldhuisen DJ; Folic Acid on Risk Diminishment After Acute Myocarial Infarction Study Group. Efficacy of folic acid when added to statin therapy in patients with hypercholesterolemia following acute myocardial infarction: a randomised pilot trial. Int J Cardiol. 2004; 93(2–3):175–9.
105. Shamsuzzaman AS, Gersh BJ, Somers VK. Obstructive sleep apnea: implications for cardiac and vascular disease. JAMA. 2003;290(14):1906–14.
106. Hamilton GS, Solin P, Naughton MT. Obstructive sleep apnoea and cardiovascular disease. Intern Med J. 2004;34(7): 420–6.
107. Parish JM, Somers VK. Obstructive sleep apnea and cardiovascular disease. Mayo Clin Proc. 2004;79(8):1036–46.
108. Svatikova A, Wolk R, Gami AS, Pohanka M, Somers VK. Interactions between obstructive sleep apnea and the metabolic syndrome. Curr Diab Rep. 2005;5(1):53–8.
109. Punjabi NM, Sorkin JD, Katzel LI, Goldberg AP, Schwartz AR, Smith PL. Sleep-disordered breathing and insulin resistance in middle-aged and overweight men. Am J Respir Crit Care Med. 2002;165(5):677–82.
110. Shamsuzzaman AS, Gersh BJ, Somers VK. Obstructive sleep apnea: implications for cardiac and vascular disease. JAMA. 2003;290(14):1906–14.
111. Narkiewicz K, van de Borne PJ, Pesek CA, Dyken ME, Montano N, Somers VK. Selective potentiation of peripheral chemoreflex sensitivity in obstructive sleep apnea. Circulation. 1999;99(9):1183–9.
112. Somers VK, Dyken ME, Clary MP, Abboud FM. Sympathetic neural mechanisms in obstructive sleep apnea. J Clin Invest. 1995;96(4):1897–904.
113. Narkiewicz K, Montano N, Cogliati C, van de Borne PJ, Dyken ME, Somers VK. Altered cardiovascular variability in obstructive sleep apnea. Circulation. 1998;98(11):1071–7.
114. Bonetti PO, Lerman LO, Lerman A. Endothelial dysfunction: a marker of atherosclerotic risk. Arterioscler Thromb Vasc Biol. 2003;23(2):168–75.
115. Phillips BG, Narkiewicz K, Pesek CA, Haynes WG, Dyken ME. Somers VK Effects of obstructive sleep apnea on endothelin-1 and blood pressure. J Hypertens. 1999;17(1): 61–6.
116. Schulz R, Schmidt D, Blum A, Lopes-Ribeiro X, Lucke C, Mayer K, et al. Decreased plasma levels of nitric oxide derivatives in obstructive sleep apnoea: response to CPAP therapy. Thorax. 2000;55(12):1046–51.
117. Meier-Ewert HK, Ridker PM, Rifai N, Regan MM, Price NJ, Dinges DF, et al. Effect of sleep loss on C-reactive protein, an inflammatory marker of cardiovascular risk. J Am Coll Cardiol. 2004;43(4):678–83.
118. Ridker PM. Clinical application of C-reactive protein for cardiovascular disease detection and prevention. Circulation. 2003;107(3):363–9.
119. Gami AS, Howard DE, Olson EJ, Somers VK. Day-night pattern of sudden death in obstructive sleep apnea. N Engl J Med. 2005;352(12):1206–14.
120. Maggard MA, Shugarman LR, Suttorp M, Maglione M, Sugarman HJ, Livingston EH, et al. Meta-analysis: surgical treatment of obesity. Ann Intern Med. 2005;142(7):547–59.
121. Lattimore JD, Celermajer DS, Wilcox I. Obstructive sleep apnea and cardiovascular disease. J Am Coll Cardiol. 2003;41(9):1429–37.
122. Caples SM, Gami AS, Somers VK. Obstructive sleep apnea. Ann Intern Med. 2005;142(3):187–97.
123. Yusuf S, Hawken S, Ounpuu S, et al. Effect of potentially modifiable risk factors associated with myocardial infarction in 52 countries (the INTERHEART study): case-control study. Lancet. 2004;364(9438):937–52.
124. Kjekshus J, Pedersen TR. Reducing the risk of coronary events: evidence from the Scandinavian Simvastatin Survival Study (4S). Am J Cardiol. 1995;76(9):64C–8.
125. Hippisley-Cox J, Coupland C. Effect of combinations of drugs on all cause mortality in patients with ischaemic heart disease: nested case-control analysis. BMJ. 2005;330(7499):1059–63.

Index

G.W. Barsness and D.R. Holmes Jr. (eds.), *Coronary Artery Disease*, DOI 10.1007/978-1-84628-712-1, © Springer-Verlag London Limited 2012

R

S